AF477958

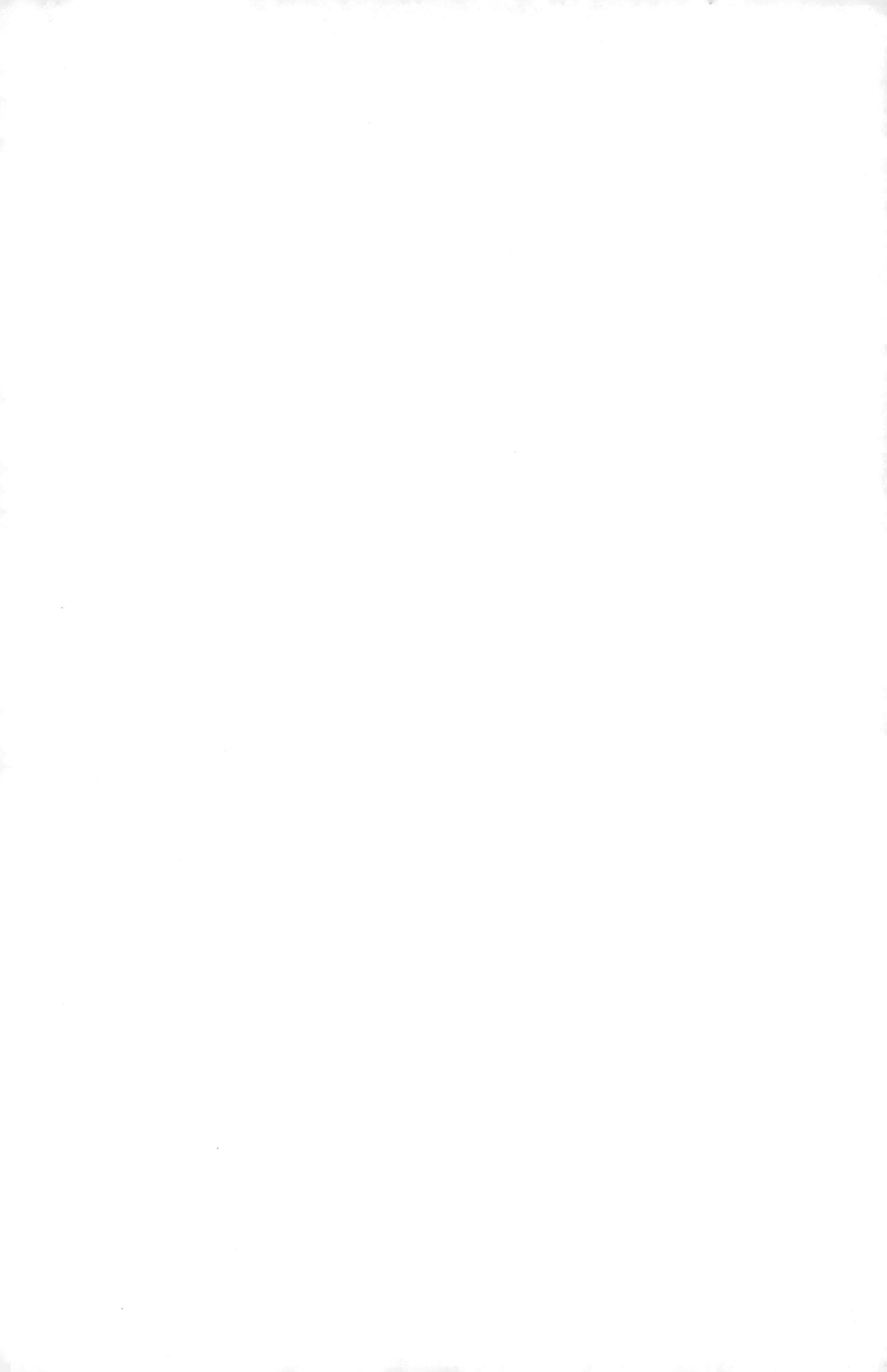

Mandibular Implant Prostheses

Elham Emami · Jocelyne Feine
Editors

Mandibular Implant Prostheses

Guidelines for Edentulous Geriatric Populations

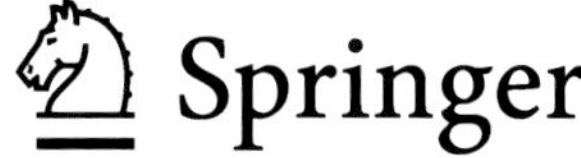

Editors
Elham Emami
Faculty of Dentistry
McGill University
Montréal
Québec
Canada

Jocelyne Feine
Faculty of Dentistry
McGill University
Montréal
Québec
Canada

Faculty of Dentistry
Université de Montréal
Montréal
Québec
Canada

ISBN 978-3-319-71179-9   ISBN 978-3-319-71181-2   (eBook)
https://doi.org/10.1007/978-3-319-71181-2

Library of Congress Control Number: 2018934959

Printed on acid-free paper

This Springer imprint is published by the registered company Springer International Publishing AG part of Springer Nature
The registered company address is: Gewerbestrasse 11, 6330 Cham, Switzerland

Preface

One of the greatest challenges for oral health-care professionals is to provide a denture that is acceptable to completely edentate individuals. This task becomes even more difficult when treating elderly patients.

The geriatric population worldwide is increasing at a significant rate, thereby creating more demand for implant prostheses from our seniors. This population may also suffer from other physical and psychological conditions or multiple chronic diseases that necessitate a comprehensive risk assessment and effective health and oral health-care management.

In the past two decades, implant technology development has produced key solutions for the management of care for patients with maladaptive issues with their dentures, especially with the mandibular denture. Mandibular implant overdentures have improved the quality of life of many patients by offering them better functional capability, stability, and comfort.

For this book, we gathered a number of internationally recognized dental specialists and scientists to share their expertise and experience with mandibular implant overdentures for the geriatric population.

The book can be used both in academia for teaching purposes and in daily clinical practice.

The principles have been classified into four parts: considerations for treatment planning, surgical phase, prosthetic phase, and treatment assessment—clinician and patient perspectives. The sequence of the parts is designed in such a way that practicing dentists and dental undergraduate and postgraduate students can use this book to understand when mandibular implant prostheses are needed and to identify various physiologic and psychosocial characteristics of elders that should be considered during treatment planning. The book will also bring readers up to date on the clinical techniques needed for a successful mandibular implant-assisted overdenture and help them to avoid the mistakes that can occur during the surgical and prosthetic phases. Dentists can also plan to maintain the functionality of such prostheses as long as possible, considering both patient-based and clinical evidence regarding important outcomes. In some chapters, pictures, illustrations and graphics have been used to help readers better understand the principles and the methods.

We are grateful to our book's co-authors for accepting our invitation and joining in this scientific journey. We thank and congratulate all of them for their unique and precious contributions to this book. We also thank their—and our—families for their forbearance and enthusiastic support.

We wish to thank Springer Nature for recognizing the need for such a
publication and for their help in the publication process.

Finally, we hope that you will enjoy this book as much as we have.

Montréal, QC, Canada
Fall 2017

Elham Emami
Jocelyne Feine

Contents

Considerations for Treatment Planning

Lyndon F. Cooper

Abstract

The worldwide prevalence of dental caries and periodontal diseases has not diminished. If edentulism is related to these leading causes of tooth loss, then it might be anticipated that the prevalence of edentulism has also not diminished. Beyond biofilm-mediated disease as a main etiology of tooth loss, the prevalence of edentulism has been and remains associated with rural dwelling, education level, and socioeconomic status. Its prevalence varies across regions and the world. As such, over-simplification fails to recognize the significant issues edentulism brings to society and health-care professions. The future of edentulism and the provision of dentures will be informed by multiple factors including the increased numbers of retained yet unrestored and diseased teeth, the impact of comorbid diseases, the chronicity of oral diseases and increased longevity, and the complex issues of access to care. Edentulism represents one symptom of adult health-care disparities that requires education, further study, and action.

The aim of this chapter is to investigate the reported knowledge regarding the epidemiology of complete tooth loss or edentulism and the current data regarding denture therapy. If there is, as predicted by epidemiological studies of edentulism and tooth loss, a dramatic decline in the incidence in edentulism, then there should be a reduction in the number of dentures provided.

Tooth loss is attributed to several causes that are frequently and primarily reported as caries, periodontal disease, and trauma. Factors associated with edentulism have repeatedly been identified and include age, socioeconomic status, and urban/rural residence. A complex interaction among these predictors varies among diverse populations [1]. Therapeutic and iatrogenic extraction of teeth has also been noted. An early epidemiological report derived from NHANES I data stated that the incidence of edentulism was correlated with baseline measures of lower income and education status, poorer oral health, self-perceptions of poor general health and oral health, absence of a regular dentist, and a lower number of remaining teeth at baseline [2]. Implied is the idea that the prevalence of these diagnosis-based causes of tooth loss can precede and predict further tooth loss and edentulism. Suggested was that the loss of teeth was a predictor of future total tooth loss or edentulism. Highlighting the level of disease in the early 1990s, Caplan and Weintraub [3] reported that 40% of individuals older than 65 years were

L. F. Cooper, D.D.S., Ph.D.
Department of Oral Biology, University of Illinois at Chicago, College of Dentistry, Chicago, IL, USA
e-mail: cooperlf@uic.edu

© Springer International Publishing AG, part of Springer Nature 2018
E. Emami, J. Feine (eds.), *Mandibular Implant Prostheses*,
https://doi.org/10.1007/978-3-319-71181-2_1

edentulous, although they further reported that in seven consecutive surveys of working US adults, the incidence of edentulism was dramatically reduced [3].

Weintraub and Burt reported that the percent edentulism for all ages based on the National Health Interview Survey of 1957–1958 (NHIS I) was 13% and of 1971 (NHIS II) was 11.2%. The National Health and Nutrition Examination Survey 1989–1991 (NHANES III) reported 10.5%, thus demonstrating a trend of declining edentulism with each 10-year cohort. Douglass et al. acknowledged the decade over decade reduction in the numbers of edentulous individuals; however, they calculated based upon estimates of population growth in the USA from 1991 to 2020 that nearly 38 million edentulous adults with 61 million edentulous arches would need one or more dentures. This indicates there would be no near-term reduction in the numbers of dentures provided for the US population.

Since the 1990s, several reports have indicated that the worldwide prevalence of dental caries and periodontal diseases has not diminished [4]. If edentulism could be related to the prevalence of caries and periodontal diseases (the leading causes of tooth loss), then it might be anticipated that the prevalence of edentulism has also not diminished. However, the burden of oral conditions (untreated caries and severe periodontitis) has actually increased in the past 20 years as the affiliated disability-adjusted life-year metric of burden due to severe tooth loss decreased. Several investigations have noted that one impact of increasing numbers of retained teeth is an increased prevalence of tooth-related disease. It may be difficult, then, to predict the prevalence of edentulism based on the prevalence of diseases that lead to tooth loss. Relating edentulism to denture use is complicated by the observation that the utilization or demand rate for dentures by edentulous was approximately 90% [5].

The Global Burden of Disease (GBD) 2010 study [6] provided estimates of tooth loss among 291 diseases that revealed significant reduction in the global burden of severe tooth loss between 1990 and 2010. Similar to the reports from the USA, this systematic review concluded globally that the age-standardized prevalence was reduced from 4.4% (95% UI: 4.1%, 4.8%) to 2.4% (95% UI: 2.2%, 2.7%). These authors concluded that a significant irony in reduced total tooth loss might be an increased prevalence and incidence of severe periodontitis and untreated dental caries. Ultimately, these conditions must be treated. Beyond biofilm-mediated disease as a main etiology of tooth loss, the prevalence of edentulism has been and remains associated with rural dwelling, education level, and socioeconomic status. Current data demonstrates that higher rates of edentulism exist in rural regions of the nation and present among the poorest of individuals [7].

When considering the need versus demand for dentures, health, social, and economic factors were acknowledged to influence demand marginally. The authors supported the previous observations that 90% of persons needing complete dentures used them. This general or average projected rate of denture use may not broadly apply across the diverse US population.

Edentulism varies among different communities within the USA. When data spanning several decades was examined for edentulism prevalence between high and low socioeconomic statuses, there existed a consistently higher prevalence of edentulism among the low socioeconomic populations that was unchanged from 1972 to 2001 [8]. Wu et al. [9] considered the data from the National Health Interview Survey recording edentulism in both the maxilla and mandible from 1994 to 2004. They observed a reduction in edentulism from 34% to 27% of those individuals surveyed. This report demonstrated that the rates of edentulism, while falling overall, differed substantially among the Native American, African-American, Caucasian, Hispanic, and Asian individuals included. A recent analysis of the 2006 Behavior Risk Factor Surveillance Survey (BRFSS) reported that 14.3% of US adults had all of their teeth removed; low socioeconomic status was associated with a 15.9 (15.8, 16.0) odds ratio (95% CI). Smoking, aging ≥65 years, reporting at least one chronic disease, and inability to work were also significant risk factors for edentulism. This study further stated that edentulous adults were 62.7% more likely to be rural

[10]. Suggested was a national condition where oral health-care and general health services are not linked. There will be variation in edentulism from community to community that reflects ethnicity, education, general wellness, and income.

Slade et al. [11] explored the estimated prevalence of edentulism by imposing age- and cohort-based effects on existing data concerning edentulism in the USA. Their analysis indicates there will be 30% fewer edentulous individuals by 2050 (8.6 million) than in 2010 (12.2 million). Over the five decades analyzed, the relative declines were 68 and 96% for the low- and high-income groups. They concluded that edentulism has been essentially cured among high-income adults by 2009–2012 [11]. This analysis further considers socioeconomic disparity in some detail with a conclusion that, accompanying the reduction in the prevalence in edentulism, there remains an absolute disparity in edentulism between low- and high-income populations. This disparity underscores the difficulty in declaring that edentulism in the USA is no longer a significant oral health-care problem. In fact, edentulism represents one symptom of adult health-care disparities that requires education, further study, and action.

Such studies of edentulism in the USA, despite highlighting the socioeconomic impact on edentulism, report aggregated statistics that do not express the disparity in oral wellness and edentulism in the USA. Data compiled nationally may not be applicable to all regions of the country, especially given the regional variation in edentulism in the USA. Studies of high prevalence of edentulism (e.g., Appalachia) indicated that there are remarkable regional differences that are not only reflective of the age structure of the regions but also related to prevention via water fluoridation, as well as poverty and access to oral health care [7]. Thus, reporting that the reduced percentage of adults in the USA is edentulous does not reflect the continued disparate distribution of total tooth loss in our population. Irrespective of the reported decade upon decade decline in edentulism, it remains problematic for select communities and oral health-care policy.

Tooth loss and edentulism may be influenced by individual and socioeconomic factors. Underlying causes of tooth loss (e.g., caries) are influenced by socioeconomic status [12]. However, the existing models used to predict tooth loss may not recognize that edentulism is often a choice selected by individuals who either cannot afford to retain teeth through restoration and prevention or do not place value in retaining natural teeth and related health. Most simply stated, given the ability to restore and preserve teeth or replace teeth with dental implants, the choice to remove teeth or all teeth may often be motivated by poverty. Indeed, tooth loss is affected by factors beyond dental disease such as patients' and dentists' attitudes, access to care, and the local prevailing philosophies of dental care [13].

There may be behavioral as well as biologic factors that influence the prevalence of edentulism in the USA. The observation that changing therapeutic concepts (e.g., extraction) influenced tooth retention suggests that the predictions of edentulism are linked to factors that influence the incidence of caries, periodontitis, and related tooth loss [11]. The historical assessment of edentulism in New Zealand provides a perspective that aside from geographic, economics, and esthetics, the culture of the day and understanding of oral disease lead to a widespread acceptance by society that extraction was a suitable means of dealing with oral disease. Strong non-discase-related social factors are acknowledged as determinants of edentulism [14]. Given the discrepancy between high- and low-income groups identified, it is entirely plausible that edentulism is a socioeconomic condition resulting from the lack of dental services that promote tooth retention [11]. In this recent analysis of the declining prevalence of edentulism, a careful discussion of the origins of edentulism was provided. It is assumed that retention of a least partial natural dentition is increasing in developed countries and associated with it is dental caries as a major oral health problem among older adults [15]. Suggested was the relationship of edentulism with conditions or factors that lead to tooth loss due to dental caries.

Several factors that could influence the future prevalence of edentulism deserve further consideration. The aged partially dentate population has poorly defined rate of failing restorations in need of replacement and may add considerably to the edentulous population of the future. A complex multidimensional perspective may be needed to predict tooth loss and to understand how non-dental factors such as physical disability contribute to the risk of tooth loss [16]. It is assumed that many teeth will be retained in our expanding, aging population; yet the access, finances, and ability of aged patients to receive tooth-preserving therapy must ultimately be reexamined. By example, a retrospective study of 491 aged participants indicated that tooth survival was influenced by caries and the use of removable prostheses that synergistically compromised tooth survival [17]. Carlsson and co-workers stated clearly that the impact of dental disease and socio-behavioral factors must be considered as significant risks for tooth loss [18].

Older, poorer individuals within the USA are believed to receive maintenance rather than preventive care, and the inability to afford or inaccessibility of dental insurance may contribute to continued edentulism in these segments of the population. Further, several investigations have demonstrated that the prevalence of edentulism is elevated in institutionalized elderly compared with the broader population [19, 20]. In a Delphi survey of geriatric dental experts convened to establish a definition of oral neglect among institutionalized elderly, the definition includes 20 oral diseases and conditions that did not include edentulism. Additionally, the condition of a "lost denture" was considered "not applicable" [21]. This can be interpreted as the lack of appreciation for denture therapy for the edentulous population and the preservation of oral health by prevention among the highest, at-risk populations. Where edentulism is prevalent, access to and importance of oral health care may be predominantly lacking.

The implications for access to care also impact dental education and may take on regional importance; areas in the USA where edentulism over 25 years of age is quite low (e.g., California <4%) may not require broad efforts and extended dental school-based education to provide adequate community oral health in the context of edentulism. Other regions where edentulism over 25 years of age remains high may continue to teach denture therapy, expand the curriculum to address the attendant individual and community health and wellness issues, or empower specialists and/or alternative health workers to provide care and expand access to the existing edentulous population. Oversimplification of the general reduced prevalence of edentulism fails to recognize the significant issues edentulism brings to society and health-care professions (Fig. 1.1).

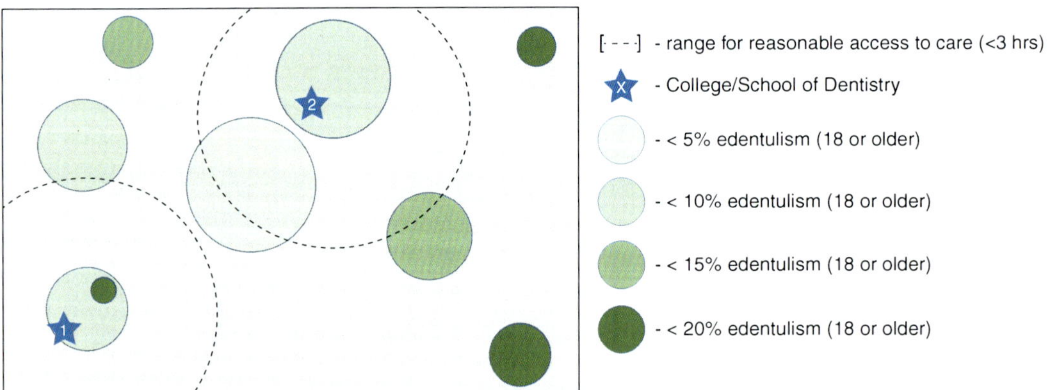

Fig. 1.1 Hypothetical representation of the disparate distribution of edentulism. This square represents any complex, large community (state, nation) where there exist two educational centers or large oral health-care provider systems. Proximal communities are urban and have highly educated populations, and the population is relatively young. More distant communities have regions with a higher prevalence of edentulism. Here, the relative size of the population is represented by the diameter of the circles, and the prevalence of edentulism is represented by color (key). The hypothetical overall prevalence of 8% edentulism in this community does not reflect the current and possible future oral wellness of the communities with higher prevalence of edentulism

Eroding support for oral health care leading to tooth loss and edentulism represents a broader societal risk. Edentulism negatively impacts individuals' social engagement and community activity [22]. Edentulism is important as a correlate of self-esteem and quality of life in older adults [1]. Rouxel et al. [23] described a more complex bidirectional longitudinal association between social capital and oral health. Functional social capital may be influenced by edentulism. Thus, localized high rates of edentulism may contribute to community wellness and should be a matter of broader concern. Overall statistics concerning edentulism, while clearly demonstrating reductions in prevalence, do not highlight the risks that poor oral health and edentulism may have on community health and wellness. Edentulism is an important hallmark of health inequity that merits continued assessment and attention. Instead of heralding opinions that educational programs should remove instruction in denture therapy, educators may reconsider our study of edentulism in terms of community health, social impact, and interprofessional education that places these issues squarely in terms of managing at-risk individuals and populations. Study of "dentures" at the technical level per se may need reconsideration or replacement by considering more broadly "edentulism."

A second factor that may impact the future prevalence of edentulism is the extent of comorbid diseases that are associated with tooth loss and edentulism. Wellness trends in the USA demonstrate striking increases in type II diabetes and obesity. The increasing rates of type 2 diabetes mellitus, a risk factor for periodontal disease and tooth loss, [24] may modestly impact the prevalence of edentulism over the next decades [1]. The influence of diseases and habits (e.g., smoking) on edentulism is clearly demonstrable. For example, in assessing a large national database, a diagnosis of diabetes was associated with greater risk of tooth loss, and current smoking risk was associated with tooth loss (OR = 4.01; 95% CI, 2.59–6.20) [25]. Felton [26] comprehensively revisited the associated comorbidities of edentulism. It is not known if increasing of prevalence of comorbid diseases such as diabetes, obesity, and mental illnesses is presently increasing or will influence the future prevalence of edentulism.

There exists a third factor that may impact the need for denture therapy when considering the prevalence of edentulism and that is, namely, the chronic nature of edentulism. Progressive changes in the alveolar bone accompany chronic denture use and edentulism [27]. This is further associated with significant oral morbidity [28]. There are aspects of managing edentulism as a chronic disorder that impact estimates of therapeutic need. Past and current epidemiological studies have not fully considered the accumulative nature of chronicity on the need for, access to, and capacity of care providers.

Lifelong management of edentulism with or without dental implants requires assessment of mucosal health (denture stomatitis and ulceration), alveolar resorption, denture hygiene (biofilm loading), esthetics, and function. Evaluation for intraoral comorbidities (including oral cancer) is suggested at least annually. Replacement of dentures may be required at approximately 5 years [29]. Denture replacement is an effective means of reducing oral biofilm risks to denture stomatitis as well as systemic disease including pneumonias [30]. The impact of management of the edentulous with dentures is acutely demonstrated in institutionalized elderly for whom denture and oral hygiene is often insufficient. Despite the reduced prevalence of edentulism, the increasing life span of individuals brings with it an increased need for managing increasingly difficult clinical scenarios of new and recurrent dental caries. In fact, with aging, it is possible that more dentures will be constructed for fewer individuals over an extended lifetime. Strategies in caring for the edentulous population require consideration of providing extended care to individuals who may need assistance in managing this chronic condition. Educational programs have an opportunity to redirect efforts to understanding, through the study of edentulism, the fundamental complexity of chronic conditions and the role of professional intervention in providing effective care.

It is broadly argued that the prevalence of edentulism is diminishing with each decade and that there is no further increase in the numbers of edentulous individuals in the USA [11]. If this is true, then the numbers of dentures constructed should be constant and falling. In an attempt to confirm if reductions in the prevalence of edentulism are reflected in the practice of clinical dentistry, several reports of denture manufacturing data were investigated. Most recently, in a published survey of denture production in the USA, 71% of respondents indicated that they expected increased denture production (not inclusive of implant-supported dentures) and denture production was anticipated to increase 6.4% for the year 2014–2015 [31]. Additional data from a 2012 report indicated that the complete denture market would grow at a 4.9% CAGR and in 2013, nearly three million complete dentures were fabricated in the USA [32]. A corporate report considering the US removable prosthesis market also indicated 1.3% growth in the complete denture market and approximately 4.5 million single dentures will be produced in the USA in 2015 [33]. This is significantly greater than the estimated incidence of edentulism or severe tooth loss and reflects previous comments concerning the need to replace dentures in managing chronic edentulism. A large denture-based DSO reported that over the decade from 2004 to 2014, annual year over year increases in the numbers of dentures provided [34]. It can be concluded from these varied reports from denture tooth manufacturers, dental laboratory industry, and denture providers that increased numbers of dentures are being been provided annually in the USA (Fig. 1.2).

When considering multiple surrogate measures to account for denture construction (sale of denture teeth, reported activity in dental laboratories, number of dentures constructed in denture-specific clinics), the past decade's management of edentulism in the USA involves the construction of dentures at an increasing annual rate, despite the reported stabilization or expected reduction in the prevalence of edentulism. This may reflect unaccounted for edentulation or improved access to care. Alternatively, the data reporting on edentulism may under-represent the edentulous population methodologically. Irrespective of interpretation, large numbers of dentures continue to be constructed annually in the USA. To place this into context, for the estimated eight million edentulous individuals, there are approximately 150,000 general dentists and 3300 prosthodontists practicing in the USA or approximately 50 patients/dentist. Edentulism is not rare, and it cannot be assumed that edentulous individuals will cease presenting for care among many clinicians in the regions of the USA where the higher prevalence of edentulism persists. These observations support Waldman's contention that prevalence of edentulism will be incrementally less in the next decade, but the need to care for a diverse edentulous population remains in the present [35].

The retention of teeth by our population requires access to dental care, and this is not without current limitations and structural challenges [36]. In the report "State of Decay. Are Older Americans Coming of Age without Oral Health Care," there exists a persistent lack of oral health coverage across much of the nation. Forty-two percent of states provide little or no dental benefits; 31 states have numerous Dental Health Provider Shortage Areas (HPSAs, meeting <40 of dental provider needs). Eight states had strikingly high rates of edentulism. Thirteen states have 60% or more residents living in communities without water fluoridation, despite recognition for 68 years that this public health measure markedly reduces dental caries. These conditions indicate there exists no safety net or little provision of community oral health care for many adults in the USA.

When adult oral health is considered at the level of caries, the rate of untreated disease is 44% among adults with income below 10% the federal poverty rate [37]. Impoverished and uninsured individuals may not have any access to denture care; in 2012, 19 state Medicaid programs did not offer denture benefits. There exists in the USA an access to care problem for adult dental care [38]. Partially edentulous individuals in need of prostheses including complete dentures may not receive appropriate oral rehabilitation. In the face of accumulated odontogenic infections, many adults may face financially realistic choice of edentulation. It remains to be determined if edentulism is largely the result of socioeconomic

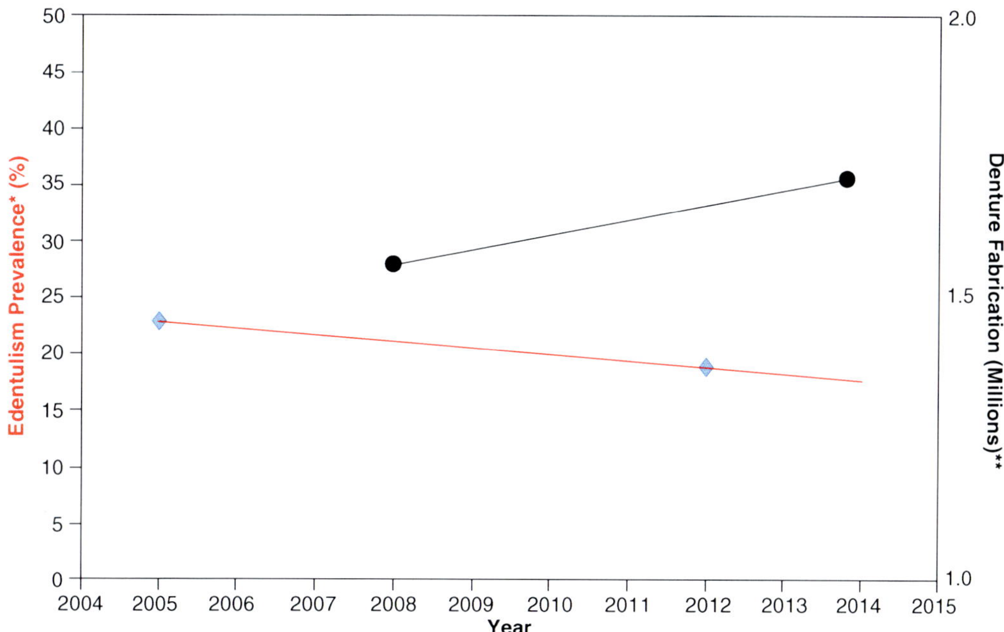

Fig. 1.2 Paradoxical increased denture delivery in the USA. *CDC/NCHC data on complete edentulism in the USA. **DataResearch, estimated denture market projected to grow at 4.9% cumulative annual growth rate (2012). Corroborating data obtained from denture tooth manufacturers, dental laboratory surveys, and denture clinics in the USA corroboratively indicate that, over the past decade, the numbers of complete dentures produced and delivered have increased at a cumulative annual growth rate of between 2 and 5%. Note this is in contrast to the reduced prevalence of edentulism in the USA reported by epidemiological studies

realities facing individuals with untreated chronic oral infections.

Current technologies that provide access to dental implant therapy have promoted the transition from a partial or failing natural dentition to an implant-supported or implant-retained prosthetic dentition. Several contemporary approaches advocate complete edentulation and replacement using multiple implants to retain fixed prostheses. The reasons for extraction to complete edentulism may include, for example, failing dental prostheses, rampant caries, and uncontrollable periodontal disease. Irrespective of the motivation for edentulation, the approach is popular and profitable. Accounting for these individuals and the associated health risks that accompany poorly managed dental implant therapy (peri-implantitis) is a novel factor that must be considered in the measurement of edentulism.

Edentulism is a chronic disability associated with important comorbid factors. The epidemiological data indicating a dramatic reduction in edentulism in the USA over the past one-half century also demonstrates that edentulism displays important health disparities and highlights the oral health access to care problem in the USA. High prevalence of edentulism in select regions or communities in the nation may be symptoms of broader wellness issues in those regions and communities. As such, dentistry must re-engage and redouble academic, clinical, and scientific activities surrounding edentulism.

References

1. Starr JM, Hall R. Predictors and correlates of edentulism in healthy older people. Curr Opin Clin Nutr Metab Care. 2010;13:19–23.
2. Eklund SA, Burt BA. Risk factors for total tooth loss in the United States; longitudinal analysis of national data. J Public Health Dent. 1994;54(1):5–14.
3. Caplan DJ, Weintraub JA. The oral health burden in the United States: a summary of recent epidemiologic studies. J Dent Educ. 1993;57(12):853–62.

4. Marcenes W, Kassebaum NJ, Bernabé E, Flaxman A, Naghavi M, Lopez A, Murray CJ. Global burden of oral conditions in 1990-2010: a systematic analysis. J Dent Res. 2013;92:592–7.

5. Redford M, Drury TF, Kingman A, Brown LJ. Denture use and the technical quality of dental prostheses among persons 18-74 years of age: United States, 1988-1991. J Dent Res. 1996;75:714–25.

6. Kassebaum NJ, Bernabé Dahiya EM, Bhandari B, Murray CJL, Marcenes W. Global burden of severe tooth loss: a systematic review and meta-analysis. J Dent Res. 2014;93(7 Suppl):20S–8S.

7. Gorsuch MM, Sanders SG, Wu B. Tooth loss in Appalachia and the Mississippi delta relative to other regions in the United States, 1999-2010. Am J Public Health. 2014;104(5):e85–91.

8. Cunha-Cruz J, Hujoel PP, Nadanovsky P. Secular trends in socio-economic disparities in edentulism: USA, 1972-2001. J Dent Res. 2007;86(2):131–6.

9. Wu B, Liang J, Plassman BL, Remle C, Luo X. Edentulism trends among middle-aged and older adults in the United States: comparison of five racial/ethnic groups. Community Dent Oral Epidemiol. 2012;40:145–53.

10. Saman DM, Lemieux A, Arevalo O, Lutfiyya MN. A population-based study of edentulism in the US: does depression and rural residency matter after controlling for potential confounders? BMC Public Health. 2014;14:65.

11. Slade GD, Akinkugbe AA, Sanders AE. Projections of U.S. Edentulism prevalence following 5 decades of decline. J Dent Res. 2014;93(10):959–65.

12. Gorsuch MM, Sander SG, Wu B. Tooth loss in Appalachia and the Mississippi delta relative to other regions in the United States, 1999–2010. Am J Public Health. 2014;104:e85–91.

13. Liang J, Wu B, Plassman B, Bennett JM, Beck J. Social stratification, oral hygiene, and trajectories of dental caries among old Americans. J Aging Health. 2014;26(6):900–23.

14. Fejerskov O, Escobar G, Jossing M, Baelum V. A functional natural dentition for all—and for life? The oral healthcare system needs revision. J Oral Rehabil. 2013;40:707–22.

15. Sussex PV, Thomson WM, Fitzgerald RP. Understanding the 'epidemic' of complete tooth loss among older New Zealanders. Gerodontology. 2010;27(2):85–95.

16. Thomson WM, Ma S. An ageing population poses dental challenges. Singapore Dental J. 2014;25:3–8.

17. Chen X, Clark JJ. Multidimensional risk assessment for tooth loss in a geriatric population with diverse medical and dental backgrounds. J Am Geriatr Soc. 2011;59(6):1116–22.

18. Chen X, Clark JJ, Naorungroj S. Length of tooth survival in older adults with complex medical, functional and dental backgrounds. J Am Dent Assoc. 2012;143:566–78.

19. Müller F, Naharro M, Carlsson GE. What are the prevalence and incidence of tooth loss in the adult and elderly population in Europe? Clin Oral Implants Res. 2007;18(Suppl 3):2–14. Review.

20. Angelillo IF, Sagliocci G, Hendricks SJ, Villari P. Tooth loss and dental caries in institutionalized elderly in Italy. Community Dentistry Oral Epidemiology. 1990;18:216–8.

21. Dolan TA, Atchison KA. Implications of access, utilization and need for oral health care by the non-institutionalized and institutionalized elderly on the dental delivery system. J Dent Educ. 1993;57(12):876–87.

22. Katz RV, Smith BJ, Berkey DB, Guset A, O'Connor MP. Defining oral neglect in institutionalized elderly: a consensus definition for the protection of vulnerable elderly people. J Am Dent Assoc. 2010;141(4):433–40.

23. Rodrigues SM, Oliveira AC, Vargas AMD, Moreira AN, Ferreira E. Implications of edentulism on quality of life among elderly. Int J Environ Res Public Health. 2012;9:100–9.

24. Rouxel P, Tsakos G, Demakakos P, Zaninotto P, Chandola T, Watt RG. Is social capital a determinant of oral health among older adults? Findings from the English longitudinal study of ageing. PLoS One. 2015;10(5):e0125557.

25. Luo H, Pan W, Sloan F, Feinglos M, Wu B. Forty-year trends in tooth loss among American adults with and without diabetes mellitus: an age-period-cohort analysis. Prev Chronic Dis. 2015;12:E211.

26. Musacchio E, Perissinotto E, Binotto P, Sartori L, Silva-Netto F, Zambon S, Manzato E, Corti MC, Baggio G, Crepaldi G. Tooth loss in the elderly and its association with nutritional status, socio-economic and lifestyle factors. Acta Odontol Scand. 2007;65(2):78–86.

27. Felton DA. Complete edentulism and comorbid diseases: an update. J Prosthodont. 2016;25(1):5–20.

28. Klemetti E. A review of residual ridge resorption and bone density. J Prosthet Dent. 1996;75(5):512–4. Review.

29. Mandali G, Sener ID, Turker SB, Ulgen H. Factors affecting the distribution and prevalence of oral mucosal lesions in complete denture wearers. Gerodontology. 2011;28(2):97–103.

30. Cooper LF. The current and future treatment of edentulism. J Prosthodont. 2009;18(2):116–22.

31. Iinuma T, Arai Y, Abe Y, Takayama M, Fukumoto M, Fukui Y, Iwase T, Takebayashi T, Hirose N, Gionhaku N, Komiyama K. Denture wearing during sleep doubles the risk of pneumonia in the very elderly. J Dent Res. 2015;94(3 Suppl):28S–36S.

32. U.S. Dental Laboratory Survey; Data reported by The Key Group, Inc.

33. DataResearch; courtesy of Ms. Pamela Johnson, Aegis Publishing.

34. Data on file, correspondence with industry December 20154.

35. Data on file; personal correspondence.

36. Waldman HB, Perlman SP, Xu L. Should the teaching of full denture prosthetics be maintained in schools of dentistry? J Dent Educ. 2007;71(4):463–6.

37. http://www.dentistryiq.com/content/dam/diq/onlinearticles/documents/2013/10/OHA_State_of_Decay_2013.PDF

38. http://files.kff.org/attachment/issue-brief-access-to-dental-care-in-medicaid-spotlight-on-nonelderly-adults

The Aging Body and Nutrition

Angus William Gilmour Walls

Abstract

Nutritional requirements change with aging; thus, the diet of older people should be nutrient dense with lower caloric intake. However, with tooth loss, dietary changes move in the opposite direction. Replacement of missing teeth results in people feeling that they can chew better but does not automatically result in dietary change unless a dietary intervention is undertaken along with improved function. Dietary intervention for people with complete dentures will result in a better "quality" diet, and this change is even greater when a lower denture is supported by mandibular implants. The "rate-limiting step" in dietary alteration appears to be what can be achieved with the least stable prosthesis. As prosthetic stability improves, dietary change can be more effective.

The amount of food that we require for maintenance and function of the body is influenced by changes associated with aging, and there are associations between nutrient intake and some of the progressive changes seen in older people. In this chapter those aspects of age change that can be affected by diet/nutrient availability will be reviewed. Following this will be a description of how oral health can influence foods choice and dietary intake, which can influence nutritional status. Finally, strategies will be described that can help patients make functional changes to alter their dietary patterns in order to benefit their health.

2.1 Alterations in Tissues with Age that may be Affected by Nutrient Intake

2.1.1 Muscle

There is a progressive loss of muscle mass and, hence, strength with increasing age (sarcopenia). The rate of loss of muscle is affected by the level of physical activity of the individual, with those who are physically inactive losing between 3 and 5% of muscle mass per decade beyond the age of 30 [1–3]. The mechanisms for the development of sarcopenia are not clear, but it is likely associated with reductions in the anabolic stimuli to muscle from growth hormone and estrogen/androgen secretion alongside changes in innervation from loss of motor neurons [4–6]. There are some data that suggest that low protein intake, as well as low intakes of vitamin D, other antioxidants, and the B-complex vitamins, may also be linked to increased rates of muscle loss [7–9]. Chronic conditions that result in lower levels of

A. W. G. Walls, Ph.D., B.D.S.
Edinburgh Dental Institute, Edinburgh, UK
e-mail: Angus.Walls@ed.ac.uk

© Springer International Publishing AG, part of Springer Nature 2018
E. Emami, J. Feine (eds.), *Mandibular Implant Prostheses*,
https://doi.org/10.1007/978-3-319-71181-2_2

exercise or increases in systemic inflammatory markers are risk factors for sarcopenia, as is smoking [6, 10, 11].

This rate of loss is reduced in those who are physically active with the reduction reflecting the extent of physical activity undertaken by the individual. However, there are very few who remain sufficiently active that they retain the bulk of their muscle mass into older age (high-performance athletes and weight lifters are best at retaining muscle into aging providing they continue to exercise regularly). The most effective forms of exercise to retain muscle mass are those which involve resistance training rather than aerobic activity per se [12, 13].

The rate of loss seems to accelerate beyond the age of 75; the reasons for this acceleration remain unclear but may simply reflect a combination of the loss of anabolic stimuli alongside an increasingly sedentary lifestyle that is often associated with advanced aging [14, 15].

Obesity can protect against some of the effects of sarcopenia in the young old, as about 25% of body weight is muscle and it takes more physical strength for an obese person to move. However, in the longer term, this protective effect is counterbalanced by a sedentary lifestyle, increasing insulin resistance associated with deposits of abdominal fat, and the production of TNFα by adipocytes, which is catabolic and may interfere with insulin receptors, resulting in greater insulin resistance [16].

Muscle is a complex tissue, and loss of muscle mass affects the various components of muscle differently. Thus, there is a disproportionally greater loss of type II fibers in proximal muscle groups; this is associated with an increase in type I collagen in the same muscle bundles. Actions that depend on fine control from by type II fiber activity are more strongly affected by increasing age. In terms of oral health, this reduced type II fiber activity would make daily oral hygiene tasks more difficult [2].

As noted above, deficiencies in protein intake and in some micronutrients are associated with increased rates of muscle loss, but there is no evidence that vitamin supplementation above recommended levels or high protein intake would result in a protective effect in the absence of resistance exercise.

There is an increased risk of protein/energy malnutrition in older people, which is driven by a combination of food choice [17]. Older people tend to exclude protein-rich foods; their appetite declines, they have difficulty digesting high protein content foods, and they fear raised cholesterol levels, thereby reducing their intake of red meat. The higher cost of protein also reduces the tendency of older people to choose these foods.

2.1.2 Gastrointestinal Tract

There is a tendency for hypo- or achlorhydria to develop with increasing age. This is associated with the development of atrophic gastritis, but it is unclear whether this is an age effect per se or a product of increasing rates of infection with *Helicobacter pylori* infection. The location of *H. pylori* infection in the stomach determines the pathology that results, so infection of the pyloric antrum occurs in people who secrete more acid naturally and serves as a stimulus for further acid secretion. This, in turn, results in gastric or duodenal ulceration. People with normal levels of gastric acid secretion develop *H. pylori* infection in the fundus of the stomach that results in an atrophic gastritis and reduction in acid secretion. Rates of hypochlorhydria and achlorhydria increase from around 24% in people aged 60–69 to 37% in those over 80 [18, 19].

Duodenal absorption of the B-complex vitamins is pH dependent, so, in those with reduced gastric pH, absorption is reduced. This is most commonly seen with vitamin B12, resulting in pernicious anemia. The prevalence of B12 deficiency is approximately 10–15%, with levels of around 35% for a combination of marginal and overt deficiency states. About 30–40% of these subjects have atrophic gastritis.

From rodent models of aging, there is some evidence of changes in structure of the small bowel that affect absorption in aged animals. However, current data for man does not support similar changes occurring, so there should be no alterations in the ability of the small bowel to absorb digested foods [20].

There are increases in gastric emptying time and colonic transit time that are likely associated with reduced sympathetic tone in older subjects. These have an effect on satiety and, therefore, on food intake. With reduced rates of gastric emptying, satiety is reached at lower levels of food intake [21].

2.1.3 The Eye

The major cause of damage to the eye is sunlight, but there are two causes of age-related damage to the eye that may also have nutritional links, cataract and age-related macular degeneration (AMD).

The evidence for cataract is stronger than for AMD, but there are associations with vitamin C status and intake of the carotenoids lutein and zeaxanthin, with increased consumption leading to a protective effect for both conditions. This evidence supports the current dietary recommendations of five portions of fruit and vegetables daily, including citrus fruits to obtain vitamin C and green leafy vegetables like spinach and kale for the carotenoids. There is also less robust evidence that some of the fat-soluble vitamins are protective against AMD.

Individuals with intermediate and advanced AMD are often given high-dose vitamin supplements, including zinc, to try to reduce the rate of progression of this disease, but there is no evidence that vitamin supplements can have a protective effect against these age-related eye diseases [22, 23].

2.2 Nutritional Requirements with Aging

Muscle is one of the principle tissues that uses sugars as a form of energy, and it is particularly important in terms of maintenance of body temperature, as sugar metabolism in muscle releases heat. To generate heat, we shiver when cold. The reduction in muscle mass associated with sarcopenia is associated with poorer thermoregulation and is why older people "feel the cold" more, as they have less capacity to generate body warmth.

As their reduced muscle mass is less metabolically active than that of younger people, older people need to reduce their energy consumption and take in fewer dietary calories for a given level of physical activity. This change is reflected in alterations in the recommended dietary reference values (DRVs) for intake of energy, as either sugars or fats with increasing age (Table 2.1). Interestingly there is marked variation between DRVs from different national organizations with variation in recommended intakes for people

Table 2.1 Recommended daily intakes of energy by age from the UK, WHO, the USA, and EU (where data were originally given in calories, these have been converted into MJoules by multiplying by 0.00418) [75–77]

| | UK/WHO | | USA | | | | EU | | | |
| | | | Sedentary[a] | | Active[b] | | Low[c] | | High[d] | |
Age	Male	Female	Male	Female	Male	Female	Male	Female	Male	Female
15–18	11.51	8.83	9.2	7.5	12.5	10.0	11.8	8.9		
19–50	10.6	8.1	10.0	7.9	12.1	9.6	11.3	8.4	12.0	9.0
51–59	10.6	8.0	8.75	6.7	10.4	8.75	11.3	8.4	12.0	9.0
60–64	9.93	7.99	8.75	6.7	10.4	8.75	8.5	7.2	9.2	7.8
65–74	9.71	7.96	8.75	6.7	10.4	8.75	8.5	7.2	9.2	7.8
75+	8.77	7.61	8.75	6.7	10.4	8.75	7.5	6.7	8.5	7.6

[a]Sedentary means a lifestyle that includes only the light physical activity associated with typical day-to-day life
[b]Active means a lifestyle that includes physical activity equivalent to walking more than 3 miles per day at 3–4 miles per hour, in addition to the light physical activity associated with typical day-to-day life
[c]Low means no physical activity, desirable body weight
[d]High means recommended physical activity normal body weight

aged over 75 of between 7.5 and 10.4 MJ/day. The direction of these differences varies across the life span and, in some countries, reflects a recognition of differing levels of physical activity.

Sugars in the diet are categorized into two major groups commonly described as "free" and "bound." Bound sugars are those that are contained within the cells of foods, while free sugars are extracellular and are often added to foods to sweeten or as a preservative. Bound sugars can be converted into free sugars through the food preparation process; for example, the sugars in an orange are regarded as bound (within the cells of the orange), whereas when the same fruit is processed to produce juice, the same sugars are regarded as "free." Normal diets contain both free and bound sugars; however, it is free sugars that are regarded as particularly harmful in terms of human disease, particularly diabetes, obesity, cardiovascular disease, and, of course, dental caries. This is reflected in the WHO recommendation and the UK government's policy that free sugars should form no more than 5% of dietary energy intake. This applies across the age span [24, 25].

While there is a reduction in the need for dietary energy as a consequence of sarcopenia, there is no evidence of any requirement for a reduction in either protein or micronutrient intake with age; indeed, there are some suggestions that protein intakes should be higher in older people than in the young. As a consequence, older people need to consume a different style of diet compared with the young that is proportionally higher in nutrients per unit of energy than the young. This dietary pattern is described as being "nutrient dense" (see, e.g., http://nihseniorhealth. gov/eatingwellasyougetolder/choosenutrient-densefoods/01.html).

The need for increased nutrient density in diet is poorly understood by consumers, and the oral health team should be aware of this when giving dietary advice to older people. Equally, the WHO/UK government recommendations in relation to free sugars are recent and need to be explained carefully to older people.

2.3 Oral Conditions That Influence Food Intake

Food intake in older people is affected by many confounding variables that can be divided into those associated with aging/lifestyle and those associated with disease (Fig. 2.1). Patterns of food consumption are largely habitual and are driven by the member of the household who buys and cooks the food. If we want to change the pattern of food consumption, we need to influence not only the person we are trying to get to change but also the person they live with if that individual is the shopper/cook. There are two oral factors that affect food consumption, alterations in taste (and smell) perception and the number of teeth that an individual has.

2.3.1 Taste and Smell

There are five basic categories of taste: salt, sweet, bitter, sour, and savory (or umami). There is a progressive reduction in taste acuity with increasing age for all of these, with the exception of savory [26–30]. The mechanisms that underpin this reduction are not well understood; however there are reductions in taste in association with specific drugs and with dry mouth either as a result of pathological gland damage or induced as a side effect of drugs used for other chronic conditions [31, 32]. There are similar reductions in the sense of smell with age, and, in combination, these result in consumers getting less enjoyment from eating food as the taste becomes progressively more bland [30, 33].

A variety of approaches have been attempted to overcome this challenge to make foods more interesting for older people. These include the use of intense (artificial) flavorings and chemicals that enhance taste perception. The most common of the latter is the addition of salt to foods, but this also has potential health consequences. Monosodium glutamate is also a very effective taste enhancer, but its use does result in people needing to drink more water as it gives a sense of dryness to foods, and it also increases the viscosity of foods, making them unpalatable [34–37].

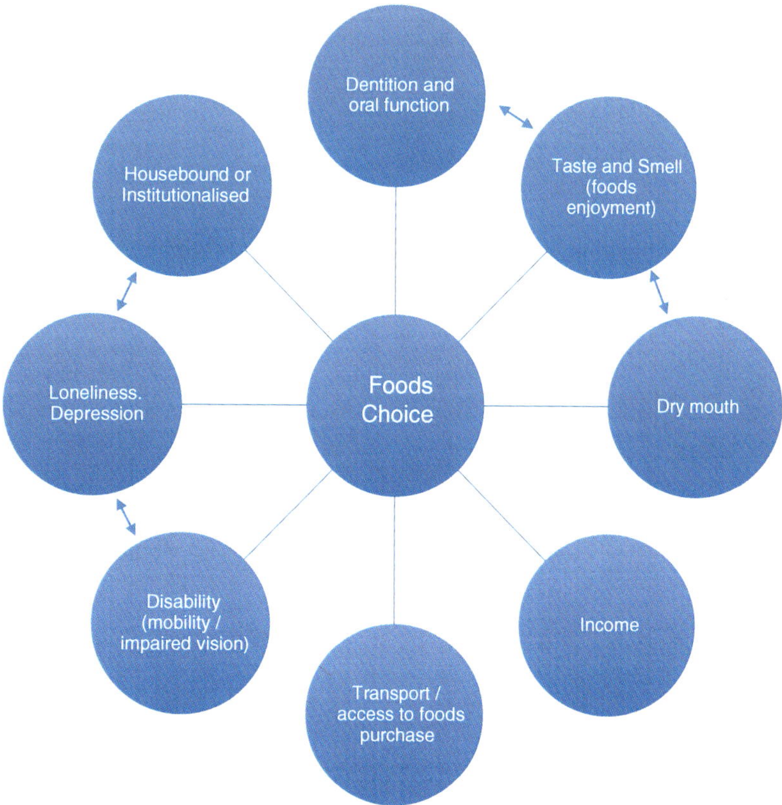

Fig. 2.1 The wide variety of factors that influence food choice in older consumers. Some factors are interrelated (arrows)

2.3.2 Saliva

Salivary flow and function remain remarkably consistent with increasing age in the medially fit and healthy individual, despite profound changes in salivary gland structure with time [38, 39]. However, dry mouth (xerostomia) is a symptom of increasing importance in older populations. Dry mouth is largely due to the side effects of many drugs used to manage the chronic diseases of older age, as well as the more rare pathological conditions that cause destruction of salivary gland tissue like Sjögren's syndrome, or as an aftermath of radiotherapy used in the management of head and neck cancer [40–43]. Reductions in both taste and smell will be compounded in people who suffer from xerostomia for two reasons:

- Both are "wet" sensations, i.e., the tastant is dissolved in water/mucin prior to its being sensed. Logically, saliva must have a taste if we consider its composition. However, it is ubiquitous, and so we ignore it when considering the taste of foods. When there is less saliva, there is less fluid bathing the taste buds into which tastes can dissolve, altering the perception for a given food.

- Saliva in xerostomic people is both sparser and has altered composition compared with that in people with normal salivary function, so the ubiquitous background "taste" is altered, driving changes in perceived taste. There is also less fluid present.

The bland taste of foods has a negative effect on food consumption, as it is not as enjoyable to eat [33, 44].

Consumers with profound xerostomia also have difficulty swallowing foods, because saliva is required to both "glue" a bolus of masticated food together and to lubricate its movement while passing through the esophagus. This problem is overcome by the consumer drinking water very frequently while eating; however water is less efficient as a lubricant/glue than saliva, due to the lack of mucins. Artificial salivas are of little value in relation to bolus formation and swallowing; they do contain bulking agents (often carboxymethylcellulose) or mucins, but, by definition, they are ineffective once swallowed unless topped up very frequently during a meal.

2.3.3 Number and Distribution of Teeth

The principle function for teeth in man is to break up foods into smaller particles to prepare the food for swallowing. The size of the particles in food that are perceived as "ready for swallowing" varies between individuals but also changes as chewing becomes less efficient, so that people with fewer or no teeth chew food less well and swallow bigger particles of food than those who have an intact dentition. This swallowing threshold is an innate characteristic.

Chewing food and mixing it with saliva have two effects: it reduces the size of the food particles in the bolus, but also enzymes in saliva (salivary amylases) start the process of digestion of starches into sugars in the oral environment. Interestingly, there is some very old and limited evidence that chewing, per se, is not required for digestion of foods with modern methods of foods preparation [45]. These data, however, were derived in young dentate volunteers, and extrapolating this to older people with fewer teeth may be inappropriate. Not only do older people have fewer teeth and, therefore, less efficient chewing; they also suffer from sarcopenia of the masticatory muscles that influence chewing force, so the composition of the food bolus is very different in a young person compared with an older one [46–49].

The efficiency of the act of chewing is affected profoundly by the number and distribution of teeth in the mouth [50–53]. In terms of research methodology, this effectiveness can be measured in one of two ways.

Study participants are given specified quantities of test foods and are told to chew them until they perceive they are ready for swallowing (the deglutition threshold). The chewed food is then removed from the mouth, and the particle size and distribution are measured either by sieving the food or using image analysis techniques. The test foods should be things that fracture into smaller pieces during chewing, like carrot or nuts, to make this process easier.

The alternative is to give people chewing gum which is in two different colors and ask them to chew for a specified number of chewing cycles. The gum is removed and analyzed in terms of the quality of mixing of the different colors, using either a visual scale or again (and more commonly) using image analysis techniques.

Both approaches have their advantages and disadvantages, but they consistently demonstrate that chewing is less efficient with fewer natural teeth, especially when the teeth do not meet in "opposing pairs." The least efficient chewing is seen in people with complete dentures that are supported by only the mucosa and bone. This is not surprising if you consider that putting a sample of food between dentures and chewing will result in the denture being displaced from its support and moving in the mouth. This is worse for a mandibular denture where the extent of support is less than for a maxillary one. In terms of chewing, the least efficient pattern of oral health is when someone has a few maxillary natural teeth and a mandibular complete denture. Chewing is only possible with dentures as a result of learned juggling of the denture by the muscles of the cheeks and tongue; for example, to incise food with upper and lower complete dentures, an individual has to stabilize the posterior of the upper denture by curling the dorsum of the tongue upward and the posterior of the lower denture by curling the sides of the tongue downward to allow pressure to be applied by the incisors without displacing the dentures. This is a complex, learned process that is compounded in humans by alerations in the fit of dentures with time. The average age of dentures worn in the UK is around 10–12 years; after this time even very slowly progressing alveolar resorption will result in a discrepancy between the fitted surface of the denture and the edentulous ridge. When there is a mismatch between the denture base and the underlying mucosa, the stabilizing adhesion and cohesion of the salivary film are less effective and so the dentures become intrinsically less stable.

This lack of fit often manifests itself when edentulous people are ill and in hospital. They commonly leave their dentures out for a period of time and then find that they can't chew as well when the denture is put back in the mouth. This is often misconstrued as the "gums having shrunk" when, in fact, it is more likely that they have forgotten how to juggle the dentures in function [54].

The effect of these changes in masticatory function with progressive tooth loss is reflected in the oral health data from the US Veterans Administration Longitudinal Study of Aging (commonly referred to as the VALDS or Veterans Administration Longitudinal Dental Survey). In this cohort, the research teams assessed diet over time with respect to tooth loss. Over an 8-year period, they showed that everyone developed a healthier diet (higher in fiber, lower in fats and cholesterol). However, in those subjects who had lost eight or more teeth during this follow-up period, the dietary changes were less marked and were characterized by dietary choices of reduced intake of foods that could be hard to chew, like raw carrot (Table 2.2) [51].

These seminal data underpin our understanding of why there are differences in diet between those with and without teeth. This is illustrated in a wide range of cross-sectional studies, for example, the VALDS, the US National Health and Nutrition Examination Survey series, and the UK National Diet and Nutrition Survey, to name but a few (Table 2.3) [52, 53, 55–57].

These data consistently demonstrate that people with fewer or no teeth consume a less healthy diet than those with more teeth. This is manifest by diets characterized as being lower in dietary fiber (lower fruit and vegetable intake) and higher in sugar and fat intake [58]. However, these associations are by no means straightforward, as the pattern of tooth loss in population studies varies markedly with socioeconomic status of the individual; thus, poorer people are more likely to have worse oral health and also make less healthy dietary choices. However,

Table 2.2 percentage of women consuming selected fruit and vegetable items one or more times per week in 1994 among women who consumed the same food one or more times per week in 1990

Food	Number consuming the food in 1990	Percent consuming the food in 1994		
		Teeth lost		
		0	1–4	≥5
Banana	37,754	86	86	91
Cantaloupe	22,360	61	60	58
Apple or pear[a]	38,984	78	76[b]	67[b]
Raw carrot[a]	34,278	79	75[b]	67[b]
Cooked carrot	34,619	68	70	72

This should be Table 4 from [51]
[a]P-value <0.05 linear trend across these three groups
[b]P-value <0.05 comparing consumption of specific food items between women who lost teeth and women who did not lose teeth after adjusting for total energy intake, age, physical activity, BMI, and smoking

Table 2.3 Intake of key nutrients with differing dental status from the US Veterans Administration Longitudinal Study of Aging and the UK National Diet and Nutrition Survey [53, 55]

	Intact		Compromised		Edentulous	
	US	UK	US	UK	US	UK
Protein (g/day)	80	72	74	67	68	60
Fiber[a] (g/day)	21[b]	16[b]	19[b]	13[b]	16[b]	11[b]
Calcium (mg/day)	773[b]	883	677[b]	812	689[b]	722[b]
Niacin (mg/day)	32	34	28	31	34	27
Vitamin C (mg/day)	156	82	146	73	127	60

[a]The numerical differences in fiber intake between the UK and US data are largely associated with different analytical techniques used for the two surveys. The US method gives a greater numerical value than the UK method
[b]These values are below the recommended daily intake values (RNIs)

when these data are analyzed and controlled for social variables, the relationship between reducing numbers of teeth and diet remains.

The most likely mechanism for the component of this change, independent of social variables, is foods choice. People with few or no teeth choose not to eat foods that are difficult to chew (e.g., raw carrot, nuts, crispy bread). There are also some unusual foods choices that are made by people with dentures who, for example, often don't eat berries (if a seed gets under the denture and the person then bites down it hurts) or green leafy vegetables (the leafy vegetable can get stuck onto the acrylic surface of the denture, which is socially embarrassing). They prefer foods that are easier to chew, so avoid hard crispy and dry food textures and prefer soft, wet, pulpy, and slimy ones [59].

There is one study that explored the relationship between food consumption and dental status that does not show this relationship. Shinkai et al. used the "healthy eating index" (HEI) as their measure of dietary quality and showed no relationship between it and numbers of teeth/edentulism [60]. HEI is a measure of overall dietary quality and does not assess individual food groups, which may explain the lack of a relationship. Also the study sample was relatively small compared with those for NHANES and the NDNS.

2.4 Does Prosthetic Intervention Affect Foods Choice?

It would be logical to think that replacing missing teeth with a prosthesis will result in people choosing to eat a better diet because their masticatory performance will improve. However, there is very little evidence to support this.

Among male health professionals there is some evidence that the use of a removable part denture to replace missing teeth results in dietary patterns similar to those in subjects with an intact dentition [61].

In a range of studies that looked at a wide range of prosthetic interventions, from fixed partial dentures through removable partial dentures, complete dentures, and implant-retained or implant-supported restorations, no changes in diet were seen subsequent to the prosthetic intervention, despite a universal trend for perceived improvements in masticatory performance. While participants reported that they could chew better/more difficult foods, they did not appear to change their diet [61–68]. An interesting study by Awad et al. showed that people with implant-supported overdentures had no differences in their overall dietary intake of nutrients compared with a control group using conventional dentures, but the implant group were more likely to derive those nutrients from fresh whole fruits and vegetables [62]. This suggests some change in dietary behavior toward a healthier diet high in fruits and vegetables intakes. There is an increasing awareness that the things we measure in terms of dietary intake, like specific micronutrients, are only a small part of the health benefits of a diet high in fruits and vegetables, as they contain so many elements that are thought or known to be beneficial to health but that are not currently recorded in dietary assessment. One example would be lycopene from tomatoes, thought to be partially responsible for the health benefits of the "Mediterranean diet," but not assessed in a formal way during these sorts of studies.

The explanation for the conundrum that people think they can chew better but do not change their foods choice involves behavior change. People do not necessarily change a behavior/habit because something is done that will allow them to make the change. Doing something that will help/allow someone to make a behavior change is known as facilitating that change. However, behaviors/habits like foods choice extend beyond the benefits of dental care and require a specific approach to induce behavior change, rather than simply to facilitate that change. Behaviors are often entrenched and require interaction with all those involved in the behavior; in relation to diet and foods choice, this includes not only the person for whom one has provided a new prosthesis but also that person's family group, as dietary change will affect all not just one.

Within behavioral change, there is a concept called "stage of change" (Fig. 2.2) [69]. This illustrates the various stages that people go through in planning for and making a change. One of the roles of the dental team when making new prostheses for patients is to help move people forward along this pathway. There are a variety of "hooks" that are available to do this, not least that one is providing something for a patient that will make chewing easier/better, that will facilitate a change. If, at the same time, the dentist talks with the person about diet and the health benefits of change, they can be helped to move them up the change ladder toward a place where change happens. This is much less likely to occur if the dentist and staff do not act as facilitators in this process.

Moynihan and colleagues have used this approach in two ways, initially with a targeted dietary intervention delivered by a dietician during the various stages of denture manufacture and, subsequently, using community nutrition assistants. Denture manufacture is a process that takes a number of stages, so lends itself to a phased approach to delivery of dietary advice linked to a formal dietary assessment. From these studies, it has been clearly demonstrated that people can and will change their diet if this change is facilitated in an appropriate manner during care. Furthermore, Moynihan et al. showed that these changes were more profound in people with implant-retained/implant-supported overdentures than in a control group with conventional dentures (Table 2.4). This study demonstrated, for the first time, that stability of the lower prosthesis was the "rate-limiting step" in terms of the magnitude of change that could be accomplished [70–73].

Bartlett et al. extended this work in a small pilot study looking at the use of denture fixatives and nutrition advice in complete denture wearers. The study used a cohort of edentulous people, all of whom received new dentures, dietary advice, and advice about the use of denture fixatives. Within the cohort, there was a marked improvement in fruit and vegetable intake and reduction of fat intake (Table 2.5). However, they were unable to differentiate between the effects of their dietary intervention alone (which comprised simply giving people some information leaflets about diet) and the

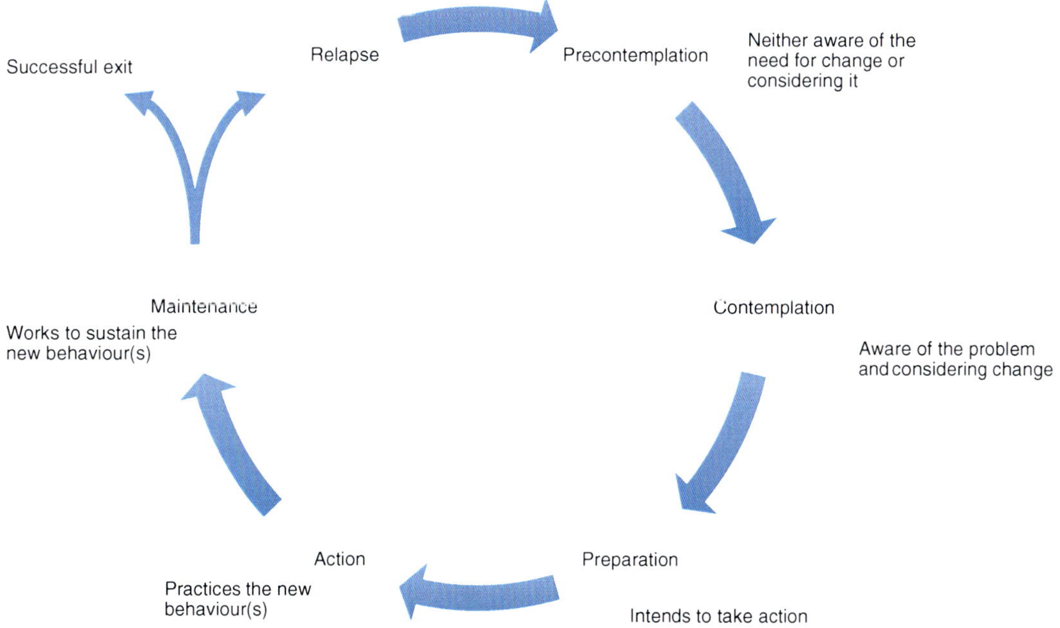

Fig. 2.2 Stages of awareness during a process of change (Adapted from Prochaska and DiClemente (1992)) [69]

Table 2.4 Changes in selected nutrient intake between conventional denture wearers and users of implant-supported overdentures after a tailored dietary intervention [73]

	Time	IOD $n = 28$		CD $n = 28$		
		Mean	95% CI	Mean	95% CI	P
Energy MJ/day	Base	7.1	6.9, 7.2	6.5	6.4, 6.6	0.001
	3/12	7.3	7.1, 7.6	7.0	7.0, 7.2	0.264
Difference		−0.27	−0.5, −0.03	−0.4	−0.7, 0.1	
Fruits and vegetables g/day	Base	445	350, 450	301	239, 363	0.013
	3/12	467	438, 626	425	281, 429	0.296
Difference		−21	−138, −35	−124	−106, −2	
Fiber g/day	Base	11.1	10.5, 11.7	10.2	9.7, 10.7	0.017
	3/12	11.7	11.2, 12.3	10.5	10.0, 10.8	0.002
Difference		−0.7	−1.3, −0.3	−0.3	−0.7, −0.2	
Saturated fatty acids (% energy)	Base	11.8	11.5, 12.2	12.0	11.6, 12.4	0.415
	3/12	11.0	10.7, 11.4	11.8	11.6, 12.1	0.004
Difference		0.8	0.34, 1.22	0.28	−0.19, 0.75	

Table 2.5 Change in food consumption associated with the use of a denture adhesive [74]

	Fruit/vegetable (servings)	Total fat (g)	Saturated fat (g)	Protein (g)	Starchy foods (servings)
n	35	35	35	35	35
Base	2.2	83.6	33.5	13.7	3.6
30 days	3.6	60.5	22.2	13.6	3.6
Change (95% CI)	1.4 (0.9, −1.9)	−23.2 (−31.4, −14.9)	−11.3 (−14.7, −7.9)	0.1 (−0.2, 4.9)	0 (−0.6, 0.6)
P	<0.0001	<0.0001	<0.0001	NS	NS

effect of use of a denture fixative. There were marked improvements in the reported chewing ability of these subjects when the fixative was used [74].

Conclusions

There are profound changes in body composition with increasing age that result in a need for an altered dietary pattern to one lower in energy but with static intake of micronutrients and protein, a "nutrient dense" dietary pattern.

Food choice is affected by the number and organization of the remaining natural teeth so that people with fewer contacting teeth or no natural teeth choose to eat foods that are easier to chew and avoid those with hard textures or that are difficult to chew.

The changes in foods choice result in reductions in intake of key nutrients especially fruits and vegetables and hence dietary fiber.

It is possible to encourage patients to improve their diet in association with denture wear/use but only if there is a dietary intervention in association with a dental one. Restoration of dental function alone does not result in improvement in dietary choice.

References

1. Janssen I, et al. Skeletal muscle cutpoints associated with elevated physical disability risk in older men and women. Am J Epidemiol. 2004;159(4):413–21.
2. Larsson L, Grimby G, Karlsson J. Muscle strength and speed of movement in relation to age and muscle morphology. J Appl Physiol Respir Environ Exerc Physiol. 1979;46(3):451–6.
3. Marcell TJ. Sarcopenia: causes, consequences, and preventions. J Gerontol A Biol Sci Med Sci. 2003;58(10):M911–6.
4. Lexell J, Downham D, Sjostrom M. Distribution of different fibre types in human skeletal muscles. Fibre type arrangement in m. vastus lateralis from three

groups of healthy men between 15 and 83 years. J Neurol Sci. 1986;72(2–3):211–22.

5. Nygaard E, Sanchez J. Intramuscular variation of fiber types in the brachial biceps and the lateral vastus muscles of elderly men: how representative is a small biopsy sample? Anat Rec. 1982;203(4):451–9.

6. Szulc P, et al. Hormonal and lifestyle determinants of appendicular skeletal muscle mass in men: the MINOS study. Am J Clin Nutr. 2004;80(2):496–503.

7. Anagnostis P, et al. Sarcopenia in post-menopausal women: is there any role for vitamin D? Maturitas. 2015;82(1):56–64.

8. Rondanelli M, et al. Novel insights on intake of meat and prevention of sarcopenia: all reasons for an adequate consumption. Nutr Hosp. 2015;32(5):2136–43.

9. Yu S, Umapathysivam K, Visvanathan R. Sarcopenia in older people. Int J Evid Based Healthc. 2014;12(4):227–43.

10. Kyle UG, et al. Body composition in 995 acutely ill or chronically ill patients at hospital admission: a controlled population study. J Am Diet Assoc. 2002;102(7):944–55.

11. Poehlman ET, et al. Sarcopenia in aging humans: the impact of menopause and disease. J Gerontol A Biol Sci Med Sci. 1995;50:73–7.

12. Rennie MJ. Control of muscle protein synthesis as a result of contractile activity and amino acid availability: implications for protein requirements. Int J Sport Nutr Exerc Metab. 2001;11(Suppl):S170–6.

13. Rennie MJ. Grandad, it ain't what you eat, it depends when you eat it—that's how muscles grow! J Physiol. 2001;535(Pt 1):2.

14. Frontera WR, et al. A cross-sectional study of muscle strength and mass in 45- to 78-yr-old men and women. J Appl Physiol (1985). 1991;71(2):644–50.

15. Hughes VA, et al. Longitudinal changes in body composition in older men and women: role of body weight change and physical activity. Am J Clin Nutr. 2002;76(2):473–81.

16. Wannamethee SG, Atkins JL. Muscle loss and obesity: the health implications of sarcopenia and sarcopenic obesity. Proc Nutr Soc. 2015;74(4):405–12.

17. Payette H. Known related effects of nutrition on aging muscle function. In: Rosenberg IH, Sastre A, editors. Nutrition and aging. Boston, MA: Karger; 2002. p. 135–50.

18. Feldman M, Cryer B, Lee E. Effects of Helicobacter pylori gastritis on gastric secretion in healthy human beings. Am J Phys. 1998;274(6 Pt 1):G1011–7.

19. Feldman M, et al. Effects of aging and gastritis on gastric acid and pepsin secretion in humans: a prospective study. Gastroenterology. 1996;110(4):1043–52.

20. Hoffmann JC, Zeitz M. Small bowel disease in the elderly: diarrhoea and malabsorption. Best Pract Res Clin Gastroenterol. 2002;16(1):17–36.

21. Shimamoto C, et al. Evaluation of gastric motor activity in the elderly by electrogastrography and the (13)C-acetate breath test. Gerontology. 2002;48(6):381–6.

22. Evans JR, Lawrenson JG. Antioxidant vitamin and mineral supplements for preventing age-related macular degeneration. Cochrane Database Syst Rev. 2012;6:CD000253.

23. Wei L, et al. Association of vitamin C with the risk of age-related cataract: a meta-analysis. Acta Ophthalmol. 2016;94(3):e170–6.

24. SACN. Carbohydrates and health. London: TSO; 2015.

25. WHO. WHO calls in countries to reduce sugars intake among adults and children. 2015 [cited 2016]; Available from: http://who.int/mediacentre/news/releases/2015/sugar-guideline/en/.

26. Finkelstein JA, Schiffman SS. Workshop on taste and smell in the elderly: an overview. Physiol Behav. 1999;66(2):173–6.

27. Mojet J, Christ-Hazelhof E, Heidema J. Taste perception with age: generic or specific losses in threshold sensitivity to the five basic tastes? Chem Senses. 2001;26(7):845–60.

28. Mojet J, Heidema J, Christ-Hazelhof E. Taste perception with age: generic or specific losses in supra-threshold intensities of five taste qualities? Chem Senses. 2003;28(5):397–413.

29. Ng K, et al. Effect of age and disease on taste perception. J Pain Symptom Manag. 2004;28(1):28–34.

30. Schiffman SS. Perception of taste and smell in elderly persons. Crit Rev Food Sci Nutr. 1993;33(1):17–26.

31. Schiffman S. Changes in taste and smell: drug interactions and food preferences. Nutr Rev. 1994;52(8 Pt 2):S11–4.

32. Schiffman SS, Graham BG. Taste and smell perception affect appetite and immunity in the elderly. Eur J Clin Nutr. 2000;54(Suppl 3):S54–63.

33. Ritchie CS. Oral health, taste, and olfaction. Clin Geriatr Med. 2002;18(4):709–17.

34. Mathey MF, et al. Flavor enhancement of food improves dietary intake and nutritional status of elderly nursing home residents. J Gerontol A Biol Sci Med Sci. 2001;56(4):M200–5.

35. Schiffman SS, et al. Taste perception of bitter compounds in young and elderly persons: relation to lipophilicity of bitter compounds. Neurobiol Aging. 1994;15(6):743–50.

36. Schiffman SS, et al. Taste perception of monosodium glutamate (MSG) in foods in young and elderly subjects. Physiol Behav. 1994;56(2):265–75.

37. Schiffman SS, Warwick ZS. Effect of flavor enhancement of foods for the elderly on nutritional status: food intake, biochemical indices, and anthropometric measures. Physiol Behav. 1993;53(2):395–402.

38. Baum BJ, Ship JA, Wu AJ. Salivary gland function and aging: a model for studying the interaction of aging and systemic disease. Crit Rev Oral Biol Med. 1992;4(1):53–64.

39. Ship JA, Baum BJ. Is reduced salivary flow normal in old people? Lancet. 1990;336(8729):1507.

40. Narhi TO, Meurman JH, Ainamo A. Xerostomia and hyposalivation: causes, consequences and treatment in the elderly. Drugs Aging. 1999;15(2):103–16.

41. Narhi TO, et al. Association between salivary flow rate and the use of systemic medication among 76-, 81-, and 86-year-old inhabitants in Helsinki. Finland J Dent Res. 1992;71(12):1875–80.

42. Ship JA, Fox PC, Baum BJ. How much saliva is enough? 'Normal' function defined. J Am Dent Assoc. 1991;122(3):63–9.

43. Ship JA, Pillemer SR, Baum BJ. Xerostomia and the geriatric patient. J Am Geriatr Soc. 2002;50(3):535–43.

44. Mattes-Kulig DA, Henkin RI. Energy and nutrient consumption of patients with dysgeusia. J Am Diet Assoc. 1985;85(7):822–6.

45. Farrell JH. The effect of mastication on the digestion of food. Br Dent J. 1956;100:149–55.

46. Kohyama K, Mioche L, Bourdiol P. Influence of age and dental status on chewing behaviour studied by EMG recordings during consumption of various food samples. Gerodontology. 2003;20(1):15–23.

47. Mioche L, et al. Changes in jaw muscles activity with age: effects on food bolus properties. Physiol Behav. 2004;82(4):621–7.

48. Mioche L, Bourdiol P, Peyron MA. Influence of age on mastication: effects on eating behaviour. Nutr Res Rev. 2004;17(1):43–54.

49. Ono T, et al. Factors influencing eating ability of old in-patients in a rehabilitation hospital in Japan. Gerodontology. 2003;20(1):24–31.

50. Akpata E, et al. Tooth loss, chewing habits, and food choices among older Nigerians in Plateau State: a preliminary study. Community Dent Oral Epidemiol. 2011;39(5):409–15.

51. Hung HC, et al. Tooth loss and dietary intake. J Am Dent Assoc. 2003;134(9):1185–92.

52. Marcenes W, et al. The relationship between dental status, food selection, nutrient intake, nutritional status, and body mass index in older people. Cad Saude Publica. 2003;19(3):809–16.

53. Sheiham A, et al. The relationship among dental status, nutrient intake, and nutritional status in older people. J Dent Res. 2001;80(2):408–13.

54. Walls AW, Murray ID. Dental care of patients in a hospice. Palliat Med. 1993;7(4):313–21.

55. Krall E, Hayes C, Garcia R. How dentition status and masticatory function affect nutrient intake. J Am Dent Assoc. 1998;129(9):1261–9.

56. Nowjack-Raymer RE, Sheiham A. Association of edentulism and diet and nutrition in US adults. J Dent Res. 2003;82(2):123–6.

57. Nowjack-Raymer RE, Sheiham A. Numbers of natural teeth, diet, and nutritional status in US adults. J Dent Res. 2007;86(12):1171–5.

58. Moynihan PJ, et al. Intake of non-starch polysaccharide (dietary fibre) in edentulous and dentate persons: an observational study. Br Dent J. 1994;177(7):243–7.

59. Kalviainen N, Salovaara H, Tuorila H. Sensory attributes and preference mapping for meusli oatflakes. J Food Sci. 2002;67(3):455–60.

60. Shinkai RS, et al. Oral function and diet quality in a community-based sample. J Dent Res. 2001;80(7):1625–30.

61. Joshipura KJ, Willett WC, Douglass CW. The impact of edentulousness on food and nutrient intake. J Am Dent Assoc. 1996;127(4):459–67.

62. Awad MA, et al. Implant overdentures and nutrition: a randomized controlled trial. J Dent Res. 2012;91(1):39–46.

63. Ettinger RL. Changing dietary patterns with changing dentition: how do people cope? Spec Care Dentist. 1998;18(1):33–9.

64. Garrett NR, et al. Veterans Administration Cooperative Dental Implant Study—comparisons between fixed partial dentures supported by blade-vent implants and removable partial dentures. Part V: comparisons of pretreatment and posttreatment dietary intakes. J Prosthet Dent. 1997;77(2):153–61.

65. Gunne HS. The effect of removable partial dentures on mastication and dietary intake. Acta Odontol Scand. 1985;43(5):269–78.

66. Gunne HS, Wall AK. The effect of new complete dentures on mastication and dietary intake. Acta Odontol Scand. 1985;43(5):257–68.

67. Hamdan NM, et al. Do implant overdentures improve dietary intake? A randomized clinical trial. J Dent Res. 2013;92(12 Suppl):146S–53S.

68. Moynihan PJ, et al. Nutrient intake in partially dentate patients: the effect of prosthetic rehabilitation. J Dent. 2000;28(8):557–63.

69. Prochaska JO, DiClemente CC. Stages of change in the modification of problem behaviors. Prog Behav Modif. 1992;28:183–218.

70. Bradbury J, et al. Nutrition counseling increases fruit and vegetable intake in the edentulous. J Dent Res. 2006;85(5):463–8.

71. Prochaska JO, Velicer WF. The transtheoretical model of health behavior change. Am J Health Promot. 1997;12(1):38–48. Review. https://www.ncbi.nlm.nih.gov/pubmed/10170434

72. Ellis JS, et al. The impact of dietary advice on edentulous adults' denture satisfaction and oral health-related quality of life 6 months after intervention. Clin Oral Implants Res. 2010;21(4):386–91.

73. Moynihan PJ, et al. Do implant-supported dentures facilitate efficacy of eating more healthily? J Dent. 2012;40(10):843–50.

74. Bartlett DW, et al. A preliminary investigation into the use of denture adhesives combined with dietary advice to improve diets in complete denture wearers. J Dent. 2013;41(2):143–7.

75. EFSA, Panel on Dietetic Products, Nutrition and Allergies (NDA). Scientific opinion on dietary reference values for protein. EFSA J. 2012;10(2):2557.

76. SACN. Dietary reference values for energy. London: TSO; 2012.

77. US Department of Health and Human Services and US Department of Agriculture. 2015–2020 dietary guidelines for americans. 8th ed; 2015.

Frauke Müller and Martin Schimmel

Abstract

Progress in medical and dental clinical practice fosters treating even very old geriatric patients with implants. Very few absolute contraindications remain nowadays, and the long-term performance of endosseous implants has largely exceeded initial expectations. In contrast to the environment in which they are placed, implants do not change. In view of the aging population, a paradigm shift in implant dentistry seems inevitable.

Physiological aging is featured by deterioration in vision, tactile sensitivity, and dexterity, rendering denture handling and oral hygiene difficult. In addition, old people often present with frailty and multimorbidity, often requiring assistance with the activities of daily living and a shift in life priorities.

F. Müller (✉)
Division of Gerodontology and Removable Prosthodontics, Department of Oral Rehabilitation, Medical Faculty, University Clinics of Dental Medicine—CUMD, University of Geneva, Geneva, Switzerland
e-mail: frauke.mueller@unige.ch

M. Schimmel, M.A.S.
Division of Gerodontology, Department of Reconstructive Dentistry and Gerodontology, Medical Faculty, School of Dental Medicine—ZMK Bern, University of Bern, Bern, Switzerland
e-mail: martin.schimmel@zmk.unibe.ch

When additional tooth loss occurs, a new restorative treatment is required. Although it is well accepted that age alone is not a contraindication for successful implant therapy, it is increasingly necessary to consider its implications in a geriatric treatment planning.

Monitoring the use and management of fixed and removable implant prostheses in geriatric patients seems mandatory. When functional decline and frailty render denture management difficult, "backing off" to a simplified and less complex restoration with or without the present implants may become necessary.

3.1 General Considerations

Dental care for elderly patients inevitably requires some adjustments in the approach used with younger adults. Firstly, physiological aging diminishes physiological reserves, and age-related changes become obvious, in terms of both physiognomy and function. Secondly, the prevalence of chronic disease and functional handicap increases with age.

Treatment planning must take into consideration the patient's physical disabilities and mental

© Springer International Publishing AG, part of Springer Nature 2018
E. Emami, J. Feine (eds.), *Mandibular Implant Prostheses*,
https://doi.org/10.1007/978-3-319-71181-2_3

handicaps, as well as a potentially declining autonomy, in managing fixed or removable dental prostheses and essential oral hygiene. The elderly patient is often not interested in long and invasive treatment procedures, like implant surgery with bone augmentation. Chronic diseases and the side effects of their treatment may also limit the range of possible surgical interventions. A dry mouth, perhaps caused by polypharmacy, increases the risk of root caries and renders the oral tissues more sensitive (Figs. 3.1 and 3.2). Muscle coordination is likely to have deteriorated, and swallowing disorders become more prevalent. Furthermore, psychological afflictions such as depression have a high prevalence in old age and may affect prosthodontic treatment outcomes and recall compliance [1]. Treatment planning should also take into account the patient's life expectancy, as well as the cost/effectiveness

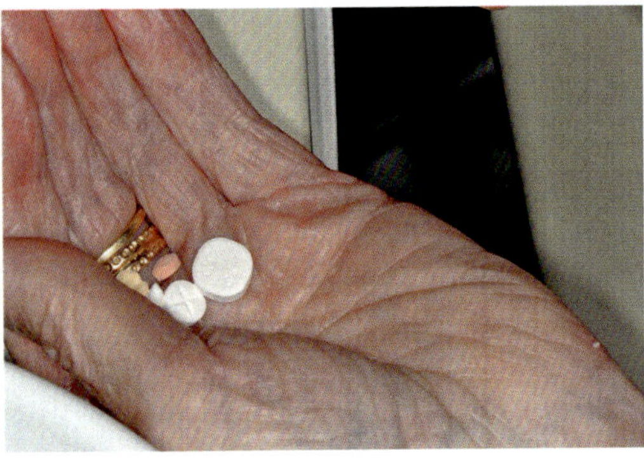

Fig. 3.1 Polypharmacy occurs along with an increase in chronic diseases. Many of those drugs will create dry mouth sensations as undesired effect

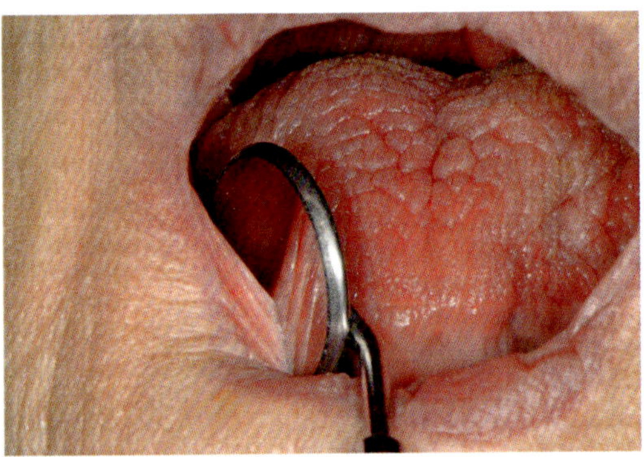

Fig. 3.2 Polypharmacy occurs along with an increase in chronic diseases. Many of those drugs will create hyposalivation and dry mouth sensations as undesired effect

of the proposed intervention. Often, the most limiting factor in treatment planning is the patients' reluctance to agree to any type of dental intervention. Many issues must be considered. How long will the patient be able to sit in the dental chair? Will he/she be able to tolerate a supine position? Can he/she open the mouth and remain still? How will working conditions be in terms of visibility and accessibility? How will the patient tolerate an impression tray? How can bedbound patients in a domiciliary setting be managed? Finally, will the patient be able to follow simple instructions, like holding an X-ray film, and be sufficiently compliant during the treatment? All of these issues need to be clarified before beginning a treatment that, once started, must be terminated. Even with many years of clinical experience, these questions remain very difficult in geriatric treatment planning.

Age-related functional and cognitive decline is not linear, and general health may deteriorate at any time. Hence, patients' medical histories must be updated regularly and their treatment adapted, if necessary. However, the potential difficulties of maintaining complex or even simple implant restorations, which were provided when the patient was still more capable physically and mentally, should not be underestimated. Even simple treatments for minor technical or biological complications may be very challenging; meticulous procedures, for example, for the treatment of peri-implantitis, will often be beyond consideration, which should be anticipated when planning the treatment of elderly patients before they become frail.

3.2 Age-Related Changes in Muscles

One of the most obvious features of physiological aging is the loss of muscle bulk (sarcopenia) described in Chap. 1; this is also true of the masticatory muscles. When studying the cross-sectional area (CSA) of the masseter and lateral pterygoid muscles, a 40% loss in CSA has been reported to occur between the ages of 25 and 85 years, and this atrophy is even more pronounced in individuals who have lost their teeth [2].

According to the physiological principle of "use it or lose it," muscles need frequent and regular training to maintain their function and bulk. The speed of atrophy following inactivity is well demonstrated when a leg is plastered after a fracture: a significant loss in muscle bulk and strength is seen after only a few weeks, and physiotherapy is required to regain normal function. For the chewing muscles, accelerated atrophy may similarly be related to a reduced "physical exercise," caused, for example, by a poor chewing activity with conventional complete dentures. Fear of denture dislodgement limits mandibular excursions, and pain in the denture-bearing tissues limits the load exerted on the replacement teeth. Denture support and retention via dental implants avoid denture displacement and limit the immediate load on the denture-bearing tissues. Hence muscle training during chewing is encouraged by the enhanced denture performance.

The presence of training and detraining effects on thigh muscle bulk was confirmed even for older and very old adults [3]. Little is known about training and detraining of masticatory muscles, especially in elderly and frail individuals. A recent case report from Schimmel and co-workers showed that 3 months of mandibular denture abstention in a 97-year-old patient induced a loss of up to 17% of masseter muscle thickness; the muscle bulk recovered during the 6 months after chewing function was restored with a mandibular implant overdenture [4] (Fig. 3.3). In a prospective randomized clinical trial, the "training effect" from implant overdentures was confirmed. The stabilization of the mandibular denture with two short interforaminal implants accounts for an increase in masseter muscle bulk, especially on the preferred chewing side [5].

The aging processes of the muscle tissues also include the motor units, which become larger with individual motor fibers disappearing and some muscle fibers being adopted by neighboring motor units. With larger motor units, movements become less precise and controlled. A very clear example for this phenomenon is the handwriting of elderly persons, which graphically depicts the age-related decline in motor control; controlling handbags or other objects like loose shoes also becomes difficult (Fig. 3.4). The mandibular closing trajectory can be more erratic, and a carefully adjusted balanced occlusion not only helps with denture retention but also gently guides the mandible to centric occlusion. A freedom-in-centric occlusal concept therefore seems most adequate for elderly

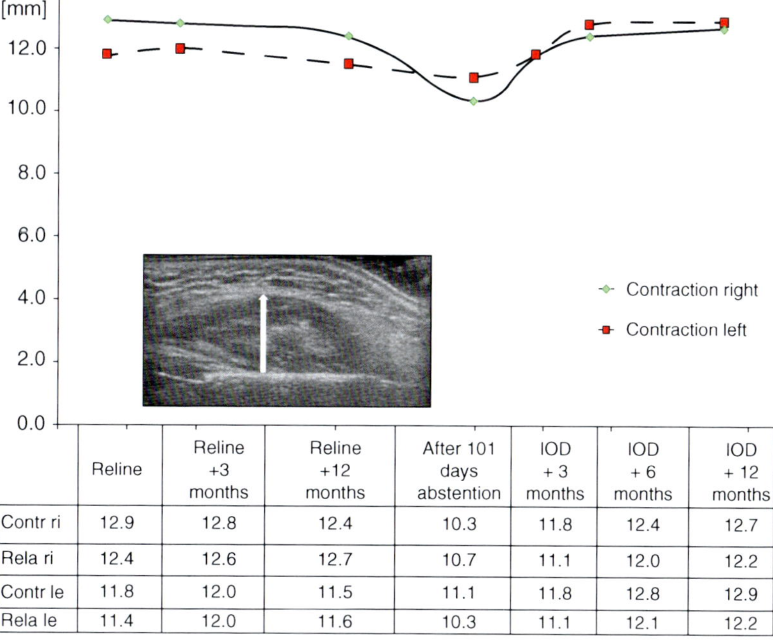

	Reline	Reline +3 months	Reline +12 months	After 101 days abstention	IOD + 3 months	IOD + 6 months	IOD + 12 months
Contr ri	12.9	12.8	12.4	10.3	11.8	12.4	12.7
Rela ri	12.4	12.6	12.7	10.7	11.1	12.0	12.2
Contr le	11.8	12.0	11.5	11.1	11.8	12.8	12.9
Rela le	11.4	12.0	11.6	10.3	11.1	12.1	12.2

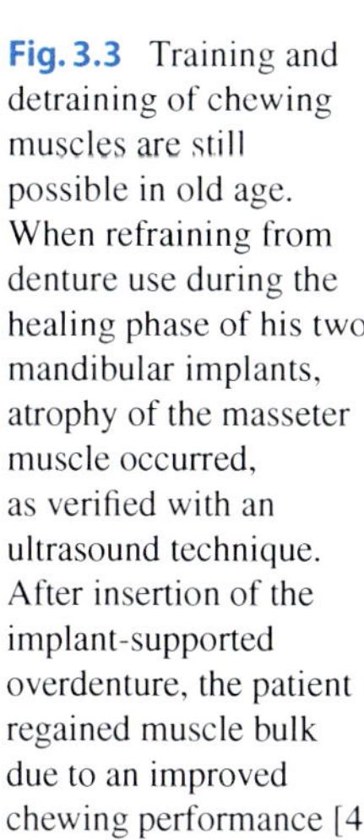

Fig. 3.3 Training and detraining of chewing muscles are still possible in old age. When refraining from denture use during the healing phase of his two mandibular implants, atrophy of the masseter muscle occurred, as verified with an ultrasound technique. After insertion of the implant-supported overdenture, the patient regained muscle bulk due to an improved chewing performance [4]

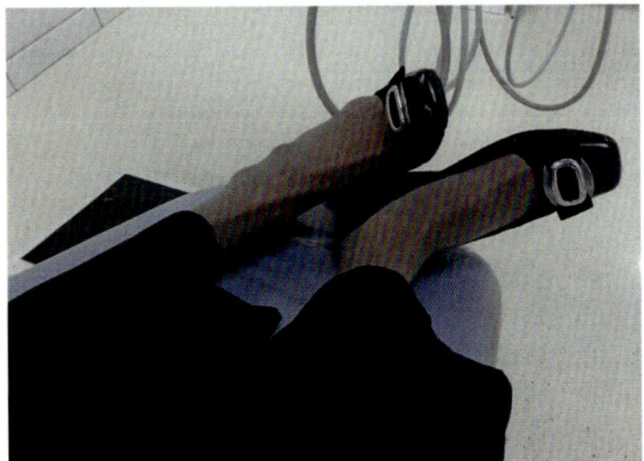

Fig. 3.4 Muscle coordination becomes more difficult in old age. Holding onto shoes, handbags, etc. may become more challenging

patients with poor motor control. Impaired muscle skill also affects denture control and retention, especially in patients with neurodegenerative diseases such as Parkinson's disease, dementia, or mandibular dyskinesia.

3.3   Age-Related Changes in Salivary Glands

Although physiological aging reduces the total amount of stimulated saliva, the quantity, which can be produced by the glands in healthy elders, should be sufficient to keep the mouth in good shape. Saliva is also important for taste; it can be noted that elderly persons tend to add more spices and more salt to their dishes. With age, when some acinar cells are replaced by connective tissue, the ratio between active cells and ducts is altered. However, rather than being age-related, the high percentage of elderly persons presenting with hyposalivation and dry mouth sensations is more related to an underlying pathology or to undesired effects of their treatment.

3.4   Age-Related Changes in Oral Mucosa

With age, the oral mucosa appears paler with a silky shine and becomes thin and delicate. Histologically, with age the epithelium becomes

thinner, with less elastic, but rather more connective tissues. Furthermore, there is a tendency toward less interstitial fluid, rendering the tissues more vulnerable to mechanical injury. A reduced number of cell bodies and increasing surface keratinization can also be noted [6]. Along with these changes, the papillae of the tongue atrophy and deep macroscopic fissures may appear in its dorsum.

3.5   Age-Related Neurological Changes

The peripheral and central nervous systems also undergo age-related physiological changes. The peripheral nerves' conduction velocity and the tactile thresholds of mechanoreceptors decrease. Large particles of food debris can often be found in the vestibular sulcus of elderly patients, as they have difficulties feeling the foreign body. However, for prosthodontics the most important age-related neurological change is reduced neuroplasticity. The insertion of a new prosthesis leads to the stimulation of differently located oral mechanoreceptors, and the modification of existing movement patterns and reflexes becomes necessary. Elderly persons with a reduced capacity of adaptation should therefore be provided with replacement dentures, which are similar in form and function to the previous well-adapted set of prostheses. Duplication techniques may be employed to transfer the desired number of successful features to the new prosthesis (Fig. 3.5). Mechanical retention may also be helpful, as neuroplasticity is less challenged when denture control does not rely on motor skills [7].

3.6   Multimorbidity and Frailty

Physiological aging, and in particular the transition from the stable stage of life (also called the "third age") to the stage featured by dependency in the activities of daily living, also named the "fourth age" or "old age," happens generally not in a linear manner. Frailty is defined by symptoms like rapid weight loss, weakness, fatigue,

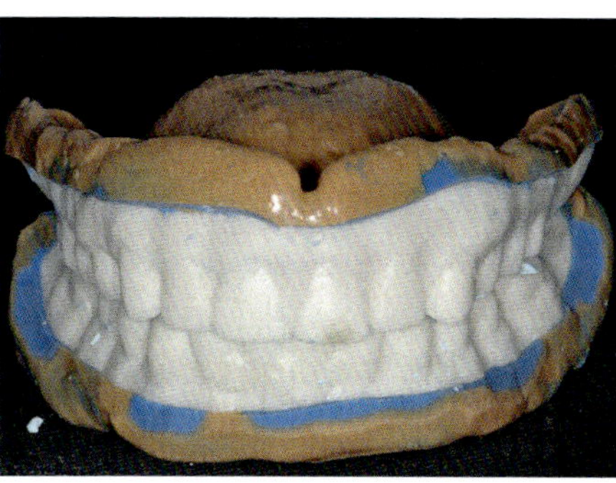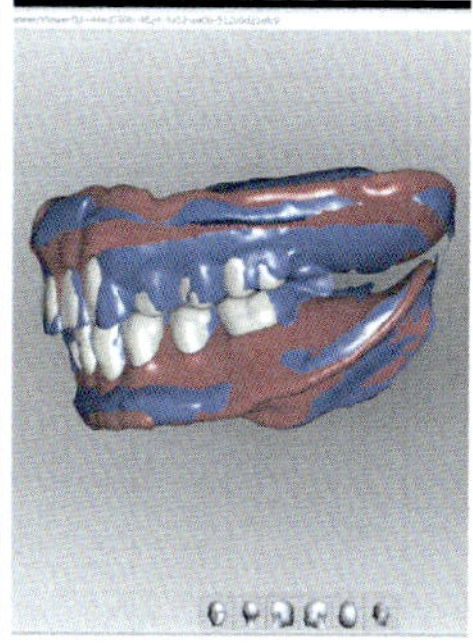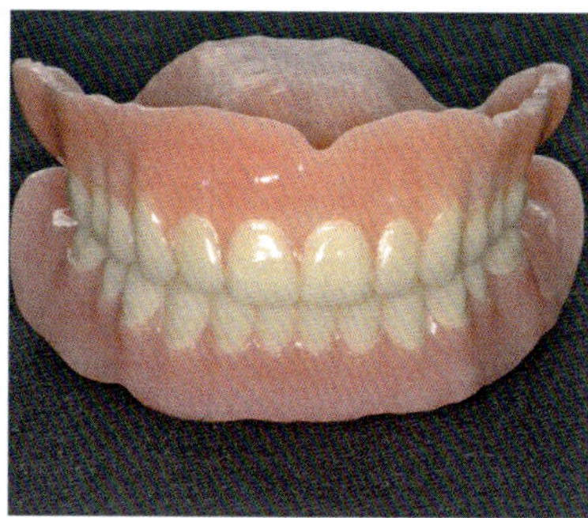

Fig. 3.5 Duplicating a successful denture helps incorporating selected features of the old to the new replacement denture. Hence, in patients with reduced neuroplasticity, adaptation is facilitated

anorexia, and physical inactivity. Clinically symptoms comprise undernutrition, sarcopenia, osteopenia, slow walking, balance problems, and poor physical fitness [8].

Whereas medical events often initiate the transition from the third to the fourth age, psychological stress or difficult life events such as the loss of a partner or moving to a new apartment can also trigger a rapid and steep functional decline. Patients may suddenly appear in the dental practice less carefully dressed, poorly shaved and washed, etc. At this point, their oral hygiene seems unusually neglected, and a severe and comprehensive periodontal breakdown may often be the consequence. Whereas young and healthy adults can regain their pre-event level of functioning, frail persons will remain permanently impaired. As frailty progresses, they will become increasingly dependent on help for the activities of daily living (ADLs). Their functional decline can be assessed and monitored by a comprehensive battery of instruments called geriatric assessment.

For a geriatric assessment in dentistry, A. Stuck, head of the geriatric medicine at the University of Bern, Switzerland, recommends only rather brief screening instruments. The final diagnosis should be completed after a comprehensive assessment by a specially trained physician.

A distinction should be made between the basic activities of daily living (ADLs), which demand less functional capacity, and the instrumental activities of daily living (IADLs). ADLs comprise issues like the mobility within the apartment, performing hygiene measures, going to the toilet, getting dressed, eating/drinking, etc. The IADLs describe more complex functions like the use of technical instruments, shopping, cooking, housekeeping, or paying bills. A short and recommendable instrument is the Katz Index of Independence in Activities of Daily Living [9] and for the IADL the brief instrumental activities of daily living measure [10].

Here, a few commonly used tests are listed as examples.

Basic activities of daily living can be evaluated by means of:

- Barthel Index for the activities of daily living [11]

The nutritional status may be evaluated by:

- Mini-Nutritional Assessment (MNA) [12]

Cognition and psychological health can be assessed by:

- Geriatric Depression Scale (GDS) [13]
- Mini-Mental State Examination (MMSE) [14]
- Clock-drawing test [15]

Although some of these tests may not seem feasible in a dental practice, the well-established but less well-documented "denture upside-down test" is easy to implement (Fig. 3.6). When a patient is handed a denture upside down and places it in the mouth without first turning it over,

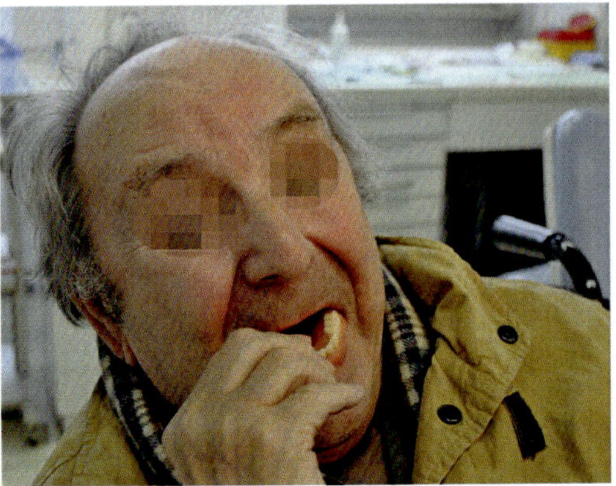

Fig. 3.6 Presenting a denture "upside down" may be a screening for cognitive performance. This patient did not realize that he tries to place the upper denture the wrong way around

this may be a sign of cognitive impairment, and the patient may benefit from an in-depth examination at a specialized memory clinic.

The most common chronic diseases in elderly adults with an average age of 84 years who live in long-term care facilities are hypertension (men, 53%; women, 56%), dementia (45%/52%), depression (31%/37%), arthritis (26%/35%), diabetes (26%/23%), reflux (23%/23%), arteriosclerosis (24%/20%), cardiac insufficiency (18%/21%), cerebrovascular diseases (24%/19%), and anemia (17%/20%) [16, 17]. In Switzerland, of 1954 inhabitants over the age of 75 years, 51.4% indicated in a survey that they had a permanent health problem [18]. This percentage is much higher in the institutionalized population.

3.7 Physical Limitations in Frail and Multimorbid Elders

Frail and multimorbid elderly persons present with physical limitations when it comes to dental treatments. Appointments have to meet individual habits: (a) not too early in the morning, as the morning toilet and dressing takes a long time; (b) not during fixed mealtimes, especially in diabetic patients, and (c) preferably during daylight. Winter months are less favorable for non-urgent treatments, as falls on slippery and icy roads all too often result in a fracture of the hip or thigh neck, an incident with a mortality of up to 20% in

old age. Appointments should be marked in writing with legible and large letters on a card with no distracting publicity. Financial agreements should also be transparent and equally made available in writing, as children and family often advise their elderly relatives, even if they are not officially appointed as legal representative. Elderly persons should be discouraged from carrying large amounts in cash when they come for their treatment, as they may become easy victims for street crime and violence. Their physical frailty may also preclude long and invasive treatment sessions. Hence, often the necessary dental treatment procedures have to be performed with high precision and in a very short time, which requires a significant degree of clinical skill and experience on the part of the operator.

3.8 Psychological and Social Aging

The U-shaped curve of psychological well-being, derived from a cohort of 340,847 participants in the United States, revealed that aging beyond the age of 50 years is accompanied by a constant increase in psychological well-being [19]. Little is known about psychological aging, although it may be an important factor in medical and dental treatment outcomes. It seems that while everything is not that perfect in old age, some suggest the elderly sport a more accepting attitude and more realistic expectations, along with lower stress levels, which tends to render elders more satisfied with their situation. On the other hand, in old age there is an increasing prevalence of depression and social isolation, as partners and friends pass away, or when relocation to a more age-adequate and "practical" accommodation reduces usual social contacts and familiar environment.

All these developments imply a certain risk that oral health will lose in priority, as oral pathologies and functional impairment are no longer correctly perceived. It is well documented that elderly persons have a lower subjective demand for improvements in their oral health or regarding their prostheses; this is in extreme contrast to the objective judgments of their treatment need by dental health professionals [20].

Of course old patients keep their right of self-determination with regard to their medical treatment. They may decide against interventions that—from a normative and professional point of view—are justified and ought to be performed. It is easy to imagine that optional interventions, especially surgical procedures, are little popular in elderly adults. The role of the health professional is to inform patients about their oral health and to propose, based on their professional knowledge and judgment, adequate treatment options, so that patients know the necessary facts to give "informed consent." Written information sheets give patients sufficient time to thoroughly reflect on the proposed treatment options and discuss them with family and friends.

3.9 The Old Patient in the Dental Practice

Treating elderly patients in a dental practice may require some particular arrangements. First, it is important that the dental practice is equipped for the physical handicaps of elders, such as reduced mobility and vision. Absence of tripping hazards, good lighting, and stable chairs that are not too deep are essential features of a dental practice. Wheelchair access may also be desirable. Administrative forms should be prepared in a legible font size, and the practice secretary or dental nurse should assist the patient in filling in the forms, if needed.

Once in the treatment room, placing the patient on the dental chair may also be a challenge; special tools are available to facilitate this task and to prevent injury to patients as well as staff. To avoid the transfer to the dental chair, simple interventions and oral examinations may even be performed with the patient still seated in the wheelchair. Radiographs are diagnostic essentials, but some elderly patients may not be able to have a panoramic radiograph taken due to their posture, reduced mobility, or fear from the small cabin or the machine itself (Fig. 3.7). In these cases, intraoral radiographs may be an alternative.

Communication with elderly persons may be difficult because of hearing problems, and it helps to not wear a face mask during conversations so

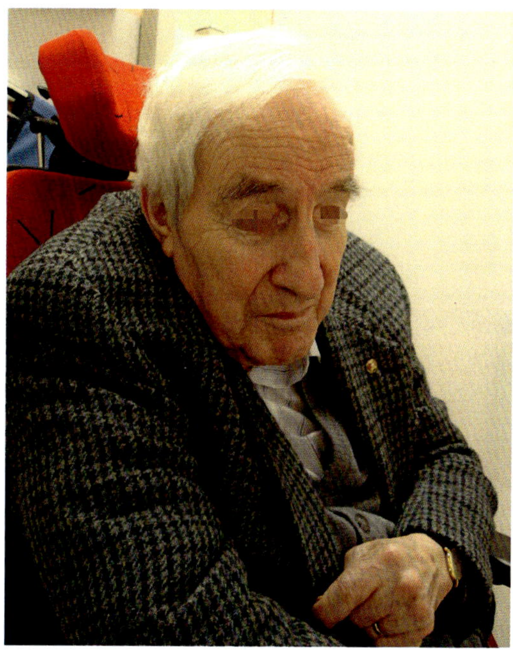

Fig. 3.7 This gentlemen's posture precluded taking an OPT radiograph. Radiological diagnostics was therefore limited to several small X-rays

they can read the lips. Furthermore, especially for dental students, it is important to be aware that old patients are a "different generation," and they have many more years of experience and different values. Technical progress, even when it concerns a dental prosthesis, may be regarded with a substantial degree of suspicion. Understanding suggested treatments and their implications is a key factor for treatment success and compliance [21]. It is important to find the right words to explain the advantages and disadvantages of a proposed treatment and to help elderly persons benefit from the recent developments in implant dentistry.

3.10 Cognitive Impairment and Legal Context

The prevalence of cognitive impairment increases with age, with more than half of the population presenting with dementia at the age of 90 years or above [22]. Several types of dementia exist, with Alzheimer's disease being the most prevalent. Clinical symptoms vary greatly between individual patients and include a progressive loss of memory accompanied by diminishing language skills, dyspraxia, impaired cognition, and a decline in executive functions. In addition, the loss of social competence is compulsory to fulfill the definition [23]. Alzheimer's disease progresses slowly, but although treatment may alleviate the symptoms, a cure does not yet exist. Impaired motor coordination is one of the clinical symptoms, and in the final stages of the disease, even chewing movements may become "deprogrammed."

Persons with dementia generally have poorer oral health and fewer teeth than healthy their cognitively healthy peers [24]. Motor control of complete dentures is also affected, even when the dentures have been previously worn successfully for many years. Weight gain seems to reduce the morbidity of the condition; hence, improving the chewing efficiency by prosthodontic means seems intuitively beneficial [25, 26]. In the final stages of the disease, dentures are rarely used, and implants may cause injury, infection, discomfort, and even pain [27]. Dental treatment becomes increasingly difficult when verbal communication is no longer effective and access to the mouth is violently refused by demented patients. Conscious sedation or even general anesthesia may become a last resort. Existing implants should be "put to sleep" in good time by connecting gingiva-level healing caps or cutting and smoothing the implant heads when one-piece systems are present. Adhesive pastes may be prescribed for denture use when necessary.

Old age and dependency for the activities of daily living do not automatically imply the loss of the individual's legal rights in terms of health decisions and financial agreements. When no official representative is appointed, old persons remain entitled to take their own financial and health decisions. However, their family may increasingly wish to be involved in and informed about any complex, costly and invasive treatment decisions. Unreasonable withholding of financial resources and psychological manipulation may constitute elder abuse.

A dentist may also be the first person to suspect the onset of a cognitive impairment. Initial suspicions can be confirmed by the abovementioned tests. Simple questions can give good first indications, especially when the patient is well-known by the practitioner. A patient may be able to recount the year he was born, but not able to calculate his or her age in the case of cognitive impairment. Another short and validated screening tool for cognitive impairment is the Ottawa 3DY test [28] (Table 3.1).

Depending on the results, a referral to a specialized memory clinic for a more comprehensive examination may be indicated. The test results, for example, a clock drawing, can be kept in the patient's file to document a responsible evaluation of the patient's cognitive function (Fig. 3.8).

Placing dental implants and fabricating a new prosthesis are never emergency treatments. It therefore seems possible to give an elderly person sufficient time (at least 1 week) to consider and

Table 3.1 The Ottawa 3DY test is a validated screening tool for cognitive impairment

Ottawa 3DY test: no answer counts as 0. Any score less than 4 is indicative of impaired cognitive function
Score: correct = 1; incorrect = 0
What is the date? /1
What day of the week is it? /1
Spell the word WORLD backward: DLROW /1
What year is it? /1

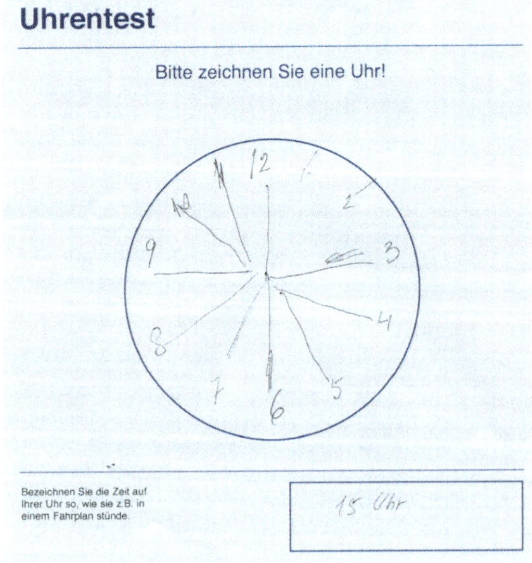

Fig. 3.8 The clock-drawing test could be a first indicator for a cognitive impairment

reconsider the proposed interventions. Written proposals with a clear statement of the financial commitment can help avoiding disagreements and conflicts. If a patient has a legal representative, it is important to know that some countries distinguish between "financial" and "other" decisions. So even if the patient's representative may have the right to take financial decisions, they may not be entitled to agree or disagree to a medical treatment. Elderly patients should also be invited to talk through the proposed treatment options with their family and friends. Only after they are completely convinced of the proposed intervention and have signed the agreement, the treatment should begin.

3.11 Reduced Dexterity and Handgrip Force

The evaluation of a patient's dexterity is essential in the planning of an implant treatment in elderly patients. For example, the Framingham study found that about one third of all elderly women present with symptomatic osteoarthritis (OA) [29], which renders handling of small objects like interdental brushes, dental floss, or even dental prostheses difficult. There is no validated screening test to predict the successful maintenance of both implants and prostheses. However, testing for the presence of osteoarthritis is strongly recommended. The grip strength can be evaluated simply by examining the patient's hands and asking for a firm handshake (Fig. 3.9). To evaluate manual dexterity, patients can also be asked to tie

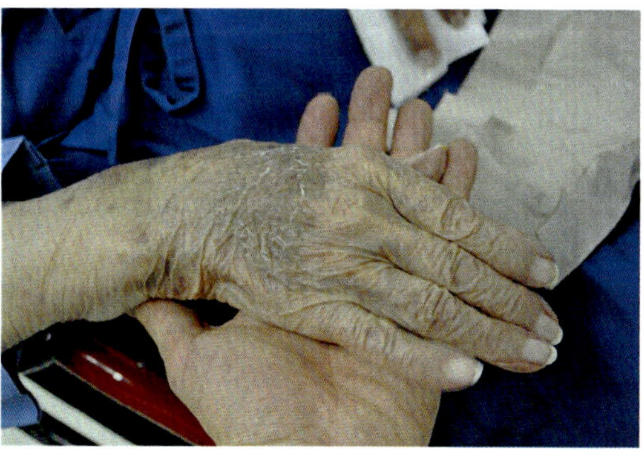

Fig. 3.9 A look at the patient's hand helps estimating their manual dexterity

a knot in the dental floss. If these tests cannot be accomplished without problems, the patient's ability to autonomously perform correct implant and denture hygiene must be questioned. By no means does this mean that implant treatment should be withheld—such patients may benefit most from treatment—but the care providers must be informed and instructed, and a close monitoring during the denture use is advised.

3.12 Prospective Treatment Planning

In general, dental prostheses for geriatric patients should not be designed any different from those for younger adults [30]. Of course, the general rules and guidelines for the construction of removable prostheses also apply to dentures for elderly and geriatric patients.

However, in addition to the general rules and guidelines, we should consider the patient's general health and any physical or cognitive impairment. Similarly important are the patient's autonomy in performing essential oral hygiene measures and the ability to manage removable dentures. Unfortunately, nursing staff often have had very little, if any, training in handling what they consider "high-tech" dentures—and even a mandibular two-implant overdenture may fall into this category.

Even for fit and active elders, prospective planning is important. There is a greater likelihood for an 80-year-old to become dependent in the following 15 years than for a 50-year-old patient. Of course, fit 80-year-old and even 95-year-old patients should not be withheld fixed implant-supported prostheses, if they wish for such a reconstruction, but these should allow for a "back-off" strategy when the onset of dependency requires simplification. Fixed implant-supported prostheses should preferably be screw-retained to facilitate replacement by a removable prosthesis later in life. In a prospective planning, implants should be placed where they could be useful even when the fixed implant prosthesis is converted to an implant-supported overdenture.

The choice of implants is equally critical. A two-piece system with a variety of available abutments is preferable, as these are easier to retrieve and replaced with another version if needed.

In short, dental prostheses for elderly adults should have the following attributes:

- Easy to insert and remove
- Easy to clean
- Freedom-in-centric occlusion, with shallow cuspal inclines
- Polished surfaces without too much detailing that would encourage biofilm adhesion

- Age-appropriate dental appearance (in agreement with the patient)
- Highest retention that still permits autonomous handling by the patient

Table 3.2 lists possible age-appropriate features, which practitioners may or may not adopt for a particular patient.

As aging and functional decline are very individual and vary from patient to patient, it is important to note that this list of features for a removable prosthesis does not apply to all old patients equally and categorically. There is no specific age

Table 3.2 Possible age-appropriate features for a partial or complete removable denture for geriatric patients

Denture design	Simple and flexible, allowing modification in case of potential future tooth loss or the onset of dependency for activities of daily living (ADLs)
Denture stability	Solid, resisting clumsy handling, without a need for immediate repair
Denture-base material	Polymethyl methacrylate (PMMA) to allow for repair, addition of teeth and other parts, and relines
Retention components	Use only the best and well-documented materials and components to reduce material failure and wear in late life
Denture surface	Polished surfaces to facilitate cleaning and avoid adhesion of biofilm and food debris (no surface details, no papilla recession)
Palatal plate	Polished, unless problems with speech or taste arise
Denture management and retention	"Removal aids" to help with the removal of the prosthesis if manual dexterity is reduced Retention only as strong as can be managed by the patients themselves Retention should be "weakened" progressively along with functional decline
Occlusal plane	Should be on or below the equator of the tongue. As for the length of the incisors, bear in mind that the upper lip becomes longer with age and the edges of the incisors should not be longer than the upper lip Occlusal breakdown with a loss in vertical dimension has to be corrected for a coherent occlusal plane
Vertical dimension	The less coordinated and controlled the mandibular movements, the smaller the occlusal vertical dimension
Occlusion	"Freedom-in-centric" concept to accommodate the increased freedom of the temporomandibular joints and poorer motor coordination Canine guidance or group function for partial dentures, balanced occlusion for complete dentures and implant-supported overdentures In difficult anatomical situations, the central bearing point method should be used for the registration of centric relation
Denture teeth	Cuspal inclination of 20° or less, preferably acrylic teeth
Abutment teeth	"Bikini design"—cover as little tooth structure as possible to allow access of saliva to the enamel Abutment teeth with severe attachment loss should be endodontically treated and decoronated for a more favorable crown/root ratio Where possible, keep healthy filled roots as overdenture abutments (except for molars)
Denture kinetics and occlusal load	The mandibular denture should be "stronger" and more stable than the maxillary denture Make an effort to keep strategically important teeth, especially mandibular canines Plan occlusal load to be transferred to denture saddles rather than abutment teeth to keep the latter for as long as possible Adopt a fail-safe principle for clasps to protect abutment teeth
Appearance	Age-appropriate appearance with abraded incisal edges and a shade of three or above
Labeling	Individual labeling of denture with name (and set) for the institutionalized patient
Comfort	Oral comfort should be assured even when the denture is not worn during the night (e.g., no sharp edges from attachments)

after which a patient is considered "geriatric" and will need a removable prosthesis!

3.13 Implants in the Geriatric Patient

When considering implants in the treatment of geriatric patients, two distinctly different scenarios have to be considered.

The first scenario is the placement of new implants, which is critical, given that in the foreseeable future the geriatric patient may increasingly lose the capability to manage implant-supported prostheses and maintain adequate oral hygiene (Fig. 3.10). The widespread assumption that patients request "tight" and firmly fitting dentures does not apply to all elderly denture wearers. Some openly admit that their oral comfort dominates their prosthodontic treatment choices. However, ethically it seems unreasonable to withhold the means of modern dentistry from a geriatric patient if implants are requested for a justified and reasonable indication. Also, there are many different varieties of "geriatric," and recommendations therefore cannot be generalized. However, when opting for implants, the circumstances should be as close to ideal as possible.

The second scenario applies to functionally declining patients who had implants placed while they were still fit, and the surgical intervention was no barrier (Figs. 3.11 and 3.12). Ideally, these patients can benefit from their implants

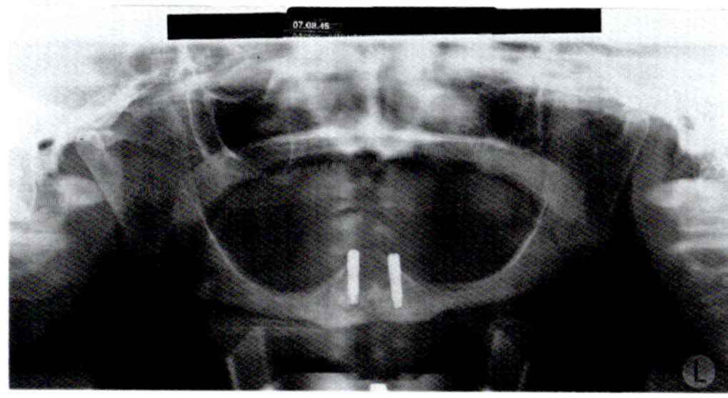

Fig. 3.10 Placing implants late in life is still possible, but given the often challenging anatomical situations and the functional decline, the treatment concepts are often limited

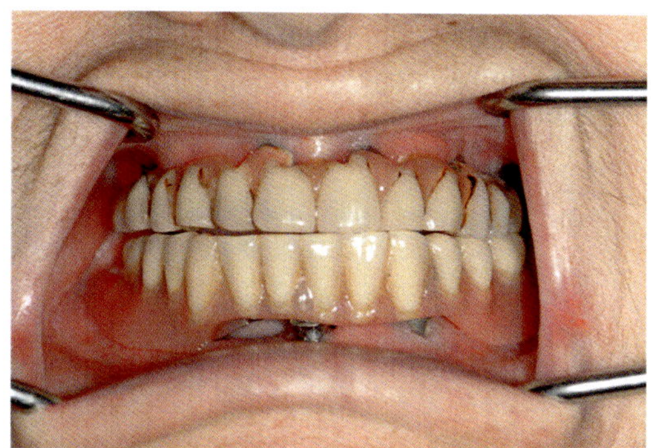

Fig. 3.11 These fixed implant dental prostheses were inserted 15 years prior to the photo. Hygiene is declining but still acceptable. When oral hygiene can no longer be managed, the implants can be used to retain a removable implant overdenture

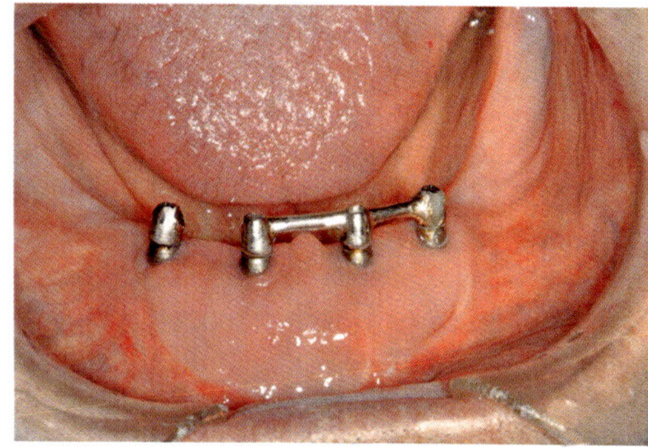

Fig. 3.12 Although this implant bar shows undeniable signs of wear and aging after 32 years in use, it still serves to retain the implant overdenture. Despite a compromised oral hygiene, the peri-implant mucosa show little signs of inflammation

until the end of their lives if maintenance of their implant-supported prosthesis is possible by the patient himself, or reliably assured through the caregiver. There is a need for an active and strict maintenance scheme, with appropriately adapted recall intervals, so as not to miss the point for "backing off" to a technically less complex prosthodontic solution [31].

In practical terms, this "back-off" strategy would, for example, imply the replacement of a fixed reconstruction by a removable prosthesis, which is easier to handle and clean for the patient or their caregiver. In doing so, great care should be taken to duplicate as many features as possible

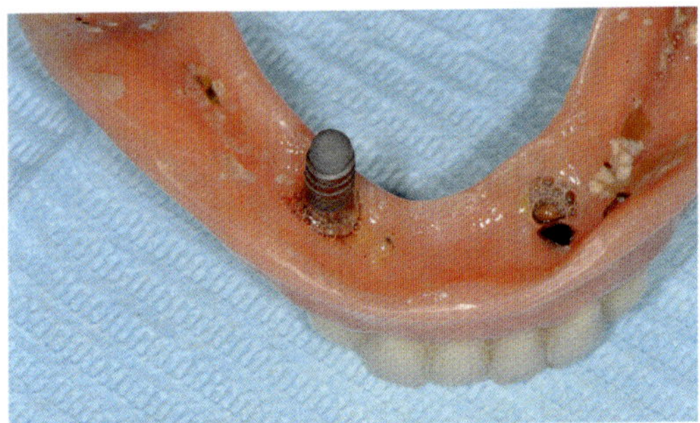

Fig. 3.13 The "backing-off" strategy implies a simplification of the implant reconstruction when functional decline occurs. Sometimes, like in this case, simplification occurs without a dental intervention

from an old fixed reconstruction to which the patient has become well adapted, to facilitate adaptation to the new prosthesis by avoiding unnecessary challenges to neuroplasticity.

Technically, in a few years' time, an existing fixed implant dental prosthesis might be scanned intraorally as basis for an identical dental arch milled or 3D-printed as a removable prosthesis. Backing off could also mean the gradual simplification of the current overdenture attachment system. For example, bar- or stud-type attachments seem more difficult to manage than ball or magnetic attachments. The last level of simplification would be the unscrewing of the attachment and its replacement by a gingiva-level healing cap.

Acknowledgments The text of this chapter is largely based on the International Team of Implantology Treatment Guide 9, Implant therapy in the Geriatric Patient (Quintessence, Berlin, 2016).

References

1. Takiguchi T, Yoshihara A, Takano N, Miyazaki H. Oral health and depression in older Japanese people. Gerodontology. 2015;33(4):439–46. https://doi.org/10.1111/ger.12177.
2. Newton J, Yemm R, Abel R, Menhinick S. Changes in human jaw muscles with age and dental state. Gerodontology. 1993;10(1):16–22.
3. Tokmakidis SP, Kalapotharakos VI, Smilios I, Parlavantzas A. Effects of detraining on muscle strength and mass after high or moderate intensity of resistance training in older adults. Clin Physiol Funct Imaging. 2009;29(4):316–9.
4. Schimmel M, Loup A, Duvernay E, Gaydarov N, Müller F. The effect of lower denture abstention on masseter muscle thickness in a 97 year-old patient: a case report. Int J Prosthodont. 2010;23:418–20.
5. Müller F, Duvernay E, Loup A, Vazquez L, Herrmann FR, Schimmel M. Implant-supported mandibular overdentures in very old adults: a randomized controlled trial. J Dent Res. 2013;92(12 Suppl):154S–60S. https://doi.org/10.1177/0022034513509630.
6. Scott J, Valentine JA, St Hill CA, Balasooriya BA. A quantitative histological analysis of the effects of age and sex on human lingual epithelium. J Biol Buccale. 1983;11(4):303–15.
7. Müller F, Link I, Fuhr K, Utz KH. Studies on adaptation to complete dentures. Part II: oral stereognosis and tactile sensibility. J Oral Rehabil. 1995;22(10):759–67.
8. Fried LP, Walston J. Frailty and failure to thrive. In: Hazzard WR, Blass JP, Jr EW, editors. Principles of geriatric medicine and gerontology. 4th ed. New York, NY: McGraw Hill; 1998. p. 1387–402.
9. Katz S, Downs TD, Cash HR, Grotz RC. Progress in development of the index of ADL. The Gerontologist. 1970;10(1):20–30.
10. Fillenbaum GG. Screening the elderly. A brief instrumental activities of daily living measure. J Am Geriatr Soc. 1985;33(10):698–706.
11. Mahoney FI, Barthel DW. Functional evaluation: the barthel index. Md State Med J. 1965;14:61–5.
12. Guigoz Y, Vellas B, Garry PJ. Mini nutritional assessment: a practical assessment tool for grading the nutritional state of elderly patients. In: The mini nutritional assessment, facts and research in gerontology, vol. Suppl I. Paris: Serdi; 1994.
13. Sheikh J, Yesavange J. Geriatric depression scale (GDS): recent evidence and development of a shorter version. In: Bring T, editor. Clinical gerontology: a guide to assessment and interventions. New York: Haworth Press; 1986. p. 165–73.
14. Folstein MF, Folstein SE, McHugh PR. "Mini-mental state". A practical method for grading the cognitive state of patients for the clinician. J Psychiatr Res. 1975;12(3):189–98.
15. Shulman KI. Clock-drawing: is it the ideal cognitive screening test? Int J Geriatr Psychiatry. 2000;15(6):548–61.
16. Moore KL, Boscardin WJ, Steinman MA, Schwartz JB. Age and sex variation in prevalence of chronic medical conditions in older residents of U.S. Nursing Homes. J Am Geriatr Soc. 2012;60(4):756–64. https://doi.org/10.1111/j.1532-5415.2012.03909.x.
17. Moore KL, Boscardin WJ, Steinman MA, Schwartz JB. Patterns of chronic co-morbid medical conditions in older residents of U.S. Nursing Homes:

differences between the sexes and across the agespan. J Nutr Health Aging. 2014;18(4):429–36. https://doi.org/10.1007/s12603-014-0001-y.

18. BFS. Medizinische Statistik der Krankenhäuser 2009—Standardtabellen. Neuchâtel: Bundesamt für Statistik; 2011.

19. Stone AA, Schwartz JE, Broderick JE, Deaton A. A snapshot of the age distribution of psychological well-being in the United States. Proc Natl Acad Sci U S A. 2010;107(22):9985–90. https://doi.org/10.1073/pnas.1003744107.

20. Locker D, Jokovic A. Using subjective oral health status indicators to screen for dental care needs in older adults. Community Dent Oral Epidemiol. 1996;24(6):398–402.

21. Müller F, Salem K, Barbezat C, Herrmann FR, Schimmel M. Knowledge and attitude of elderly persons towards dental implants. Gerodontology. 2012;29(2):e914–23.

22. Graves AB, Larson EB, Edland SD, Bowen JD, McCormick WC, McCurry SM, Rice MM, Wenzlow A, Uomoto JM. Prevalence of dementia and its subtypes in the Japanese American population of King County, Washington state. The Kame Project. Am J Epidemiol. 1996;144(8):760–71.

23. American Psychiatry Association. Diagnostic and statistical manual of mental disorders 4th edn. Washington, DC: APA; 1994.

24. Syrjala AM, Ylostalo P, Ruoppi P, Komulainen K, Hartikainen S, Sulkava R, Knuuttila M. Dementia and oral health among subjects aged 75 years or older. Gerodontology. 2012;29(1):36–42. https://doi.org/10.1111/j.1741-2358.2010.00396.x.

25. Faxen-Irving G, Basun H, Cederholm T. Nutritional and cognitive relationships and long-term mortality in patients with various dementia disorders. Age Ageing. 2005;34(2):136–41. https://doi.org/10.1093/ageing/afi023.

26. White H. Weight change in Alzheimer's disease. J Nutr Health Aging. 1998;2(2):110–2.

27. Taji T, Yoshida M, Hiasa K, Abe Y, Tsuga K, Akagawa Y. Influence of mental status on removable prosthesis compliance in institutionalized elderly persons. Int J Prosthodont. 2005;18(2):146–9.

28. Wilding L, Eagles D, Molnar F, O'Brien JA, Dalziel WB, Moors J, Stiell I. Prospective validation of the Ottawa 3DY Scale by Geriatric Emergency Management Nurses to Identify Impaired Cognition in Older Emergency Department Patients. Ann Emerg Med. 2016;67(2):157–63. https://doi.org/10.1016/j.annemergmed.2015.09.008.

29. Zhang Y, Niu J, Kelly-Hayes M, Chaisson CE, Aliabadi P, Felson DT. Prevalence of symptomatic hand osteoarthritis and its impact on functional status among the elderly: the Framingham Study. Am J Epidemiol. 2002;156(11):1021–7.

30. Müller F, Rentsch A. Les prothèses de recouvrement supraradiculaires. Titane. 2010;7(4):249–57.

31. Müller F, Schimmel M. GUEST EDITORIAL: revised success criteria: a vision to meet frailty and dependency in implant patients. JOMI. 2016;31(1):15.

Pharmacological Risk Assessment for Dental Implants

Xixi Wu and Faleh Tamimi

Abstract

The process of osseointegration around dental implants is similar to the biological events occurring during bone repair and fracture healing. Therefore, bone metabolic activity plays a crucial role on the success of osseointegration, and dysregulation of bone metabolism can have a negative impact on bone healing and implant osseointegration. Accordingly, it could be hypothesized that drugs interfering with healing and bone metabolism could affect osseointegration and implant survival. Looking into the relationship between pharmacology, osseointegration, and dental implant drugs can open the door for new pharmacological innovations to improve implant success and avoid unnecessary complications, and it is also of special interest because most implant patients are elder adults that are often polymedicated. In this commentary we discuss the discoveries made by us as well as by other researchers regarding the effect of several drugs on bone, osseointegration, and implant survival. Of particular interest is the growing evidence showing that commonly used drugs such as nonsteroidal anti-inflammatories, serotonin reuptake inhibitors, and proton pump inhibitors could lead to implant failure.

Osseointegrated dental implants are considered one of the most important innovations in oral rehabilitation [1, 2]. Despite this importance and many advances in techniques, materials, and implant design, the potential for clinical failure remains a significant concern for both dentists and patients [1]. Osseointegrated dental implant success is dependent on the successful osseointegration [3]. Osseointegration is the direct structural and functional connection between the living bone and the dental implant surface, with a physiological process that resembles bone fracture healing [3]. Therefore, bone metabolic activities play crucial roles on the success of osseointegration [3].

Bone is continuously remodeling throughout life [4]. Osteoblastic bone formation and osteoclastic bone resorption are closely coordinated by a variety of local and systemic pathways that maintain bone mass constant [4]. Some pharmacological agents can interfere with the pathways that regulate bone metabolism and subsequently affect bone turnover, osseointegration, and ultimately implant survival. In addition, a large proportion of the population suffering from diseases or conditions are under medical management, but

X. Wu · F. Tamimi (✉)
Faculty of Dentistry, McGill University,
Montreal, QC, Canada
e-mail: xixi.wu@mail.mcgill.ca; faleh.
tamimimarino@mcgill.ca

© Springer International Publishing AG, part of Springer Nature 2018
E. Emami, J. Feine (eds.), *Mandibular Implant Prostheses*,
https://doi.org/10.1007/978-3-319-71181-2_4

"""

relatively little is known about the effects of these medications on osseointegrated dental implants. Therefore, in this chapter we list the main groups of drugs known to affect bone metabolism and discuss their impact on bone metabolism, osseointegration, and implant success (Table 4.1).

4.1 Drugs Targeting the Central Nervous System

The central nervous system (CNS) is a main regulator of bone metabolism [5]. For this reason, neurological drugs can have an effect on bone accrual, bone healing, osseointegration, and implant survival. Underneath we discuss four types of neurological drug that have been found to affect bone and even osseointegrated implants, including selective serotonin reuptake inhibitors (SSRIs), acetylcholinesterase inhibitors (AChEIs), melatonin, antiepileptic drugs (AEDs), and opioids.

4.1.1 Selective Serotonin Reuptake Inhibitors (SSRIs)

There is evidence from cohort studies indicating that SSRIs could have negative effects on implant survival [6] and bone fracture [7]. SSRIs, such as Celexa, Paxil, Lexapro, Prozac, and Zoloft, are drugs designed to inhibit the reuptake of serotonin and boost its levels to treat depression [5, 8]. Because of their unique effectiveness in depression treatment, SSRIs have become the most widely used antidepressants all over the world [9].

Serotonin, also called 5-hydroxytryptamine (5-HT), is a monoamine neurotransmitter [10], which is popularly thought to be a contributor to feelings of well-being and happiness [11]. Biochemically derived from tryptophan, serotonin is primarily found not only in the nervous tissue but also in peripheral tissues such as the digestive tract, blood platelets, and bones of animals, including humans [11]. Accordingly, SSRIs can affect the function of the digestive, cardiovascular, and skeletal systems [9]. In the skeletal

system, serotonin regulates bone cells by acting on 5-HT1B, 5-HT2B, 5-HT2C receptors and serotonin transporters (5-HTTs) in osteoblasts and osteoclasts [9]. SSRIs block 5-HTTs on bone cells, resulting in a direct negative effect on bone formation [12, 13] and metabolism [9] by increasing osteoclast differentiation [14] and inhibiting osteoblast proliferation [9]. As a result, SSRIs decrease bone mass and bone mineral density (BMD) [12–14], at an annual reduction rate of 0.60%–0.93% [12, 13], increasing the risk of osteoporosis [15] and bone fracture [5], especially osteoporotic fracture [15]. In the retrospective cohort study conducted by Tamimi research group on 490 patients treated with 916 dental implants, we found that SSRI could be significantly associated with an increased risk of dental implants failure [6].

4.1.2 Acetylcholinesterase Inhibitors (AChEIs)

Clinical evidence from case-control studies, retrospective cohort studies, and in vitro studies shows that the use of AChEIs, such as rivastigmine, donepezil, galantamine, etc., is associated with lower risk of fracture and enhanced fracture healing by affecting osteoblasts and osteoclasts [16, 17]. AChEIs, also called anticholinesterase, are drugs that inhibit the acetylcholinesterase, the enzyme responsible for breaking down acetylcholine, thereby increasing both the level and duration of action of the neurotransmitter acetylcholine [18]. AChEIs have been widely used for the treatment of Alzheimer's disease (AD), Lewy body dementia, Parkinson's disease, and other dementias [19, 20]. Recent research has revealed the presence of acetylcholine receptors (AChRs) subunits in bone tissues, highly expressed on osteoblasts, especially during the osteoblast differentiation stage, which may play a possible role in regulating alkaline phosphatase (ALP) activity [21, 22]. Accordingly, AChEIs can affect the proliferation and differentiation of osteoblasts [22, 23] and subsequently exert positive effects on bone mass and fracture healing [16, 17]. It is also shown that AChEIs would suppress bone

Table 4.1 Impact of drugs on bone and implants

			Effects on the bone							Effects on implants	
Drug category	Drug name	Mechanism[a]	BMD[b]	Bone formation[b]	Bone resorption[b]	Bone turnover[b]	Fracture risk[c]	Osteoporosis[c]	Bone/fracture healing[c]	Osseointegration[b]	Implant survival[c]
Drugs targeting the central nervous system	SSRIs	↑OC ↑RANKL	↓	↓	↑		↑	↑			↓
	AChEIs	↑OB ↓OC ↑Calcification ↑ALP		↑	↓		↓		↑		
	Melatonin	↑OB ↓OC	↑	↑	↓				↑	↑	
	AEDs	↓OB ↑PTH ↓Vitamin D	↓				↑				
	Opioids	↓Gonadotrophins	↓				↓				
Antihypertensive drugs	β-Blockers	↑OB ↓OC ↑β-receptor inhibition ↑Bone accrual	↑	↑	↓		↓	↓	↑	↑	↑
	Thiazide diuretics	↑OB ↑RUNX2 ↑Osteopontin ↑Serum calcium	↑	↑	↓	↓	↓				↑
	ACE inhibitors	↓OC ↑PTH ↑Calcium	↑	↑	↓		↓				↑
	ARBs	↑OB ↓OC	↑	↑	↓		↓		↑		↑
	CCBs	↑OB ↓OC ↕Calcium homeostasis ↑Vitamin D			↓						
Antidiabetic drugs	Metformin	↑OB ↑AMP ↑BMP-2 ↑ALP		↑	↓		↓				
	GLP-1	↑OB ↓OC ↑Calcitonin	↑	↑	↓	↑					
	DPP-4 inhibitors	↑OB ↓OC ↑Calcitonin	↑	↑	↓		↓				
	Thiazolidinedione	↑Osteoclastogenesis ↓ALP ↓PTH			↑		↑	↑	↓		

(continued)

Table 4.1 (continued)

			Effects on the bone							Effects on implants	
Drug category	Drug name	Mechanism[a]	BMD[b]	Bone formation[b]	Bone resorption[b]	Bone turnover[b]	Fracture risk[c]	Osteoporosis[c]	Bone/fracture healing[c]	Osseointegration[b]	Implant survival[c]
Gastrointestinal drugs	PPIs	↓OB ↓OC ↓BMP-2, BMP-4 ↓PHOSPHO1 ↓ALP ↓Calcium level ↓Apoptosis	↓	↓	↑	↓	↑		↓	↓	↓
Immunosuppressants	Calcineurin inhibitors	↓OB ↑OC ↕Calcineurin/NFAT	↓	↓	↑		↑	↑			
	Cyclosporine	Immunosuppressive	↓	↓	↑	↑	↑	↑	↓	↓	
Antineoplastics	Anti-VEGF	↓OC ↓Angiogenesis				↓		↓		↓	
	Radium-223	↓OB									
	Exemestane	↑ALP ↑PINP ↑Osteocalcin ↑CTX ↑NTX	↓			↑	↑	↑			
Chemotherapy		↓Bone cells		↓					↓		
Anti-inflammatories	NSAIDs	↓OB ↓OC	↓	↓			↑	↓	↓	↓	↓
	Glucocorticoids	↑OC ↓Vitamin D		↓	↑		↑	↑			
Hormone replacement therapy	Thyroid	↑OB ↑IGF-1 ↑Calcitonin ↑Growth factor		↑			↓	↓			
	GIP	↑OB ↑Calcium ↓Apoptosis		↑	↓			↓			
	Sex steroids	↓OC ↑RANKL/ RANK/OPG	↑	↑	↓	↓		↓			
Anti-osteoporosis	PTH	↕Calcium homeostasis	↑	↑	↓			↓	↑	↑	
	Calcitonin	↓OC	↑		↓			↓	↓		
	Bisphosphonate	↓OC			↓	↓		↓	↓		
	Sclerostin inhibitors	↓LRP5/6 ↓Wnt signaling	↑	↑				↓			

Hypercholesterolemia medications	Statins	↑OB ↓OC ↑BMP ↑COLLIA1 ↑Osteocalcin ↓RANKL	↑				↓	↓		↑	
Antihistamines		↓RANKL	↑		↓				↓		
HIV therapy	Antiretrovirals	↑OC	↓		↑		↑	↑			
Anticoagulants	Heparin	↓OB ↑OC	↓	↓	↑		↑	↑			
Alcohol		↓OC impair immune system	↓	↓				↑	↓	↓	↓

↑ = increase; ↓ = decrease; ↕ = two-way regulate

OB osteoblasts, *OC* osteoclasts, *BMD* bone mineral density, *SSRIs* selective serotonin reuptake inhibitors, *AChEIs* acetylcholinesterase inhibitors, *AEDs* antiepileptic drugs, *ACE inhibitors* angiotensin-converting enzyme inhibitors, *ARBs* angiotensin II receptor blockers, *CCBs* calcium channel blockers, *GLP-1* glucagon-like peptide-1, *DPP-4 inhibitors* dipeptidyl peptidase-4 inhibitors, *PPIs* proton pump inhibitors, *Anti-VEGF* anti-vascular endothelial growth factor, *NSAIDs* nonsteroidal anti-inflammatory drugs, *PTH* parathyroid hormone, *GIP* gastric inhibitory polypeptide, *ERT* estrogen replacement therapy, *RANKL* the receptor activator of nuclear factor κB ligand, *ALP* alkaline phosphatase, *RUNX2* runt-related transcription factor 2, *AMP* thymidine kinase, *BMP-2* bone morphogenetic protein-2, *PHOSPHO1* phosphoethanolamine/phosphocholine phosphatase, *NFAT* nuclear factor of activated T cells, *PINP* procollagen type 1 amino-terminal propeptide, *CTX* C-telopeptide, *NTX* N-telopeptide, *IGF-1* insulin-like growth factors, *RANK* the receptor activator of nuclear factor κB, *OPG* osteoprotegerin, *LRP* low-density lipoprotein receptor-related protein, *COLLIA1* candidate genes 136–41 collagen

[a]Mechanism is based on in vitro studies

[b]From clinical evidence

[c]From in vivo evidence

resorption rate by promoting osteoclasts apoptosis [23]. In summary, AChEIs may accelerate calcification at the fracture site, favor bone mass, minimize healing complication, and have a beneficial effect on bone turnover that could translate into reduction of bone fracture risk [16, 17]. However, future studies are needed to assess if AChEIs have effects on osseointegration and dental implants.

4.1.3 Melatonin

In vivo [24, 25] and in vitro [26] studies reveal that melatonin has positive effects on bone and implant osseointegration and promotes bone fracture healing [27]. Melatonin, also known as the sleep hormone, is a tryptophan-derived indolamine secreted by the pineal gland that plays an important role in the biologic regulation of circadian rhythms, sleep, aging, tumor growth, reproduction [28], and bone physiology [29]. Studies indicate that bone marrow cells are capable of synthesizing melatonin, leading to high concentrations of melatonin in bone marrow [30].

Melatonin binds specifically to its membrane-bound G protein-coupled receptors (MT1 and MT2), found in many cells including osteoblasts and osteoclasts [31]. Melatonin can promote osteoblastic proliferation and differentiation, increase production of osteoblastic protein osteoprotegerin, and inhibit osteoclastic activities, leading to bone strengthening [26, 29, 32]. Moreover, melatonin administration releases growth hormone, a very important hormone for normal longitudinal bone growth in both rats and humans [33, 34].

Melatonin can also have therapeutic activity in bone by affecting calcium uptake [29]. Suppression of melatonin secretion in newborn rats lowers serum calcium concentration, while melatonin treatment prevents serum calcium decrease [29]. Researchers speculated that melatonin might interact with calcium-calmodulin signaling [35], because it can reduce systolic blood pressure in humans by increasing serum calcium level [36–38].

Therefore, it is suggested that melatonin supplement could improve the health of bones, acting as an antiaging and anti-osteoporosis therapy for bone deterioration. Besides, melatonin could also be a potential agent to stimulate the peri-implant bone response and osseointegration during implant placement, which may need more research to confirm.

4.1.4 Antiepileptic Drugs (AEDs)

There is evidence from epidemiological studies, in vivo studies, and also in vitro studies suggesting that AEDs can increase bone fracture and reduce BMD and bone mass by affecting bone mineralization and calcium metabolism [39]. AEDs, including phenobarbital, carbamazepine, valproate, oxcarbazepine, gabapentin, etc., are usually required as long-term treatment for people with epilepsy, which is a common chronic neurological disorder, with episodes that can vary from brief and nearly undetectable to long periods of vigorous shaking [40, 41].

The association between AEDs use and increased risk of fracture has been widely recognized [39, 42, 43]. It is reported that patients chronically taking AEDs suffer from clinical bone disorders, including altered calcium metabolism and radiographic rickets [44–46]. The reason of AEDs-associated bone diseases and complications remains controversial. The possible mechanisms contributing to AEDs-induced bone problems include vitamin D inactivation, altered calcium metabolism, increased parathyroid, vitamin K deficiency, decreased calcitonin, and/or osteoblast inhibition, etc. [39]. More specifically, AEDs are more proven to induce cytochrome p450 enzymes (CYP450), such as phenytoin and phenobarbital, leading to changes in calcium metabolism due to increased vitamin D degradation and vitamin D deficiency [47].

Given their overwhelming negative effect on bone, it could be speculated that AEDs could also have a negative effect on bone healing and osseointegration. However, future studies will be needed to assess the gap in knowledge in regard to the impact of AEDs on bone healing, osseointegration, and dental implants.

4.1.5 Opioids

Opioids, acting on opioid receptors medically to relieve pain, have been shown to be associated with a decreased BMD [48], possibly related to a suppression of the gonadotrophins (luteinizing hormone and follicle-stimulating hormone) and thus sex steroid deficiency in vivo and clinically [49]. Increased risk of fractures has been observed with the use of opioids, although significant differences may exist between different types [50]. One mechanism behind the increased risk of fractures is falls, which may be related to dizziness and altered postural balance related to the CNS effects of opioids [51]. However, changes in bone structure and thus bone biomechanical competence are also a possibility [52].

4.2 Antihypertensive Drugs

Antihypertensive medications, such as β-blockers, thiazide diuretics, angiotensin-converting-enzyme (ACE) inhibitors, angiotensin II receptor blockers (ARBs), and calcium channel blockers (CCBs), are the most commonly prescribed drugs for people suffering from hypertension, a chronic medical condition in which the blood pressure in the arteries is elevated [53]. Antihypertension medications are observed to be associated with oral tori and an increased survival rate of osseointegrated implants due to their bone-stimulating properties [54–56].

4.2.1 β-Blockers

Evidence from epidemiological studies, in vivo studies, and in vitro studies suggests that β-blockers reduce the risk of bone fracture and also increase BMD, BM, bone healing, osseointegration, and dental implant survival rate, by stimulating bone formation and inhibiting bone resorption [54, 57–61]. β-Blockers are among the most widely used treatments for hypertension. They exert their effect on blood pressure by inhibiting the sympathetic β-adrenergic receptors [62]. Besides their

cardiovascular effects, it appears that stimulation of these β-receptors may also have catabolic actions on bone cells [63], leading to increased bone resorption by stimulation of osteoclastic differentiation, proliferation, and activity [64, 65]. On the other hand, the activation of β2-adrenergic receptors, the only β-adrenergic receptors known to be expressed by osteoblasts, results in the downregulation of bone formation [63, 66, 67].

The potential mechanism by which β-blockers affect bone may be similar to the leptin-sympathetic nervous system pathway [64]. In animal models, leptin deficiency results in a low sympathetic tone, and genetic or pharmacological ablation of adrenergic signaling leads to leptin resistance and high bone mass [64]. β-Blockers, as anti-sympathetic agents, increase bone mass via the same pathway, which acts locally through β2-adrenergic receptors on bone osteoblasts [57, 64]. It is proven that bone resorption can be inversely decreased by β-blockers [68]. Furthermore, there is evidence that propranolol, a commonly used β-blockers, increases cross-linking of type 1 collagen in tissues, enhancing the tensile strength [69]. Taken together, in vivo and in vitro results suggest that β-blocker use has a beneficial effect on bone health. This is also confirmed by clinical studies showing that β-blockers seem to be associated with lower risk of bone fracture and exert beneficial effects on bone structure, metabolism, fracture healing, osseointegration, and implant survival [54, 57–59, 61, 64, 70].

4.2.2 Thiazide Diuretics

Observational studies and in vitro studies showed that thiazide diuretics reduce the risk of bone fracture [71], increase BMD [72], and reduce bone loss [73]. Thiazide diuretics control high blood pressure by inhibiting the thiazide-sensitive sodium chloride cotransporter (NCC) in the distal tubules of the kidney reducing renal calcium excretion and subsequently enhance calcium uptake [74]. Thiazide diuretics can also affect bone through the following potential mechanism:

1. Decreased urinary calcium excretion leading to increased serum calcium levels that could in turn lead to reduced parathyroid hormone (PTH) levels, which result in reduced bone turnover and increased BMD [75].
2. Thiazide diuretics may have a direct positive homeostatic effect on bone by blocking the NCC expressed on osteoblasts and osteoblast-like cells [76, 77].
3. Thiazide diuretics also exert effects on bone by stimulating osteoblast differentiation through osteoblast differentiation markers, runt-related transcription factor 2 (RUNX2) and osteopontin [78].

The abovementioned mechanisms could be the reason why in a recent cohort study [54] an association was found between usage of antihypertensive medication, including thiazide diuretics, and lower risk of dental implant failure, although in vivo studies in more depth are required to confirm the effect of the drugs on implant osseointegration.

4.2.3 Angiotensin-Converting Enzyme (ACE) Inhibitors

Cohort studies, case-control studies, randomized clinical trials, as well as in vivo and in vitro studies indicate that ACE inhibitors are associated with higher BMD and lower risk of bone fracture, by acting on the renin-angiotensin-aldosterone system (RAAS) locally in bone [79–82]. ACE inhibitors are among the primary prescriptions for hypertension [83]. They inhibit the production of ACE, an enzyme responsible for the conversion of angiotensin I converting to angiotensin II in RAAS [83]. RAAS operates systemically and locally in several tissues including bone [84]. Osteoblasts and osteoclasts express angiotensin II type 1 receptors, suggesting the existence of local RAAS [85]. Moreover, angiotensin II induces the expression of receptor activator of NF-kappaB ligand (RANKL) in osteoblasts, leading to the activation of osteoclasts resulting in bone resorption and detrimen-

tal effects on bone [86, 87]. In addition, angiotensin II can also affect bone by interfering with the calcium metabolism; angiotensin II decreases plasma ionic calcium levels resulting in a concomitant increase in PTH levels [88]. Therefore, by hindering the angiotensin II production, ACE inhibitors seem to have positive effects on bone metabolism both directly and indirectly. However, future in vivo studies are needed to assess the effect of ACE inhibitors on osseointegration and dental implants.

4.2.4 Angiotensin II Receptor Blockers (ARBs)

Just as ACE inhibitors, there are epidemiological, in vivo, and in vitro studies indicating that angiotensin II receptor blockers (ARBs) exert protective effects on relative fracture risk over time, by acting on the RAAS locally in bone [79–82, 89]. ARBs, also known as angiotensin II receptor antagonists, sartans, or AT_1-receptor antagonists, are a group of pharmaceuticals used to treat hypertension when patients are intolerant to ACE inhibitor therapy [90]. ARBs target the RAAS (see in ACE inhibitors) and inhibit angiotensin II production in bone by blocking angiotensin II AT_1 receptors, leading to protective effects bone metabolism [83].

Animal studies confirmed that ARBs, including telmisartan, olmesartan, and losartan, could reduce bone loss [91] and attenuate the ovariectomy-induced decrease in BMD by inhibiting the activity of tartrate-resistant acid phosphatase, an enzyme responsible for bone resorption [86]. Moreover, telmisartan promotes fracture healing and protects from bone loss by actively blocking thiazolidinedione-induced anti-osteoblastic activity via maintaining peroxisome proliferator-activated receptor-γ (PPAR-γ) serine 112 phosphorylation [92, 93]. Overall, ARBs seem to increase bone strength, mass, and trabecular connections [94, 95], which can lead to interesting investigations about their effects on osseointegration and dental implant survival in the future.

4.2.5 Calcium Channel Blockers (CCBs)

In vivo and in vitro studies demonstrated that CCBs seem to inhibit bone resorption by suppressing osteoclast function and stimulating the growth and differentiation of osteoblasts [96–98]. CCBs are a group of medications that inhibit the voltage-activated inward influx of calcium from the extracellular medium, exerting potent cardiovascular effects that are very useful for the treatment of hypertension [99]. Through similar ways, CCBs also influence bone homeostatics [85]. During bone resorption, osteoclasts can sense changes in ambient calcium concentration, which triggers a sharp cytosolic calcium increase through both calcium release and calcium influx [85]. The change in cytosolic calcium is transduced into inhibition of bone resorption, regulating growth and differentiation of osteoblasts and stimulating the function of these cells [96]. Although epidemiological studies show increased vitamin D levels in patients taking CCBs [100], there is no literature indicating if CCB use is associated with bone fractures, bone healing, osseointegration, and/or dental implants, which needs future studies to assess.

4.3 Antidiabetic Drugs

Worldwide, more than 171 million people have diabetes, and its prevalence is expected to double by 2030 [101]. And many antidiabetic drugs are now used to control hyperglycemia. These drugs might have positive or negative effects on bone metabolism and subsequently implants. According to available studies, metformin, glucagon-like peptide-1 (GLP-1), and dipeptidyl peptidase-4 inhibitors (DPP-4 inhibitors) seem to exert positive effects on bone, but thiazolidinedione can have negative effects on bone.

4.3.1 Metformin

Metformin inhibits bone loss in vivo, and it has osteogenic potency in vitro. It is also noted that the use of metformin may be associated with reduced bone fractures [102]. Metformin is an antidiabetic agent widely used for the treatment of type 2 diabetes as adjunct to insulin therapy in selected patients of type 1 diabetes since the late 1950s [103]. Metformin acts primarily by suppressing glucose production by the liver [103], but several recent studies have reported the positive effects of this agent on bone metabolism by activating thymidine kinase (AMP) signaling pathway, upregulating endothelial nitric oxide synthase, and expressing bone morphogenetic protein-2 (BMP-2) [104, 105], thereby exerting a direct inhibition on bone loss in vivo [103]. In vitro metformin promotes the osteogenic action of osteoblasts, including cell proliferation, type 1 collagen production, ALP activity, mineral deposition, and osteoblast-like cells differentiation [104]. Based on these findings, metformin may exert a positive effect on bone. Therefore, it is necessary to investigate whether metformin has positive effects on bone healing, osseointegration, and dental implant survival.

4.3.2 Glucagon-Like Peptide-1 (GLP-1)

In vivo and in vitro studies demonstrated that GLP-1 seems to have anabolic effects on bone as a bone turnover modulator that increases BMD by inducing osteoblast differentiation and inhibiting osteoclastic activity [106–108]. GLP-1, also known as incretin, is a neuropeptide derived from the transcription product of the proglucagon gene, exerting insulin-like effects upon glucose transport and/or metabolism [109, 110]. GLP-1 also affects bone by directly stimulating the secretion of calcitonin, a potent inhibitor of osteoclastic bone resorption [111, 112]. It is believed that GLP-1 mainly targets calcitonin to modulate bone turnover because genetic loss of GLP-1 receptor signaling increases osteoclastic bone resorption activity, without affecting bone formation, leading to a significant reduction in trabecular separation and an increase in bone strength [108]. In summary, GLP-1 might be useful as a pharmacological agent for improving bone formation and bone structure; however, there is no literature on its effects on bone fracture, bone healing, osseointegration, and dental implant survival which needs to be addressed in future studies.

4.3.3 Dipeptidyl Peptidase-4 Inhibitors (DPP-4 Inhibitors)

In vitro studies suggest that drugs capable of increasing incretin levels, such as DPP-4 inhibitors, could exert beneficial effects on the bone, and epidemiological studies indicate that DPP-4 inhibitors are associated with decreased bone fractures [113]. Inhibitors of dipeptidyl peptidase-4, also known as gliptins, are a class of oral hypoglycemics that block DPP-4, and they are used to treat diabetes mellitus type 2 [114]. Treatments with DPP-4 inhibitors for type 2 diabetes patients could have a protective effect on bone and have been associated with a reduced risk of bone fractures. These drugs affect bone metabolism by increasing the circulating levels of GLP-1 and gastric intestinal polypeptide, both involved in the regulation of bone metabolism [107, 108, 113, 115–118]. Despite their positive effects on bone metabolism, the effects of DPP-4 inhibitors on osseointegration and dental implant survival have not been investigated and require future researches.

4.3.4 Thiazolidinedione

Thiazolidinedione, glucose-lowering agent, has been reported to reduce BMD, increase bone loss, delay bone healing, and increase the incidence of fractures [119–123]. Thiazolidinedione, also known as glitazones, are a class of medications used in the treatment of diabetes mellitus type 2 with a beneficial effect on insulin sensitivity [124]. Thiazolidinedione exerts their antidiabetic effects by activating PPAR-γ nuclear receptor, which controls glucose and fatty acid metabolism, and is also a key regulator of bone cell development and activity in the skeleton [125]. In bone, PPAR-γ controls differentiation of cells of mesenchymal and hematopoietic lineages, and its activation by thiazolidinedione leads to unbalanced bone remodeling [125].

In vivo, thiazolidinedione induces bone loss by affecting the bone remodeling process, suppressing new bone formation by osteoblasts, and increasing bone resorption by osteoclasts, which leads to significantly decreased BMD, bone volume, and changed bone microarchitecture [126, 127]. The observed bone loss was associated with changes in the structure and function of the bone marrow, including a decreased number of osteoblasts, decreased osteoblastic function, an increased number of adipocytes, promoted osteoclast differentiation, and increased osteoclastogenesis [123, 128–130]. It is also reported that thiazolidinedione has a negative effect on markers of bone formation such as ALP and PTH [131–133]. Overall, thiazolidinedione seems to exert an adverse effect on bone health, so further studies are necessary to assess the effects of thiazolidinedione on osseointegration and dental implants.

4.4 Gastrointestinal Drugs

Given the skeletal requirements of calcium, amino acids, and energy for bone turnover and renewal, it is not surprising that the gastrointestinal tract is of major importance for skeletal integrity [134]. So far proton pump inhibitors (PPIs) have been found to affect bone [135–137], but given the importance of gastrointestinal function in bone, it could be speculated that more gastrointestinal drugs would be found to affect bone in the future.

4.4.1 Proton Pump Inhibitors (PPIs)

In vivo, in vitro, and clinical studies indicate that PPI usage is associated with decreased bone healing, bone accrual, bone turnover, and osseointegration, as well as increased risk of bone fracture and dental implant failure, by affecting osteoblasts, osteoclasts, and calcium balance [135–137]. PPIs are a group of drugs that are rapidly becoming the third most prescribed pharmaceutical products worldwide [138]. This type of medication, including omeprazole, lansoprazole, pantoprazole, dexlansoprazole, esomeprazole, rabeprazole, etc., is very effective in both prevention and treatment of gastrointestinal acid-related conditions, such as peptic ulcer, gastroesophageal reflux disease (GERD or GORD), dyspepsia, *Helicobacter pylori* infections, eosinophilic esophagitis, gastrinomas, and stress gastritis [138]. In the past 20 years, a marked increase of PPI exposure has been observed [139], and besides occasional use of this medication, millions of individuals are also using PPIs as a continuous or long-term therapy [140]. This is of particular relevance because a relationship between PPI administration and bone metabolism has been acknowledged by the US Food and Drug Administration [141].

PPIs suppress gastric acidity by inhibiting the functions of the proton pump (H+/K+ ATPase) [142, 143]. The proton pump can also be found in bones, and its inhibition in osteoclasts can decrease their activities, leading to reduced cortical thickness, bone weight, and bone biomechanical properties [144, 145]. In addition to their effects on osteoclastic behavior, PPIs might also interfere with osteoblastic cells, by inhibiting phosphoethanolamine/phosphocholine phosphatase (PHOSPHO1) and ALP in bone [146–148]. Other mechanisms suggest indirectly negative effects of PPIs on bone metabolism by affecting calcium homeostasis [141, 149]. Specifically, PPIs impair calcium absorption in the gastrointestinal track by increasing the pH in the small intestine and thus reducing calcium availability for incorporation in bone, thereby decreasing its mineral density [141, 149]. Clinically, observational studies have shown an association between the use of PPIs and high risk of bone loss and bone fractures [150]. Our recent in vivo and epidemiological studies also confirmed the negative effect of PPIs on bone healing and implants [136, 137]. Indeed, usage of PPIs reduces osseointegration, delays bone healing, and is associated with increased dental implant failure [136, 137].

4.5 Immunosuppressants

Bone remodeling is strongly influenced by the immune system [151, 152]. Accordingly, dysregulation of the immune system by some drugs might be associated with bone loss and fracture [152]. It is worth mentioning that RANKL, a crucial signal for osteoclast function, is expressed by several immune cells (e.g., CD8, CD4, TH1, TH2) [153, 154]. Moreover, T cells can suppress osteoclastogenesis through expression of interferon-γ (INF-γ), IL-4, or T lymphocyte protein 4, which in turn suggests a protective effects of T cells on bone [155].

4.5.1 Calcineurin Inhibitors

In vivo and in vitro studies indicate that calcineurin inhibitors have adverse effects on bone, leading to increased bone loss and decreased BMD [156]. Calcineurin is a calcium- and calmodulin-dependent serine/threonine protein phosphatase [157]. And inhibitors of calcineurin are immunosuppressant agents used to prevent organ transplant rejection and to treat autoimmune diseases and some non-autoimmune inflammatory diseases [158]. Patients treated with the calcineurin inhibitors develop osteopenia and have an increased incidence of fractures [159–162]. It is suggested that calcineurin inhibitors suppress bone formation and stimulate bone resorption by hindering osteoblast differentiation and promoting osteoclast activity [163]. And it is possible that calcineurin inhibitors affect bone metabolism through the regulation of calcineurin/nuclear factor of activated T cell (NFAT) signaling pathway, which is necessary for osteoclastogenesis [163]. However, no data is yet available on the effects of calcineurin inhibitors on bone healing, osseointegration, as well as dental implants, and this might need more investigation in the future.

4.5.2 Cyclosporine

Cyclosporine A (CsA) is an immunosuppressant drug widely used in organ transplantation to prevent rejection [164]. It reduces the activity of the immune system by interfering with the activity and growth of T cells [165]. In vivo and in vitro studies indicate that CsA might have anti-anabolic effects in bone remodeling by suppressing the critical role of T lymphocytes, leading to increased bone turnover and bone loss and increased risk of osteopenia, bone fracture, and osteoporosis [166–168]. It is suggested the reason why CsA affects bone metabolism may be related to its immunosuppressive mechanisms mediated by cytokines, but the specific mechanism is still unclear [169].

Moreover, in vivo studies also demonstrated that the use of CsA might delay bone healing and hinder osseointegration around dental implants [170–172]. Given the negative effects of CsA on bone metabolism, it might be reconsidered that patients with CsA therapy undergo implant placement. However, clinical studies are needed to confirm the effects of CsA on dental implants survival.

4.6 Antineoplastic Drugs

Osseointegration and bone healing require cell proliferation, differentiation, and angiogenesis. Antineoplastic drugs act mainly by inhibiting cell proliferation and angiogenesis. Therefore, it is expected that this type of medication would have negative effects on bone healing, osseointegration, and implants. Underneath we discuss some antineoplastic drugs known to have negative effects on bone.

4.6.1 Anti-vascular Endothelial Growth Factor (Anti-VEGF)

In vivo and in vitro studies suggest adverse effects of anti-vascular endothelial growth factor (anti-VEGF) on bone turnover, bone healing, and osseo-integration by hindering angiogenesis and osteoclasts [173, 174]. Vascular endothelial growth factor (VEGF), originally known as vascular permeability factor (VPF), is a signal protein produced by cells that stimulates vasculogenesis and angiogenesis [175]. VEGF is considered a key regulator in blood vessel growth associated with angiogenesis that is crucial for bone repair and also can stimulate bone turnover through osteoclast chemotaxis and activity [176]. Therefore, VEGFs inhibition by some medications can have a negative impact on bone health [173]. These include inhibition of bone growth, decrease of bone turnover, and impairments in wound healing, because of the inhibition of newly formed blood vessels [177], which lead to delayed bone healing and less osseointegration for Ti implants [173]. However, epidemiological studies are needed to confirm this.

4.6.2 Radium-223

The principal use of radium-223 (Ra-223, ^{223}Ra) is to treat metastatic cancers in bone as a radio-pharmaceutical, with the advantages of its chemical similarity to calcium and the short range of the alpha radiation it emits [178]. ^{223}Ra, an isotope of radium with an 11.4-day half-life, is a targeted α-particle emitter that selectively targets bone metastases with high energy [179]. As a calcium mimetic, ^{223}Ra has a natural bone-seeking capability and preferentially binds to newly formed bone matrix, targeting osteoblastic metastatic lesions [180]. The high-energy, short-range α-particle radiation predominantly induces irreparable double-stranded DNA breaks resulting in potent cytotoxic activity localized to target areas while minimizing damage to bone marrow and adjacent healthy tissue [180, 181]. Despite its effect on bone, no data is yet available on the effects of ^{223}Ra on bone fracture, bone healing, osseointegration, and/or dental implants, which might need more investigations in future studies.

4.6.3 Exemestane

In vitro and clinical studies suggest that exemestane treatment reduces BMD, increases osteoporosis, accelerates bone turnover, and increases bone fracture risk [182–184]. Exemestane is an aromatase inhibitor, and it is used in the treatment of early and advanced breast cancer, acting by substantially reducing estrogen synthesis [185]. Exemestane has an anabolic effect on bone metabolism, increasing both markers of bone formation (i.e., bone alkaline phosphatase (BAP), procollagen type 1 amino-terminal propeptide (PINP), and osteocalcin) and bone resorption (i.e., C-telopeptide (CTX) and N-telopeptide (NTX)) [182]. The fact that not only bone resorption but also bone formation is increased in patients treated with exemestane is interesting, and it may be because the enhanced bone degradation could lead to enhanced synthesis per se [186]. Nevertheless, future studies are needed to look into the effects of exemestane on osseointegration and dental implants.

4.7 Chemotherapeutic Agents

Chemotherapy is a treatment using chemotherapeutic agents (cytostatic or cytotoxic agents) to treat cancer by preventing the proliferation of cancer cells [187]. The problem of using chemotherapeutic agents is their lack of selectivity, which might lead to actions on normal cells that have an accelerated cell cycle, including bone cells [187]. In vivo studies indicate that the use of chemotherapeutic agents is associated with delayed bone healing and less osseointegration [187]. On the other hand, studies report no detrimental effects of chemotherapeutic agents on osseointegration and dental survival [188]. So it seems that there is no available evidence to prove that patients undergo chemotherapy cannot take dental implant placement. However, given the negative effects of postoperative chemotherapy on bone formation, we should be aware of the risk to place implants on patients who are using chemotherapeutic agents.

4.8 Anti-inflammatories

Anti-inflammatories are a group of drugs that used to treat or reduce inflammation or swelling [189]. Underneath we discuss the anti-inflammatories known to affect bone and/or dental implants.

4.8.1 Nonsteroidal Anti-inflammatory Drugs (NSAIDs)

In vivo, in vitro, and clinical studies indicate that nonsteroidal anti-inflammatory drugs (NSAIDs) inhibit bone healing, decrease BMD, inhibit newly formed bone, and increase the risk of bone fracture, playing a detrimental role in bone metabolism [190, 191]. NSAIDs, such as ibuprofen, indomethacin, aspirin, ketorolac, and naproxen, are widely used to relieve pain and inflammation, particularly for symptoms associated with osteoarthritis and other chronic musculoskeletal conditions [192]. NSAIDs reduce pain and inflammation by inhibiting the synthesis of prostaglandin [193]. However, NSAIDs present negative side effects on bone since prostaglandin plays an important role in bone metabolism [194].

One particular situation in which NSAIDs can have a negative impact on bone is in procedure involving bone healing [195]. Bone injuries result in the local production and release of prostaglandins [195]. This release of prostaglandins triggers inflammation and increases the activity of osteoblasts and osteoclasts, all of which are ultimately required for proper bone healing [193]. NSAIDs inhibit this production of prostaglandins and thereby interfering directly with the proper process of bone healing [195–198].

Our epidemiological study [137] also discovers that NSAIDs exert adverse effects on osseointegrated dental implants (HR = 2.47; 95% CI = 1.09–5.58), and this might be exacerbated by the fact that patients who need NSAIDs therapy are often given co-therapy of gastro-protectants (i.e., PPIs), as prevention for gastroesophageal side effects [199], which also has negative effects on bone. However, in vivo studies also confirm that loss of osseointegration and delayed peri-implant bone healing are observed after NSAID administration [200, 201]. Therefore, it may be advisable to avoid NSAID prescription before or after bone surgeries and/or implant placement [202].

4.8.2 Glucocorticoids

Glucocorticoids, such as cortisone, are a class of corticosteroids that are highly effective in the treatment of inflammatory and autoimmune conditions [203]. In vivo, in vitro, and clinical studies indicate that glucocorticoids affect bone by increasing bone resorption and decreasing bone formation, mediated by direct actions on bone cells, leading to increased osteoporosis and risk of bone fracture [204, 205]. Glucocorticoids act directly on differentiated osteoclasts to extend their life span and on osteoblasts to stimulate their apoptosis [206] and also reduce vitamin D plasma level [207]. Glucocorticoids cause bone loss in two phases: a rapid, early phase in which bone mass is lost due to excessive bone resorption and a slower, later phase in which bone is lost due to inadequate bone formation [206, 208].

Regarding the effects of glucocorticoids on osseointegration and dental implants in vivo, there are conflicting results. Some studies report that delayed implant healing and decreased osseointegration are associated with glucocorticoids treatment [209, 210]. But others suggest no association between glucocorticoids users and nonusers [211, 212]. However, given their negative effects on bone metabolism, clinical studies should be carried out to address the influence of glucocorticoids on bone healing, osseointegration, and dental implants.

4.9 Hormone Replacement Therapy

Hormones are chemicals made by glands that travel throughout the body and have effects on growth, maturation, energy, weight, and bone strength [213]. Sex hormones (estrogen made in the ovary of females and testosterone made by the testes in males) control ability to reproduce and also lead to increased bone strength especially in early teenage years [213]. Other hormones come from the thyroid gland, the parathyroid gland, the pituitary gland near the brain, and the brain itself. These hormones control levels of calcium in the blood, energy levels, and ability to grow [214]. They act the same in both genders. Underneath we discuss some of the main hormones and hormone replacement therapy.

4.9.1 Thyroid Hormone

The thyroid is one of the largest endocrine glands in the body, controlling energy sources, protein synthesis, and the sensitivity to other hormones [215]. It participates in these processes by producing thyroid hormones, thyroxine (T_4) and triiodothyronine (T_3), synthesized from iodine and tyrosine [215]. In vivo, in vitro, and clinical studies show that T_3 is essential for the normal development of endochondral and intramembranous bone and plays an important role in the linear growth and maintenance of bone mass [216]. T_3 deficiency or excess results in severe skeletal abnormalities in childhood, and thyrotoxicosis is associated with osteoporosis and an increased risk of fracture in adults [217]. In the growth plate, T_3 inhibits chondrocyte proliferation and promotes hypertrophic differentiation, matrix synthesis, mineralization, and angiogenesis [218]. It also promotes osteoblastic proliferation, differentiation, and apoptosis, by its induction of IL-6, PGs, and RANKL, and also promotes osteoclast formation and activation [219]. Besides, thyroid hormones may act on bone cells indirectly by increasing secretion of growth hormone and insulin-like growth factor-1 (IGF-1) and also producing calcitonin that is crucial in calcium homeostasis [215, 219]. Future studies should address the influence of thyroid hormone on bone healing, osseointegration, and dental implants.

4.9.2 Gastric Inhibitory Polypeptide (GIP)

In vivo and in vitro studies indicate that gastric inhibitory polypeptide (GIP) exerts a protective effect on bone with decreased bone resorption and increased bone formation, by favoring osteoblast function, hindering apoptosis, and improving calcium intake [220, 221]. GIP is a gastrointestinal peptide hormone that is released from duodenal endocrine K cells after absorption of glucose or fat [222]. GIP is used for the treatment of type 2 diabetes, as well as obesity-related glucose intolerance and the alleviation of insulin resistance [223].

Besides gastric tissues, GIP receptor is also expressed in osteoblasts regulating bone turnover [224], and its activation with GIP protects osteoblasts from apoptosis and increases their function, leading to promoted osteoblastic bone formation [220, 224]. GIP also promotes the efficient storage of ingested calcium into bone, playing a positive physiological role in calcium homeostasis in vivo [220]. Therefore, the elevation of blood GIP levels elicited by meals plays a crucial role on preventing osteoporosis pathogenesis and development [220]. Given its positive effects on bone metabolism, further research is required to elucidate the role of GIP on fracture risk, bone healing, osseointegration, and dental implants.

4.9.3   Sex Steroids

In vivo, in vitro, and clinical studies indicate that sex steroids, the steroid hormones that interact with vertebrate androgen or estrogen receptors, play a major role in the regulation of bone turnover [225]. This is why gonadectomy in either sex is associated with increased bone remodeling, increased bone resorption, decreased BMD, and a relative deficit in bone formation, resulting in accelerated bone loss and increased risk of bone fracture [226].

The effects of cellular and molecular mediators of sex steroid on the bone-forming osteoblasts and bone-resorbing osteoclasts can be explained by the fact that both estrogen and androgens inhibit bone resorption via the RANKL/RANK/osteoprotegerin system, as well as by reducing the production of pro-resorptive cytokines, along with their direct effects on osteoclast activity and life span [225].

Also studies show that serum osteoprotegerin (OPG) and RANKL concentrations might be influenced by menopause [227]. Therefore, it is indicated that estrogen replacement therapy exerts beneficial effects in preventing and treating osteoporosis in postmenopausal women, increasing BMD, and decreasing the risk of fracture [228–230]. As abovementioned, estrogen depletion is an important risk factor for the development of osteoporosis [231], so it is important to consider the estrogen replacement therapy as a possible underlying factor for bone-related diseases [228]. Regarding to dental field, estrogen deficiency results in significant loss of interproximal bone density, and the use of estrogen replacement therapy led to increased density in the crestal and subcrestal regions of the alveolar bone [232].

However, currently there is no literature available on the effects of sex steroid or estrogen replacement therapy on bone healing, osseointegration, and dental implant survival, especially for aged women, and future research is needed on this.

4.10   Anti-osteoporosis Drugs

Osteoporosis is a skeletal disorder characterized by compromised bone strength predisposing to an increased risk of fracture [233]. Bone strength primarily reflects the integration of bone density and bone quality [234]. Many pharmacological agents are approved for the treatment of osteoporosis [233]. We find that grouping them into anti-catabolic and anabolic classes based on the mechanisms of their actions on bone remodeling [233] that we discuss underneath.

4.10.1   Sex Steroids (See section 4.9.3)

4.10.1.1   Parathyroid Hormone (PTH)

PTH, an 84-amino acid peptide secreted by the parathyroid glands, is essential for the maintenance of calcium homeostasis, and its actions can regulate bone remodeling [235]. PTH regulates calcium homeostasis because the signal for its production and secretion is a reduced extracellular ionized calcium concentration, while the signal for its reduction is an increase in extracellular ionized calcium concentration [236]. In vivo, in vitro, and clinical studies prove that PTH has direct effects on osteoblasts and osteocytes and indirect actions on osteoclasts, exerting either anabolic or catabolic effects depending on the duration and periodicity of PTH exposure [236]. The intermittent administration of PTH has anabolic effects on the skeleton, while the catabolic actions can be seen upon continuous exposure to PTH [237]. With continuous PTH infusion, PTH receptor signaling in osteoblasts and osteocytes can increase the RANKL/OPG ratio, thereby stimulating bone resorption [238]. In contrast, PTH induces bone formation due to its ability to downregulate SOST/sclerostin expression in osteocytes, unleashing the anabolic Wnt signaling pathway, and also stimulate the expression of runx2, osteocalcin, ALP, and collagen type 1 alpha 1 (COL1A1), which are all typical signals of bone formation [238].

Preclinical and clinical studies indicate that PTH given intermittently has beneficial effects by improving BMD and bone mass, reducing fracture risk (both osteoporotic and nonosteoporotic) and osteoporosis, while also improving fracture healing [235]. Actually, PTH is considered to be the only osteoanabolic therapy currently available for osteoporosis and bone fracture healing [235, 239]. In vivo studies also indicate that PTH administration increases bone density around implants and enhances implant anchorage and early fixation, which might lead to improved clinical results in future studies [240].

4.10.1.2 Calcitonin

Standard treatment for postmenopausal osteoporosis usually includes calcium supplementation and exercise along with the prescription of antiresorptive drugs, such as calcitonin [241]. Besides its use for treatment of postmenopausal osteoporosis, calcitonin is also used to treat hypercalcemia, Paget's disease, and other bone-related conditions [241]. The hormone participates in calcium and phosphorus metabolism, counteracting PTH [241]. In vivo, in vitro, and clinical studies demonstrated that calcitonin is a physiologic endogenous inhibitor of bone resorption that can decrease osteoclast number and osteoclast activity, leading to decreased bone resorption, increased BMD, reduced osteoporosis, and reduced risk of bone fractures [242, 243]. Due to its positive effects on bone metabolism, future studies should address the influence of calcitonin on bone healing, osseointegration, and dental implants.

4.10.1.3 Bisphosphonate

Bisphosphonates, such as clodronate and zoledronic acid, are used to inhibit bone resorption by regulating osteoclast function, particularly in the management of osteoporosis and Paget's disease [244]. In vivo, in vitro, and clinical studies indicate that bisphosphonates are used successfully in the treatment of osteoporosis to reduce bone resorption and hypercalcemia and prevent pathologic bone fractures [244]. Specifically, bisphosphonates bind to hydroxyapatite crystals and inhibit crystal growth and dissolution [245]. Besides, bisphosphonates also act directly on osteoclasts and interfere with specific intracellular biochemical processes such as isoprenoid biosynthesis and subsequent protein prenylation to inhibit cell activity [246]. However, there is growing concern regarding the fact that bisphosphonates, particularly nitrogen-containing bisphosphonates, may be associated with bisphosphonate-related osteonecrosis of the jaw (BRONJ) by inhibiting osteoclasts activity and over-suppressing bone remodeling [247]. BRONJ is an area of uncovered bone in the maxillofacial region that did not heal within 8 weeks after identification by healthcare provider, in a patient who was receiving or had been exposed to bisphosphonate therapy without previous radiation therapy to the craniofacial region [248]. Literature is conflict regarding the association between BRONJ and dental implants. In 2007, the American Association of Oral and Maxillofacial Surgeons recommended that dental implants should be avoided in patients receiving bisphosphonates treatment because an increased risk of BRONJ is associated with dental implants [249]. But other studies observed no association or found out a late complication of BRONJ in those dental implant patients but not related to the oral surgery [250]. However, it is necessary for the need of an extended follow-up of patients who are taking bisphosphonates and also undergo dental implant placement, and their dental implants should be removed only if the antibiotic treatment fails to alleviate the signs and symptoms of BRONJ [250]. Future studies are necessary for the deeper explanation on this topic, as well as the effects of bisphosphonates on bone healing, osseointegration, and dental implants.

4.10.1.4 Sclerostin Inhibitors

Sclerostin is a protein encoded by the symbol for the protein sclerostin (SOST) gene. Sclerostin is a secreted glycoprotein with a C-terminal cysteine knot-like (CTCK) domain and sequence similarity to the DAN (differential screening-selected gene aberrative in neuroblastoma) family of BMP antagonists [251]. In vivo and in vitro studies indicate that sclerostin is produced by the osteocyte and has anti-anabolic effects on bone formation by binding to low-density lipoprotein receptor-related protein 5/6 (LRP5/6) and inhibiting Wnt signaling [252]. The absence of sclerostin results in the high bone mass clinical disorder sclerosteosis [252]. Antibodies to sclerostin increase bone formation dramatically and improve bone strength without affecting bone resorption [252]. Therefore, sclerostin inhibitors are currently being explored as a potential anabolic treatment of osteoporosis [253]. However, future studies are still needed to confirm the effects of sclerostin inhibitors on bone healing, osseointegration, and implants.

4.11 Hypercholesterolemia Medications

Hypercholesterolemia, also called dyslipidemia, is the presence of high levels of cholesterol in the blood, which needs anticholesterol drugs for the treatment [254]. Underneath we discuss statins, the medication widely used for hypercholesterolemia which also can exert effects on bone and dental implants.

4.11.1 Statins

Statins, also known as 3-hydroxy-3-methylglutaryl-coenzyme A (HMG-CoA) reductase inhibitors, are a class of lipid-lowering medications that reversibly inhibit the enzyme HMG-CoA reductase which plays a central role in the production of cholesterol [255]. Statins are currently used for clinical treatment of hypercholesterolemia [255]. Besides their action as lipid-lowering agents, statins can also regulate bone metabolism [256].

In vivo, in vitro, and clinical studies have shown that administration of statins presents anabolic effects on bone by promoting osteoblast activity and suppressing osteoclasts, resulting in increased bone formation, increased BMD, improved fracture healing, decreased risk of bone fracture, and prevention of osteoporosis [257, 258]. Statins stimulate the expression of anabolic genes, such as BMP-2, COLLIA1, and osteocalcin, and also suppress osteoclast activity by decreasing RANKL/OPG ratio, leading to beneficial effects on bone [259, 260]. Moreover, in vivo studies also indicate that statins can promote osseointegration and bone healing around titanium implants, even in osteoporotic animals [261, 262]. However, its impact on implant success needs to be confirmed in epidemiological studies.

4.12 Antihistamine Drugs

Antihistamines are a type of pharmaceutical drug that opposes the activity of histamine receptors in the body and are used to treat allergic diseases [263]. In vivo, in vitro, and clinical studies indicate that antihistamine drugs can cause increased BMD and decreased bone resorption, but it inhibits bone healing [264]. Antihistamines increase the levels of serum calcitriol and directly enhance bone formation by stimulating calcitriol synthesizing enzyme [265]. Histamine seems to mediate the osteoclastic pathway by expression of RANKL in osteoblasts and bone marrow stromal cells [266–268]. Antihistamines then stimulate RANKL expression, but cannot develop osteoclastogenesis, resulting in increased BMD but delayed bone healing [265]. No data indicating there is association between antihistamines and increased risk of bone fracture, so more researches are needed for further investigation on this, as well as the association between antihistamines and other procedures, such as osseointegration and dental implant survival.

4.13　HIV Infection Therapy

Human immunodeficiency virus infection and acquired immune deficiency syndrome (HIV/AIDS) is a spectrum of conditions caused by infection with the human immunodeficiency virus (HIV). Antiretroviral therapy is currently the most commonly used treatment for HIV/AIDS and also exerts effects on bone metabolism that are discussed underneath.

4.13.1　Antiretroviral Therapies

It seems that the use of antiretroviral therapies causes increased bone loss, decreased BMD, increased osteoporosis, and increased fracture rate, according to in vivo and clinical studies [269]. Patients with HIV/AIDS are living longer due to the success of highly active antiretroviral therapy [270], with dramatically reduced morbidity and mortality rates from the HIV infection [271]. There have been anecdotal reports of bone disorders such as avascular necrosis of the hip and compression fracture in HIV-infected patients receiving antiretroviral therapies, which are recognized complications of severe osteoporosis [271, 272]. The mechanisms underlying the bone loss with antiretroviral therapies initiation are not clear, because of the inability to replicate in vivo effects of that in vitro [273]. It might be because that these drugs increase osteoclastogenesis, induce osteoclastic function, and lead to increased bone resorption and loss [207, 271]. Future studies are needed to confirm the mechanism in vitro and also the effects of antiretroviral therapies on bone healing, osseointegration, and dental implants.

4.14　Anticoagulants

Anticoagulants are a class of drugs that work to prevent blood coagulation (clotting), among which heparin is one of the most frequently prescribed drugs. Heparin also has been proven to affect bone metabolism that is discussed underneath.

4.14.1　Heparin

Heparin, which works by activating antithrombin III and blocking thrombin from clotting blood, is a widely used injectable anticoagulant, to treat and prevent deep vein thrombosis and pulmonary embolism (collectively known as venous thromboembolism), and is also used as part of the treatment of myocardial infarction and unstable angina [274].

Epidemiological, in vivo, and in vitro studies reveal that heparin decrease BMD, increase bone fractures, and develop osteoporosis by enhancing bone resorption and hindering bone formation [275]. Heparin treatment leads to a reduction in bone density and an increased risk of fractures because it stimulates BMP signaling and possibly Wnt signaling, which results in enhanced mineralization in vitro [275]. Previous published protein data on the decoy effects of heparin on OPG binding to RANKL suggests that heparin stimulates osteoclastogenesis by downregulating the expression of OPG [276–278]. There is no significant correlation between bone density and the dose or duration of heparin [279]. Also there is no literature talking about the effects of heparin on bone healing, osseointegration, and dental implant survival, which may bring out more insight, especially that patients who receive heparin appear to have an increased risk of overall and major bleeding events [280].

4.15　Alcohol

Alcohol is a central nervous system depressant with detrimental systemic effects on central nervous system, gastrointestinal tract, immune system, cardiovascular system, and bone tissue [281, 282]. In vivo, in vitro, and clinical studies indicate that alcohol exert negative effects on bone metabolism by inhibiting osteoclast activities, leading to delayed bone healing and increased risk of osteoporosis and bone fracture [282, 283].

Studies also discover the negative effects of alcohol on osseointegration and dental implants in vivo, with less bone density around implants and reduced direct bone-to-implant contact [284].

Clinically, alcohol addiction seems to be significantly associated with higher risk of dental implant failure [285]. The possible mechanism might be due to suppression of T lymphocytes and impaired mobility, adhesion, and phagocytic capabilities of the innate immune system [286].

4.16 Final Remarks

In the above we have summarized the literature on drugs we know could affect bone and osseointegration. However, we cannot rule out many other possible drugs that have not been investigated yet. There are over 1400 FDA-approved drugs that are being used routinely all around the world. And future studies will have to be done to explain the effects of other drugs on bone, osseointegration, and implants.

References

1. Misch CE. Dental implant prosthetics: Elsevier Health Sciences; 2014.
2. Takanashi Y, Penrod JR, Lund JP, Feine JS. A cost comparison of mandibular two-implant overdenture and conventional denture treatment. J Prosthet Dent. 2004;92(2):199.
3. Bonsignore LA, Anderson JR, Lee Z, Goldberg VM, Greenfield EM. Adherent lipopolysaccharide inhibits the osseointegration of orthopedic implants by impairing osteoblast differentiation. Bone. 2013;52(1):93–101.
4. Hadjidakis DJ, Androulakis II. Bone remodeling. Ann N Y Acad Sci. 2006;1092(1):385–96.
5. Liu B, Anderson G, Mittmann N, To T, Axcell T, Shear N. Use of selective serotonin-reuptake inhibitors or tricyclic antidepressants and risk of hip fractures in elderly people. Lancet. 1998;351(9112):1303–7.
6. Wu X, Al-Abedalla K, Rastikerdar E, Nader SA, Daniel N, Nicolau B, et al. Selective serotonin reuptake inhibitors and the risk of osseointegrated implant failure: a cohort study. J Dent Res. 2014;93(11):1054–61. https://doi.org/10.1177/0022034514549378.
7. Schwan S, Hallberg P. SSRIs, bone mineral density, and risk of fractures—a review. Eur Neuropsychopharmacol. 2009;19(10):683–92.
8. Nutt DJ, Forshall S, Bell C, Rich A, Sandford J, Nash J, et al. Mechanisms of action of selective serotonin reuptake inhibitors in the treatment of psychiatric disorders. Eur Neuropsychopharmacol. 1999;9:S81–S6.
9. Tsapakis E, Gamie Z, Tran G, Adshead S, Lampard A, Mantalaris A, et al. The adverse skeletal effects of selective serotonin reuptake inhibitors. Eur Psychiatry. 2012;27(3):156–69.
10. Gustafsson B, Thommesen L, Stunes AK, Tommeras K, Westbroek I, Waldum H, et al. Serotonin and fluoxetine modulate bone cell function in vitro. J Cell Biochem. 2006;98(1):139–51.
11. Young SN. How to increase serotonin in the human brain without drugs. J Psychiatry Neurosci. 2007;32(6):394.
12. Diem SJ, Blackwell TL, Stone KL, Yaffe K, Haney EM, Bliziotes MM, et al. Use of antidepressants and rates of hip bone loss in older women: the study of osteoporotic fractures. Arch Intern Med. 2007;167(12):1240.
13. Yadav VK, Ryu J-H, Suda N, Tanaka KF, Gingrich JA, Schütz G, et al. Lrp5 controls bone formation by inhibiting serotonin synthesis in the duodenum. Cell. 2008;135(5):825–37.
14. Battaglino R, Fu J, Späte U, Ersoy U, Joe M, Sedaghat L, et al. Serotonin regulates osteoclast differentiation through its transporter. J Bone Miner Res. 2004;19(9):1420–31.
15. Verdel BM, Souverein PC, Egberts TC, Van Staa TP, Leufkens HG, de Vries F. Use of antidepressant drugs and risk of osteoporotic and non-osteoporotic fractures. Bone. 2010;47(3):604–9.
16. Tamimi I, Ojea T, Sanchez-Siles JM, Rojas F, Martin I, Gormaz I, et al. Acetylcholinesterase inhibitors and the risk of hip fracture in Alzheimer's disease patients: a case-control study. J Bone Miner Res. 2012;27(7):1518–27.
17. Eimar H, Perez Lara A, Tamimi I, Márquez Sánchez P, Gormaz Talavera I, Rojas Tomba F, et al. Acetylcholinesterase inhibitors and healing of hip fracture in Alzheimer's disease patients: a retrospective cohort study. J Musculoskelet Neuronal Interact. 2013;
18. Pohanka M. Acetylcholinesterase inhibitors: a patent review (2008–present). Expert Opin Ther Pat. 2012;22(8):871–86.
19. Massoud F, Gauthier S. Update on the pharmacological treatment of Alzheimer's disease. Curr Neuropharmacol. 2010;8(1):69–80
20. Taylor D, Paton C, Kapur S. The Maudsley prescribing guidelines in psychiatry: Wiley; 2015.
21. Genever P, Birch M, Brown E, Skerry T. Osteoblast-derived acetylcholinesterase: a novel mediator of cell-matrix interactions in bone? Bone. 1999;24(4):297–303.
22. Sato T, Abe T, Chida D, Nakamoto N, Hori N, Kokabu S, et al. Functional role of acetylcholine and the expression of cholinergic receptors and components in osteoblasts. FEBS Lett. 2010;584(4):817–24.
23. En-Nosse M, Hartmann S, Trinkaus K, Alt V, Stigler B, Heiss C, et al. Expression of non-neuronal cholinergic system in osteoblast-like cells and its involvement in osteogenesis. Cell Tissue Res. 2009;338(2):203–15.

24. Tresguerres IF, Clemente C, Blanco L, Khraisat A, Tamimi F, Tresguerres JA. Effects of local melatonin application on implant osseointegration. Clin Implant Dent Relat Res. 2012;14(3):395–9.
25. Tresguerres IF, Tamimi F, Eimar H, Barralet JE, Prieto S, Torres J, et al. Melatonin dietary supplement as an anti-aging therapy for age-related bone loss. Rejuvenation Res. 2014;17(4):341–6.
26. Roth JA, Kim B-G, Lin W-L, Cho M-I. Melatonin promotes osteoblast differentiation and bone formation. J Biol Chem. 1999;274(31):22041–7.
27. Halıcı M, Öner M, Güney A, Canöz Ö, Narin F, Halıcı C. Melatonin promotes fracture healing in the rat model. Eklem Hastalik Cerrahisi. 2010;21(3):172–7.
28. Cardinali DP, Pévet P. Basic aspects of melatonin action. Sleep Med Rev. 1998;2(3):175–90.
29. Cardinali DP, Ladizesky MG, Boggio V, Cutrera RA, Mautalen C. Melatonin effects on bone: experimental facts and clinical perspectives. J Pineal Res. 2003;34(2):81–7.
30. Conti A, Conconi S, Hertens E, Skwarlo-Sonta K, Markowska M, Maestroni GJ. Evidence for melatonin synthesis in mouse and human bone marrow cells. J Pineal Res. 2000;28(4):193–202.
31. Slominski RM, Reiter RJ, Schlabritz-Loutsevitch N, Ostrom RS, Slominski AT. Melatonin membrane receptors in peripheral tissues: distribution and functions. Mol Cell Endocrinol. 2012;351(2):152–66.
32. Koyama H, Nakade O, Takada Y, Kaku T, Lau KHW. Melatonin at pharmacologic doses increases bone mass by suppressing resorption through down-regulation of the RANKL-mediated osteoclast formation and activation. J Bone Miner Res. 2002;17(7):1219–29.
33. Ostrowska Z, Kos-Kudla B, Swietochowska E, Marek B, Kajdaniuk D, Ciesielska-Kopacz N. Influence of pinealectomy and long-term melatonin administration on GH-IGF-I axis function in male rats. Neuroendocrinol Lett. 2001;22(4):255–62.
34. Forsling ML, Wheeler M, Williams A. The effect of melatonin administration on pituitary hormone secretion in man. Clin Endocrinol. 1999;51(5):637–42.
35. Lusardi P, Piazza E, Fogari R. Cardiovascular effects of melatonin in hypertensive patients well controlled by nifedipine: a 24-hour study. Br J Clin Pharmacol. 2000;49(5):423–7.
36. Gómez-Moreno G, Guardia J, Ferrera M, Cutando A, Reiter R. Melatonin in diseases of the oral cavity. Oral Dis. 2010;16(3):242–7.
37. Paulis L, Pechanova O, Zicha J, Barta A, Gardlik R, Celec P, et al. Melatonin interactions with blood pressure and vascular function during l-NAME-induced hypertension. J Pineal Res. 2010;48(2):102–8.
38. Hakanson DO, Bergstrom WH. Pineal and adrenal effects on calcium homeostasis in the rat. Pediatr Res. 1990;27(6):571–3.
39. Valsamis HA, Arora SK, Labban B, McFarlane SI. Antiepileptic drugs and bone metabolism. Nutr Metab. 2006;3(1):1.
40. Lennox WG. Epilepsy and related disorders. Boston: Little, Brown; 1960.
41. Rogawski MA, Porter RJ. Antiepileptic drugs: pharmacological mechanisms and clinical efficacy with consideration of promising developmental stage compounds. Pharmacol Rev. 1990;42(3):223–86.
42. Kruse R. Osteopathies in antiepileptic long-term therapy (preliminary report). Monatsschrift fur Kinderheilkunde. 1968;116(6):378–81.
43. Vestergaard P, Rejnmark L, Mosekilde L. Fracture risk associated with use of antiepileptic drugs. Epilepsia. 2004;45(11):1330–7.
44. Hunter J, Maxwell J, Stewart D, Parsons V, Williams R. Altered calcium metabolism in epileptic children on anticonvulsants. Br Med J. 1971;4(5781):202–4.
45. Valmadrid C, Voorhees C, Litt B, Schneyer CR. Practice patterns of neurologists regarding bone and mineral effects of antiepileptic drug therapy. Arch Neurol. 2001;58(9):1369–74.
46. Petty SJ, O'brien T, Wark J. Anti-epileptic medication and bone health. Osteoporos Int. 2007;18(2):129–42.
47. Hahn TJ, Hendin BA, Scharp CR, Boisseau VC, Haddad JG Jr. Serum 25-hydroxycalciferol levels and bone mass in children on chronic anticonvulsant therapy. N Engl J Med. 1975;292(11):550–4.
48. Kinjo M, Setoguchi S, Schneeweiss S, Solomon DH. Bone mineral density in subjects using central nervous system-active medications. Am J Med. 2005;118(12):1414. e7–e12.
49. Daniell HW. Hypogonadism in men consuming sustained-action oral opioids. J Pain. 2002;3(5):377–84.
50. Vestergaard P, Rejnmark L, Mosekilde L. Fracture risk associated with the use of morphine and opiates. J Intern Med. 2006;260(1):76–87.
51. Vestergaard P. Pain-relief medication and risk of fractures. Curr Drug Saf. 2008;3(3):199–203.
52. Vestergaard P, Hermann P, Jensen J-E, Eiken P, Mosekilde L. Effects of paracetamol, non-steroidal anti-inflammatory drugs, acetylsalicylic acid, and opioids on bone mineral density and risk of fracture: results of the Danish Osteoporosis Prevention Study (DOPS). Osteoporos Int. 2012;23(4):1255–65.
53. Ong KL, Cheung BM, Man YB, Lau CP, Lam KS. Prevalence, awareness, treatment, and control of hypertension among United States adults 1999–2004. Hypertension. 2007;49(1):69–75.
54. Wu X, Al-Abedalla K, Eimar H, Arekunnath Madathil S, Abi-Nader S, Daniel NG, et al. Antihypertensive medications and the survival rate of osseointegrated dental implants: a cohort study. Clin Implant Dent Relat Res. 2016;18(6):1171–82.
55. Morrison MD, Tamimi F. Oral tori are associated with local mechanical and systemic factors: a case-control study. J Maxillofac Oral Surg. 2013;71(1):14–22.
56. Torres García-Denche J, Wu X, Martinez PP, Eimar H, Ikbal DJA, Hernández G, et al. Membranes over the lateral window in sinus augmentation procedures:

a two-arm and split-mouth randomized clinical trials. J Clin Periodontol. 2013;40(11):1043–51.

57. Yang S, Nguyen ND, Center JR, Eisman JA, Nguyen TV. Association between beta-blocker use and fracture risk: the Dubbo Osteoporosis Epidemiology Study. Bone. 2011;48(3):451–5.

58. Togari A, Arai M. Pharmacological topics of bone metabolism: the physiological function of the sympathetic nervous system in modulating bone resorption. J Pharmacol Sci. 2008;106(4):542–6.

59. Pierroz DD, Bonnet N, Bianchi EN, Bouxsein ML, Baldock PA, Rizzoli R, et al. Deletion of β-adrenergic receptor 1, 2, or both leads to different bone phenotypes and response to mechanical stimulation. J Bone Miner Res. 2012;27(6):1252–62.

60. Levasseur R, Dargent-Molina P, Sabatier JP, Marcelli C, Bréart G. Beta-blocker use, bone mineral density, and fracture risk in older women: results from the epidemiologie de l'ostéoporose prospective study. J Am Geriatr Soc. 2005;53(3):550–2.

61. Al-Subaie AE, Laurenti M, Abdallah MN, Tamimi I, Yaghoubi F, Eimar H, et al. Propranolol enhances bone healing and implant osseointegration in rats tibiae. J Clin Periodontol. 2016;43(12):1160–70.

62. Perez-Castrillon JL, Justo I, Sanz-Cantalapiedra A, Pueyo C, Hernandez G, Dueñas A. Effect of the antihypertensive treatment on the bone mineral density and osteoporotic fracture. Curr Hypertens Rev. 2005;1(1):61–6.

63. Moore RE, Smith CK, Bailey CS, Voelkel EF, Tashjian AH. Characterization of beta-adrenergic receptors on rat and human osteoblast-like cells and demonstration that beta-receptor agonists can stimulate bone resorption in organ culture. Bone Miner. 1993;23(3):301–15.

64. Takeda S, Elefteriou F, Levasseur R, Liu X, Zhao L, Parker KL, et al. Leptin regulates bone formation via the sympathetic nervous system. Cell. 2002;111(3):305–17.

65. Schlienger RG, Kraenzlin ME, Jick SS, Meier CR. Use of β-blockers and risk of fractures. JAMA. 2004;292(11):1326–32.

66. Ma Y, Nyman JS, Tao H, Moss HH, Yang X, Elefteriou F. β2-Adrenergic receptor signaling in osteoblasts contributes to the catabolic effect of glucocorticoids on bone. Endocrinology. 2011;152(4):1412–22.

67. Bouxsein M, Devlin M, Glatt V, Dhillon H, Pierroz D, Ferrari SL. Mice lacking β-adrenergic receptors have increased bone mass but are not protected from deleterious skeletal effects of ovariectomy. Endocrinology. 2009;150(1):144–52.

68. Kondo H, Togari A. Continuous treatment with a low-dose β-agonist reduces bone mass by increasing bone resorption without suppressing bone formation. Calcif Tissue Int. 2011;88(1):23–32.

69. Minkowitz B, Boskey AL, Lane JM, Pearlman HS, Vigorita VJ. Effects of propranolol on bone metabolism in the rat. J Orthop Res. 1991;9(6):869–75.

70. Cherruau M, Facchinetti P, Baroukh B, Saffar J. Chemical sympathectomy impairs bone resorption in rats: a role for the sympathetic system on bone metabolism. Bone. 1999;25(5):545–51.

71. Aung K, Htay T. Thiazide diuretics and the risk of hip fracture. Cochrane Database Syst Rev. 2011;(10):CD005185.

72. Sigurdsson G, Franzson L. Increased bone mineral density in a population-based group of 70-year-old women on thiazide diuretics, independent of parathyroid hormone levels. J Intern Med. 2001;250(1):51–6.

73. Wasnich R, Davis J, Ross P, Vogel J. Effect of thiazide on rates of bone mineral loss: a longitudinal study. BMJ. 1990;301(6764):1303–5.

74. Bazzini C, Vezzoli V, Sironi C, Dossena S, Ravasio A, De Biasi S, et al. Thiazide-sensitive NaCl-cotransporter in the intestine possible role of hydrochlorothiazide in the intestinal Ca2+ uptake. J Biol Chem. 2005;280(20):19902–10.

75. Bolland M, Ames R, Horne A, Orr-Walker B, Gamble G, Reid I. The effect of treatment with a thiazide diuretic for 4 years on bone density in normal postmenopausal women. Osteoporos Int. 2007;18(4):479–86.

76. Barry E, Gesek F, Kaplan M, Hebert S, Friedman P. Expression of the sodium-chloride cotransporter in osteoblast-like cells: effect of thiazide diuretics. Am J Phys Cell Phys. 1997;272(1):C109–C16.

77. Aubin R, Menard P, Lajeunesse D. Selective effect of thiazides on the human osteoblast-like cell line MG-63. Kidney Int. 1996;50(5):1476–82.

78. Dvorak MM, De Joussineau C, Carter DH, Pisitkun T, Knepper MA, Gamba G, et al. Thiazide diuretics directly induce osteoblast differentiation and mineralized nodule formation by interacting with a sodium chloride co-transporter in bone. J Am Soc Nephrol. 2007;18(9):2509–16.

79. Lynn H, Kwok T, Wong S, Woo J, Leung P. Angiotensin converting enzyme inhibitor use is associated with higher bone mineral density in elderly Chinese. Bone. 2006;38(4):584–8.

80. Rejnmark L, Vestergaard P, Mosekilde L. Treatment with beta-blockers, ACE inhibitors, and calcium-channel blockers is associated with a reduced fracture risk: a nationwide case–control study. J Hypertens. 2006;24(3):581–9.

81. Shimizu H, Nakagami H, Osako MK, Nakagami F, Kunugiza Y, Tomita T, et al. Prevention of osteoporosis by angiotensin-converting enzyme inhibitor in spontaneous hypertensive rats. Hypertens Res. 2009;32(9):786–90.

82. Ma L, Ji J, Ji H, Yu X, Ding L, Liu K, et al. Telmisartan alleviates rosiglitazone-induced bone loss in ovariectomized spontaneous hypertensive rats. Bone. 2010;47(1):5–11.

83. Kwok T, Leung J, Zhang Y, Bauer D, Ensrud K, Barrett-Connor E, et al. Does the use of ACE inhibitors or angiotensin receptor blockers affect bone loss in older men? Osteoporos Int. 2012;23(8):2159–67.

84. Nakagami H, Osako MK, Morishita R. Potential effect of angiotensin II receptor blockade in adipose tissue and bone. Curr Pharm Des. 2013;19(17): 3049–53.

85. Ghosh M, Majumdar SR. Antihypertensive medications, bone mineral density, and fractures: a review of old cardiac drugs that provides new insights into osteoporosis. Endocrine. 2014;46(3):397–405.

86. Shimizu H, Nakagami H, Osako MK, Hanayama R, Kunugiza Y, Kizawa T, et al. Angiotensin II accelerates osteoporosis by activating osteoclasts. FASEB J. 2008;22(7):2465–75.

87. Wiens M, Etminan M, Gill S, Takkouche B. Effects of antihypertensive drug treatments on fracture outcomes: a meta-analysis of observational studies. J Intern Med. 2006;260(4):350–62.

88. Grant FD, Mandel SJ, Brown EM, Williams GH, Seely EW. Interrelationships between the renin-angiotensin-aldosterone and calcium homeostatic systems. J Clin Endocrinol Metabol. 1992;75(4):988–92.

89. Solomon DH, Mogun H, Garneau K, Fischer MA. Risk of fractures in older adults using antihypertensive medications. J Bone Miner Res. 2011;26(7): 1561–7.

90. Chobanian AV, Bakris GL, Black HR, Cushman WC, Green LA, Izzo JL Jr, et al. The seventh report of the joint national committee on prevention, detection, evaluation, and treatment of high blood pressure: the JNC 7 report. JAMA. 2003;289(19):2560–71.

91. Kang KY, Kang Y, Kim M, Kim Y, Yi H, Kim J, et al. The effects of antihypertensive drugs on bone mineral density in ovariectomized mice. J Korean Med Sci. 2013;28(8):1139–44.

92. Kolli V, Stechschulte LA, Dowling AR, Rahman S, Czernik PJ, Lecka-Czernik B. Partial agonist, telmisartan, maintains PPARγ serine 112 phosphorylation, and does not affect osteoblast differentiation and bone mass. PLoS One. 2014;9(5):e96323.

93. Zhao X, J-x W, Y-f F, Z-x W, Zhang Y, Shi L, et al. Systemic treatment with telmisartan improves femur fracture healing in mice. PLoS One. 2014;9(3):e92085.

94. Donmez BO, Ozdemir S, Sarikanat M, Yaras N, Koc P, Demir N, et al. Effect of angiotensin II type 1 receptor blocker on osteoporotic rat femurs. Pharmacol Rep. 2012;64(4):878–88.

95. Rajkumar D, Faitelson A, Gudyrev O, Dubrovin G, Pokrovski M, Ivanov A. Comparative evaluation of enalapril and losartan in pharmacological correction of experimental osteoporosis and fractures of its background. J Osteoporos. 2013;2013

96. Kosaka N, Uchii M. Effect of benidipine hydrochloride, a dihydropyridine-type calcium antagonist, on the function of mouse osteoblastic cells. Calcif Tissue Int. 1998;62(6):554–6.

97. Gradosova I, Zivna H, Palicka V, Hubena S, Svejkovska K, Zivny P. Protective effect of amlodipine on rat bone tissue after orchidectomy. Pharmacology. 2012;89(1–2):37–43.

98. Ushijima K, Liu Y, Maekawa T, Ishikawa E, Motosugi Y, Ando H, et al. Protective effect of amlodipine against osteoporosis in stroke-prone spontaneously hypertensive rats. Eur J Pharmacol. 2010;635(1):227–30.

99. Himori N, Taira N. Differential effects of the calcium-antagonistic vasodilators, nifedipine and verapamil, on the tracheal musculature and vasculature of the dog. Br J Pharmacol. 1980;68(4):595–7.

100. Ay SA, Karaman M, Cakar M, Balta S, Arslan E, Bulucu F, et al. Amlodipine increases vitamin D levels more than valsartan in newly diagnosed hypertensive patients: pointing to an additional effect on bone metabolism or a novel marker of inflammation? Ren Fail. 2013;35(5):691–6.

101. Padwal R, Majumdar SR, Johnson JA, Varney J, McAlister FA. A systematic review of drug therapy to delay or prevent type 2 diabetes. Diabetes Care. 2005;28(3):736–44.

102. Vestergaard P, Rejnmark L, Mosekilde L. Relative fracture risk in patients with diabetes mellitus, and the impact of insulin and oral antidiabetic medication on relative fracture risk. Diabetologia. 2005;48(7):1292–9.

103. Gao Y, Li Y, Xue J, Jia Y, Hu J. Effect of the anti-diabetic drug metformin on bone mass in ovariectomized rats. Eur J Pharmacol. 2010;635(1):231–6.

104. Cortizo AM, Sedlinsky C, McCarthy AD, Blanco A, Schurman L. Osteogenic actions of the anti-diabetic drug metformin on osteoblasts in culture. Eur J Pharmacol. 2006;536(1):38–46.

105. Kanazawa I, Yamaguchi T, Yano S, Yamauchi M, Sugimoto T. Metformin enhances the differentiation and mineralization of osteoblastic MC3T3-E1 cells via AMP kinase activation as well as eNOS and BMP-2 expression. Biochem Biophys Res Commun. 2008;375(3):414–9.

106. Nuche-Berenguer B, Moreno P, Esbrit P, Dapía S, Caeiro JR, Cancelas J, et al. Effect of GLP-1 treatment on bone turnover in normal, type 2 diabetic, and insulin-resistant states. Calcif Tissue Int. 2009;84(6):453–61.

107. Sanz C, Vazquez P, Blazquez C, Barrio P, Alvarez MDM, Blazquez E. Signaling and biological effects of glucagon-like peptide 1 on the differentiation of mesenchymal stem cells from human bone marrow. Am J Physiol Endocrinol Metab. 2010;298(3):E634–E43.

108. Yamada C, Yamada Y, Tsukiyama K, Yamada K, Udagawa N, Takahashi N, et al. The murine glucagon-like peptide-1 receptor is essential for control of bone resorption. Endocrinology. 2008;149(2):574–9.

109. Toft-Nielsen M-B, Madsbad S, Holst J. Determinants of the effectiveness of glucagon-like peptide-1 in type 2 diabetes. J Clin Endocrinol Metabol. 2001;86(8): 3853–60.

110. Valverde I, Morales M, Clemente F, López-Delgado MI, Delgado E, Perea A, et al. Glucagon-like peptide 1: a potent glycogenic hormone. FEBS Lett. 1994;349(2):313–6.

111. Crespel A, De Boisvilliers F, Gros L, Kervran A. Effects of glucagon and glucagon-like peptide-

1-(7-36) amide on C cells from rat thyroid and medullary thyroid carcinoma CA-77 cell line. Endocrinology. 1996;137(9):3674–80.

112. Lamari Y, Boissard C, Moukhtar M, Jullienne A, Rosselin G, Garel J-M. Expression of glucagon-like peptide 1 receptor in a murine C cell line regulation of calcitonin gene by glucagon-like peptide 1. FEBS Lett. 1996;393(2–3):248–52.

113. Monami M, Dicembrini I, Antenore A, Mannucci E. Dipeptidyl peptidase-4 inhibitors and bone fractures: a meta-analysis of randomized clinical trials. Diabetes Care. 2011;34(11):2474–6.

114. McIntosh CH, Demuth H-U, Pospisilik JA, Pederson R. Dipeptidyl peptidase IV inhibitors: how do they work as new antidiabetic agents? Regul Pept. 2005;128(2):159–65.

115. Monami M, Dicembrini I, Antenore A, Mannucci E. Dipeptidyl peptidase-4 inhibitors and bone fractures: a meta-analysis of randomized clinical trials. Diabetes Care. 2011; 34: 2474–2476. Diabetes Care. 2014;37(1):312.

116. Nuche-Berenguer B, Moreno P, Portal-Nuñez S, Dapía S, Esbrit P, Villanueva-Peñacarrillo ML. Exendin-4 exerts osteogenic actions in insulin-resistant and type 2 diabetic states. Regul Pept. 2010;159(1):61–6.

117. Baggio LL, Drucker DJ. Biology of incretins: GLP-1 and GIP. Gastroenterology. 2007;132(6):2131–57.

118. Seino Y, Fukushima M, Yabe D. GIP and GLP-1, the two incretin hormones: similarities and differences. J Diabetes Invest. 2010;1(1–2):8–23.

119. Grey A. Thiazolidinedione-induced skeletal fragility–mechanisms and implications. Diabetes Obes Metab. 2009;11(4):275–84.

120. Yaturu S, Bryant B, Jain SK. Thiazolidinedione treatment decreases bone mineral density in type 2 diabetic men. Diabetes Care. 2007;30(6): 1574–6.

121. Kahn SE, Zinman B, Lachin JM, Haffner SM, Herman WH, Holman RR, et al. Rosiglitazone-associated fractures in type 2 diabetes an analysis from a diabetes outcome progression trial (ADOPT). Diabetes Care. 2008;31(5):845–51.

122. Home PD, Pocock SJ, Beck-Nielsen H, Curtis PS, Gomis R, Hanefeld M, et al. Rosiglitazone evaluated for cardiovascular outcomes in oral agent combination therapy for type 2 diabetes (RECORD): a multicentre, randomised, open-label trial. Lancet. 2009;373(9681):2125–35.

123. Lecka-Czernik B. Bone loss in diabetes: use of antidiabetic thiazolidinediones and secondary osteoporosis. Curr Osteoporos Rep. 2010;8(4):178–84.

124. Schwartz AV, Sellmeyer DE, Vittinghoff E, Palermo L, Lecka-Czernik B, Feingold KR, et al. Thiazolidinedione use and bone loss in older diabetic adults. J Clin Endocrinol Metabol. 2006;91(9):3349–54.

125. Lecka-Czernik B. PPARs in bone: the role in bone cell differentiation and regulation of energy metabolism. Curr Osteoporos Rep. 2010;8(2):84–90.

126. Rzonca S, Suva L, Gaddy D, Montague D, Lecka-Czernik B. Bone is a target for the antidiabetic compound rosiglitazone. Endocrinology. 2004;145(1):401–6.

127. Lazarenko OP, Rzonca SO, Hogue WR, Swain FL, Suva LJ, Lecka-Czernik B. Rosiglitazone induces decreases in bone mass and strength that are reminiscent of aged bone. Endocrinology. 2007;148(6):2669–80.

128. Wan Y, Chong L-W, Evans RM. PPAR-γ regulates osteoclastogenesis in mice. Nat Med. 2007;13(12):1496–503.

129. Ali AA, Weinstein RS, Stewart SA, Parfitt AM, Manolagas SC, Jilka RL. Rosiglitazone causes bone loss in mice by suppressing osteoblast differentiation and bone formation. Endocrinology. 2005;146(3):1226–35.

130. Soročéanu MA, Miao D, Bai X-Y, Su H, Goltzman D, Karaplis AC. Rosiglitazone impacts negatively on bone by promoting osteoblast/osteocyte apoptosis. J Endocrinol. 2004;183(1):203–16.

131. Grey A, Bolland M, Gamble G, Wattie D, Horne A, Davidson J, et al. The peroxisome proliferator-activated receptor-γ agonist rosiglitazone decreases bone formation and bone mineral density in healthy postmenopausal women: a randomized, controlled trial. J Clin Endocrinol Metabol. 2007;92(4): 1305–10.

132. Glintborg D, Andersen M, Hagen C, Heickendorff L, Hermann AP. Association of pioglitazone treatment with decreased bone mineral density in obese premenopausal patients with polycystic ovary syndrome: a randomized, placebo-controlled trial. J Clin Endocrinol Metabol. 2008;93(5):1696–701.

133. Berberoglu Z, Gursoy A, Bayraktar N, Yazici AC, Bascil Tutuncu N, Guvener Demirag N. Rosiglitazone decreases serum bone-specific alkaline phosphatase activity in postmenopausal diabetic women. J Clin Endocrinol Metabol. 2007;92(9):3523–30.

134. Keller J, Schinke T. The role of the gastrointestinal tract in calcium homeostasis and bone remodeling. Osteoporos Int. 2013;24(11):2737–48.

135. Wright MJ, Proctor DD, Insogna KL, Kerstetter JE. Proton pump-inhibiting drugs, calcium homeostasis, and bone health. Nutr Rev. 2008;66(2):103–8.

136. Al Subaie A, Emami E, Tamimi I, Laurenti M, Eimar H, Tamimi F. Systemic administration of omeprazole interferes with bone healing & implant osseointegration: an in vivo study on rat tibiae. J Clin Periodontol. 2016;

137. Wu X, Al-Abedalla K, Abi-Nader S, Daniel NG, Nicolau B, Tamimi F. Proton pump inhibitors and the risk of osseointegrated dental implant failure: a cohort study. Clin Implant Dent Relat Res. 2016;

138. Lodato F, Azzaroli F, Turco L, Mazzella N, Buonfiglioli F, Zoli M, et al. Adverse effects of proton pump inhibitors. Best Pract Res Clin Gastroenterol. 2010;24(2):193–201.

139. McCarthy DM. Adverse effects of proton pump inhibitor drugs: clues and conclusions. Curr Opin Gastroenterol. 2010;26(6):624–31.

140. Jacobson BC, Ferris TG, Shea TL, Mahlis EM, Lee TH, Wang TC. Who is using chronic acid suppression therapy and why&quest. Am J Gastroenterol. 2003;98(1):51–8.

141. Ye X, Liu H, Wu C, Qin Y, Zang J, Gao Q, et al. Proton pump inhibitors therapy and risk of hip fracture: a systematic review and meta-analysis. Eur J Gastroenterol Hepatol. 2011;23(9):794–800.

142. Stedman C, Barclay M. Review article: comparison of the pharmacokinetics, acid suppression and efficacy of proton pump inhibitors. Aliment Pharmacol Ther. 2000;14(8):963–78.

143. Yang Y-X. Chronic proton pump inhibitor therapy and calcium metabolism. Curr Gastroenterol Rep. 2012;14(6):473–9.

144. Ngamruengphong S, Leontiadis GI, Radhi S, Dentino A, Nugent K. Proton pump inhibitors and risk of fracture: a systematic review and meta-analysis of observational studies. Am J Gastroenterol. 2011;106(7):1209–18.

145. Costa-Rodrigues J, Reis S, Teixeira S, Lopes S, Fernandes MH. Dose-dependent inhibitory effects of proton pump inhibitors on human osteoclastic and osteoblastic cell activity. FEBS J. 2013;280(20):5052–64.

146. Narisawa S, Harmey D, Yadav MC, O'Neill WC, Hoylaerts MF, Millán JL. Novel inhibitors of alkaline phosphatase suppress vascular smooth muscle cell calcification. J Bone Miner Res. 2007;22(11):1700–10.

147. Delomenède M, Buchet R, Mebarek S. Lansoprazole is an uncompetitive inhibitor of tissue-nonspecific alkaline phosphatase. Acta Biochim Pol. 2009;56(2):301.

148. Roberts S, Narisawa S, Harmey D, Millán JL, Farquharson C. Functional involvement of PHOSPHO1 in matrix vesicle–mediated skeletal mineralization. J Bone Miner Res. 2007;22(4):617–27.

149. O'Connell MB, Madden DM, Murray AM, Heaney RP, Kerzner LJ. Effects of proton pump inhibitors on calcium carbonate absorption in women: a randomized crossover trial. Am J Med. 2005;118(7):778–81.

150. Abrahamsen B, Vestergaard P. Proton pump inhibitor use and fracture risk—effect modification by histamine H1 receptor blockade. Observational case–control study using National Prescription Data. Bone. 2013;57(1):269–71.

151. Charles JF, Nakamura MC. Bone and the innate immune system. Curr Osteoporos Rep. 2014;12(1):1–8.

152. Schett G, David J-P. The multiple faces of autoimmune-mediated bone loss. Nat Rev Endocrinol. 2010;6(12):698–706.

153. Usuda N, Arai H, Sasaki H, Hanai T, Nagata T, Muramatsu T, et al. Differential subcellular localization of neural isoforms of the catalytic subunit of calmodulin-dependent protein phosphatase (calcineurin) in central nervous system neurons: immunohistochemistry on Formalin-fixed paraffin sections employing antigen retrieval by microwave irradiation. J Histochem Cytochem. 1996;44(1):13–8.

154. Norris CM, Kadish I, Blalock EM, Chen K-C, Thibault V, Porter NM, et al. Calcineurin triggers reactive/inflammatory processes in astrocytes and is upregulated in aging and Alzheimer's models. J Neurosci. 2005;25(18):4649–58.

155. Aramburu J, Rao A, Klee CB. Calcineurin: from structure to function. Curr Top Cell Regul. 2001;36:237–95.

156. Sun L, Blair HC, Peng Y, Zaidi N, Adebanjo OA, Wu XB, et al. Calcineurin regulates bone formation by the osteoblast. Proc Natl Acad Sci U S A. 2005;102(47):17130–5.

157. Klee C, Draetta G, Hubbard M, Meister A. Advances in enzymology and related areas of molecular biology. Adv Enzymol Relat Areas Mol Biol. 1988;61:149–200.

158. Naesens M, Kuypers DR, Sarwal M. Calcineurin inhibitor nephrotoxicity. Clin J Am Soc Nephrol. 2009;4(2):481–508.

159. Katz IA, Epstein S. Perspectives: posttransplantation bone disease. J Bone Miner Res. 1992;7(2):123–6.

160. Rodino MA, Shane E. Osteoporosis after organ transplantation. Am J Med. 1998;104(5):459–69.

161. Sprague SM. Mechanism of transplantation-associated bone loss. Pediatr Nephrol. 2000;14(7):650–3.

162. Sprague SM, Josephson MA. Bone disease after kidney transplantation. In: Seminars in nephrology: Elsevier; 2004.

163. Winslow MM, Pan M, Starbuck M, Gallo EM, Deng L, Karsenty G, et al. Calcineurin/NFAT signaling in osteoblasts regulates bone mass. Dev Cell. 2006;10(6):771–82.

164. Laupacis A, Keown P, Ulan R, McKenzie N, Stiller C. Cyclosporin A: a powerful immunosuppressant. Can Med Assoc J. 1982;126(9):1041.

165. Cantrell DA, Smith KA. The interleukin-2 T-cell system: a new cell growth model. Science. 1984;224(4655):1312–6.

166. El Hadary AA, Yassin HH, Mekhemer ST, Holmes JC, Grootveld M. Evaluation of the effect of ozonated plant oils on the quality of osseointegration of dental implants under the influence of cyclosporin a: an in vivo study. J Oral Implantol. 2011;37(2):247–57.

167. Schlosberg M, Movsowitz C, Epstein S, Ismail F, Fallon M, Thomas S. The effect of cyclosporin A administration and its withdrawal on bone mineral metabolism in the rat. Endocrinology. 1989;124(5):2179–84.

168. Av C, Wysolmerski J, Simpson C, Mitnick MA, Gundberg C, Kliger A, et al. Posttransplant bone disease: evidence for a high bone resorption state. Transplantation. 2000;70(12):1722–8.

169. Sakakura CE, Lopes B, Margonar R, Queiroz TP, Nociti F, Marcantonio E. Cyclosporine-A and bone density around titanium implants: a histometric study in rabbits. J Osseointegr. 2011;3:25–9.

170. Sakakura CE, Margonar R, Holzhausen M, Nociti FH Jr, Alba RC Jr, Marcantonio E Jr. Influence of cyclosporin A therapy on bone healing around tita-

nium implants: a histometric and biomechanic study in rabbits. J Periodontol. 2003;74(7):976–81.

171. Duarte PM, Nogueira Filho GR, Sallum EA, Toledo S, Sallum AW, Nociti FH Jr. The effect of an immunosuppressive therapy and its withdrawal on bone healing around titanium implants. A histometric study in rabbits. J Periodontol. 2001;72(10): 1391–7.

172. Sakakura CE, Marcantonio E, Wenzel A, Scaf G. Influence of cyclosporin A on quality of bone around integrated dental implants: a radiographic study in rabbits. Clin Oral Implants Res. 2007;18(1):34–9.

173. Al Subaie AE, Eimar H, Abdallah MN, Durand R, Feine J, Tamimi F, et al. Anti-VEGFs hinder bone healing and implant osseointegration in rat tibiae. J Clin Periodontol. 2015;42(7):688–96.

174. Zhang L, Zhang L, Lan X, Xu M, Mao Z, Lv H, et al. Improvement in angiogenesis and osteogenesis with modified cannulated screws combined with VEGF/PLGA/fibrin glue in femoral neck fractures. J Mater Sci Mater Med. 2014;25(4):1165–72.

175. Senger DR, Galli SJ, Dvorak AM, Perruzzi CA, Harvey VS, Dvorak HF. Tumor cells secrete a vascular permeability factor that promotes accumulation of ascites fluid. Science. 1983;219(4587):983–5.

176. Cui Q, Dighe AS, Irvine J, James N. Combined angiogenic and osteogenic factor delivery for bone regenerative engineering. Curr Pharm Des. 2013;19(19):3374–83.

177. Semeraro F, Morescalchi F, Parmeggiani F, Arcidiacono B, Costagliola C. Systemic adverse drug reactions secondary to anti-VEGF intravitreal injection in patients with neovascular age-related macular degeneration. Curr Vasc Pharmacol. 2011;9(5):629–46.

178. Bauman G, Charette M, Reid R, Sathya J, TRGG of Cancer. Radiopharmaceuticals for the palliation of painful bone metastases—a systematic review. Radiother Oncol. 2005;75(3):258. E1-. E13

179. Bruland ØS, Nilsson S, Fisher DR, Larsen RH. High-linear energy transfer irradiation targeted to skeletal metastases by the α-emitter 223Ra: adjuvant or alternative to conventional modalities? Clin Cancer Res 2006;12(20):6250s–7s.

180. Henriksen G, Breistøl K, Bruland ØS, Fodstad Ø, Larsen RH. Significant antitumor effect from bone-seeking, α-particle-emitting 223Ra demonstrated in an experimental skeletal metastases model. Cancer Res. 2002;62(11):3120–5.

181. Sartor O, Coleman R, Nilsson S, Heinrich D, Helle SI, O'Sullivan JM, et al. Effect of radium-223 dichloride on symptomatic skeletal events in patients with castration-resistant prostate cancer and bone metastases: results from a phase 3, double-blind, randomised trial. Lancet Oncol. 2014;15(7):738–46.

182. Lønning PE, Geisler J, Krag LE, Erikstein B, Bremnes Y, Hagen AI, et al. Effects of exemestane administered for 2 years versus placebo on bone mineral density, bone biomarkers, and plasma lipids in patients with surgically resected early breast cancer. J Clin Oncol. 2005;23(22):5126–37.

183. Coleman RE, Banks LM, Girgis SI, Kilburn LS, Vrdoljak E, Fox J, et al. Skeletal effects of exemestane on bone-mineral density, bone biomarkers, and fracture incidence in postmenopausal women with early breast cancer participating in the Intergroup Exemestane Study (IES): a randomised controlled study. Lancet Oncol. 2007;8(2):119–27.

184. McCloskey E. Effects of third-generation aromatase inhibitors on bone. Eur J Cancer. 2006;42(8):1044–51.

185. Coombes R, Kilburn L, Snowdon C, Paridaens R, Coleman R, Jones S, et al. Survival and safety of exemestane versus tamoxifen after 2–3 years' tamoxifen treatment (Intergroup Exemestane Study): a randomised controlled trial. Lancet. 2007;369(9561):559–70.

186. Heaney RP, Recker RR, Saville PD. Menopausal changes in bone remodeling. J Lab Clin Med. 1978;92(6):964–70.

187. López BC, Esteve CG, Pérez MGS. Dental treatment considerations in the chemotherapy patient. J Clin Exp Dent. 2011;3(1):31–42.

188. Kovács AF. Influence of chemotherapy on endosteal implant survival and success in oral cancer patients. Int J Oral Maxillofac Surg. 2001;30(2):144–7.

189. Alia B, Bashir A, Tanira M. Anti-inflammatory, antipyretic, and analgesic effects of Lawsonia inermis L.(henna) in rats. Pharmacology. 1995;51(6):356–63.

190. Chuang P-Y, Shen S-H, Yang T-Y, Huang T-W, Huang K-C. Non-steroidal anti-inflammatory drugs and the risk of a second hip fracture: a propensity-score matching study. BMC Musculoskelet Disord. 2016;17(1):1.

191. Konstantinidis I, N Papageorgiou S, Kyrgidis A, Tzellos G, Kouvelas D. Effect of non-steroidal anti-inflammatory drugs on bone turnover: an evidence-based review. Rev Recent Clin Trials. 2013;8(1):48–60.

192. Griffin MR. Epidemiology of nonsteroidal anti-inflammatory drug–associated gastrointestinal injury. Am J Med. 1998;104(3):23S–9S.

193. Harder AT, An YH. The mechanisms of the inhibitory effects of nonsteroidal anti-inflammatory drugs on bone healing: a concise review. J Clin Pharmacol. 2003;43(8):807–15.

194. Wheeler P, Batt M. Do non-steroidal anti-inflammatory drugs adversely affect stress fracture healing? A short review. Br J Sports Med. 2005;39(2):65–9.

195. Su B, O'Connor JP. NSAID therapy effects on healing of bone, tendon, and the enthesis. J Appl Physiol. 2013;115(6):892–9.

196. Wittenberg JM, Wittenberg RH. Release of prostaglandins from bone and muscle after femoral osteotomy in rats. Acta Orthop Scand. 1991;62(6): 577–81.

197. Kawaguchi H, Pilbeam CC, Harrison JR, Raisz LG. The role of prostaglandins in the regulation of bone metabolism. Clin Orthop Relat Res. 1995; 313:36–46.

198. Raisz L, Martin T. Prostaglandins in bone and mineral metabolism. Bone Miner Res. 1984;2: 286–310.

199. Sostres C, Gargallo CJ, Arroyo MT, Lanas A. Adverse effects of non-steroidal anti-inflammatory drugs (NSAIDs, aspirin and coxibs) on upper gastrointestinal tract. Best Pract Res Clin Gastroenterol. 2010;24(2):121–32.

200. Ribeiro FV, Nociti FH Jr, Sallum EA, Casati MZ. Effect of aluminum oxide-blasted implant surface on the bone healing around implants in rats submitted to continuous administration of selective cyclooxygenase-2 inhibitors. Int J Oral Maxillofac Implants. 2009;24(2)

201. Pablos AB, Ramalho SA, König B Jr, Furuse C, de Araújo VC, Cury PR. Effect of meloxicam and diclofenac sodium on peri-implant bone healing in rats. J Periodontol. 2008;79(2):300–6.

202. Ouanounou A, Hassanpour S, Glogauer M. The influence of systemic medications on osseointegration of dental implants. J Can Dent Assoc. 2016;82(g7): 1488–2159.

203. Henneicke H, Gasparini SJ, Brennan-Speranza TC, Zhou H, Seibel MJ. Glucocorticoids and bone: local effects and systemic implications. Trends Endocrinol Metab. 2014;25(4):197–211.

204. O'Brien CA, Jia D, Plotkin LI, Bellido T, Powers CC, Stewart SA, et al. Glucocorticoids act directly on osteoblasts and osteocytes to induce their apoptosis and reduce bone formation and strength. Endocrinology. 2004;145(4):1835–41.

205. Amiche M, Albaum J, Tadrous M, Pechlivanoglou P, Lévesque L, Adachi J, et al. Fracture risk in oral glucocorticoid users: a Bayesian meta-regression leveraging control arms of osteoporosis clinical trials. Osteoporos Int. 2016;27(5):1709–18.

206. Weinstein RS, Chen J-R, Powers CC, Stewart SA, Landes RD, Bellido T, et al. Promotion of osteoclast survival and antagonism of bisphosphonate-induced osteoclast apoptosis by glucocorticoids. J Clin Invest. 2002;109(8):1041–8.

207. Mazziotti G, Canalis E, Giustina A. Drug-induced osteoporosis: mechanisms and clinical implications. Am J Med. 2010;123(10):877–84.

208. Weinstein RS, Jia D, Powers CC, Stewart SA, Jilka RL, Parfitt AM, et al. The skeletal effects of glucocorticoid excess override those of orchidectomy in mice. Endocrinology. 2004;145(4):1980–7.

209. Smith RA, Berger R, Dodson TB. Risk factors associated with dental implants in healthy and medically compromised patients. Int J Oral Maxillofac Implants. 1992;7(3)

210. Cranin A. Endosteal implants in a patient with corticosteroid dependence. J Oral Implantol. 1991; 17(4):414.

211. Bencharit S, Reside GJ, Howard-Williams EL. Complex prosthodontic treatment with dental implants for a patient with polymyalgia rheumatica: a clinical report. Int J Oral Maxillofac Implants. 2010;25(6)

212. Werner S, Tessler J, Guglielmotti M, Cabrini R. Effect of dexamethasone on osseointegration: a preliminary experimental study. J Oral Implantol. 1995;22(3–4):216–9.

213. LeBlanc ES, Janowsky J, Chan BK, Nelson HD. Hormone replacement therapy and cognition: systematic review and meta-analysis. JAMA. 2001;285(11):1489–99.

214. Ardawi M-S, Sibiany A, Bakhsh T, Qari M, Maimani A. High prevalence of vitamin D deficiency among healthy Saudi Arabian men: relationship to bone mineral density, parathyroid hormone, bone turnover markers, and lifestyle factors. Osteoporos Int. 2012;23(2):675–86.

215. Nachiappan AC, Metwalli ZA, Hailey BS, Patel RA, Ostrowski ML, Wynne DM. The thyroid: review of imaging features and biopsy techniques with radiologic-pathologic correlation. Radiographics. 2014;34(2):276–93.

216. Bassett JD, Williams GR. The molecular actions of thyroid hormone in bone. Trends Endocrinol Metab. 2003;14(8):356–64.

217. Weiss RE, Refetoff S. Effect of thyroid hormone on growth: lessons from the syndrome of resistance to thyroid hormone. Endocrinol Metab Clin N Am. 1996;25(3):719–30.

218. Stevens DA, Hasserjian RP, Robson H, Siebler T, Shalet SM, Williams GR. Thyroid hormones regulate hypertrophic chondrocyte differentiation and expression of parathyroid hormone-related peptide and its receptor during endochondral bone formation. J Bone Miner Res. 2000;15(12):2431–42.

219. Milne M, Quail JM, Rosen CJ, Baran DT. Insulin-like growth factor binding proteins in femoral and vertebral bone marrow stromal cells: expression and regulation by thyroid hormone and dexamethasone. J Cell Biochem. 2001;81(2):229–40.

220. Tsukiyama K, Yamada Y, Yamada C, Harada N, Kawasaki Y, Ogura M, et al. Gastric inhibitory polypeptide as an endogenous factor promoting new bone formation after food ingestion. Mol Endocrinol. 2006;20(7):1644–51.

221. Finkelstein JS, Hayes A, Hunzelman JL, Wyland JJ, Lee H, Neer RM. The effects of parathyroid hormone, alendronate, or both in men with osteoporosis. N Engl J Med. 2003;349(13):1216–26.

222. Henriksen DB, Alexandersen P, Bjarnason NH, Vilsbøll T, Hartmann B, Henriksen EE, et al. Role of gastrointestinal hormones in postprandial reduction of bone resorption. J Bone Miner Res. 2003;18(12): 2180–9.

223. Gault VA, Irwin N, Green BD, McCluskey JT, Greer B, Bailey CJ, et al. Chemical ablation of gastric inhibitory polypeptide receptor action by daily (Pro3) GIP administration improves glucose tolerance and ameliorates insulin resistance and abnormalities of islet structure in obesity-related diabetes. Diabetes. 2005;54(8):2436–46.

224. Bollag RJ, Zhong Q, Ding K, Phillips P, Zhong L, Qin F, et al. Glucose-dependent insulinotropic peptide is

an integrative hormone with osteotropic effects. Mol Cell Endocrinol. 2001;177(1):35–41.

225. Syed F, Khosla S. Mechanisms of sex steroid effects on bone. Biochem Biophys Res Commun. 2005;328(3):688–96.

226. Adinoff AD, Hollister JR. Steroid-induced fractures and bone loss in patients with asthma. N Engl J Med. 1983;309(5):265–8.

227. Liu J, Zhao H, Ning G, Zhao Y, Chen Y, Zhang Z, et al. Relationships between the changes of serum levels of OPG and RANKL with age, menopause, bone biochemical markers and bone mineral density in Chinese women aged 20-75. Calcif Tissue Int. 2005;76(1):1–6.

228. Cauley JA, Seeley DG, Ensrud K, Ettinger B, Black D, Cummings SR. Estrogen replacement therapy and fractures in older women. Ann Intern Med. 1995;122(1):9–16.

229. Lane NE, Haupt D, Kimmel DB, Modin G, Kinney JH. Early estrogen replacement therapy reverses the rapid loss of trabecular bone volume and prevents further deterioration of connectivity in the rat. J Bone Miner Res. 1999;14(2):206–14.

230. Ettinger B, Genant HK, Cann CE. Long-term estrogen replacement therapy prevents bone loss and fractures. Ann Intern Med. 1985;102(3):319–24.

231. Lindsay R. Sex steroids in the pathogenesis and prevention of osteoporosis. In: Osteoporosis: etiology, diagnosis and management. New York: Raven Press; 1988. p. 333–58.

232. Ronderos M, Jacobs DR, Himes JH, Pihlstrom BL. Associations of periodontal disease with femoral bone mineral density and estrogen replacement therapy: cross-sectional evaluation of US adults from NHANES III. J Clin Periodontol. 2000;27(10):778–86.

233. Riggs BL, Parfitt AM. Drugs used to treat osteoporosis: the critical need for a uniform nomenclature based on their action on bone remodeling. J Bone Miner Res. 2005;20(2):177–84.

234. Consensus A. Consensus development conference: diagnosis, prophylaxis, and treatment of osteoporosis. Am J Med. 1993;94(6):646–50.

235. Ellegaard M, Jørgensen N, Schwarz P. Parathyroid hormone and bone healing. Calcif Tissue Int. 2010;87(1):1–13.

236. Silva BC, Bilezikian JP. Parathyroid hormone: anabolic and catabolic actions on the skeleton. Curr Opin Pharmacol. 2015;22:41–50.

237. Iwaniec U, Moore K, Rivera M, Myers S, Vanegas S, Wronski T. A comparative study of the bone-restorative efficacy of anabolic agents in aged ovariectomized rats. Osteoporos Int. 2007;18(3):351–62.

238. Kanzawa M, Sugimoto T, Kanatani M, Chihara K. Involvement of osteoprotegerin/osteoclastogenesis inhibitory factor in the stimulation of osteoclast formation by parathyroid hormone in mouse bone cells. Eur J Endocrinol. 2000;142(6):661–4.

239. Neer RM, Arnaud CD, Zanchetta JR, Prince R, Gaich GA, Reginster J-Y, et al. Effect of parathyroid hormone (1-34) on fractures and bone mineral density in postmenopausal women with osteoporosis. N Engl J Med. 2001;344(19):1434–41.

240. Shirota T, Tashiro M, Ohno K, Yamaguchi A. Effect of intermittent parathyroid hormone (1-34) treatment on the bone response after placement of titanium implants into the tibia of ovariectomized rats. J Oral Maxillofac Surg. 2003;61(4):471–80.

241. Eddy D, Cummings S, Dawson-Hughes B, Johnston C, Lindsay R, Melton L. Guidelines for the prevention, diagnosis and treatment of osteoporosis: cost-effectiveness analysis and review of the evidence. Osteoporos Int. 1998;8(Suppl. 4):1–88.

242. Nieves JW, Komar L, Cosman F, Lindsay R. Calcium potentiates the effect of estrogen and calcitonin on bone mass: review and analysis. Am J Clin Nutr. 1998;67(1):18–24.

243. Knopp JA, Diner BM, Blitz M, Lyritis GP, Rowe BH. Calcitonin for treating acute pain of osteoporotic vertebral compression fractures: a systematic review of randomized, controlled trials. Osteoporos Int. 2005;16(10):1281–90.

244. Fleisch H. Bisphosphonates in bone disease: from the laboratory to the patient: Academic; 2000.

245. Russell RG, Mühlbauer R, Bisaz S, Williams D, Fleisch H. The influence of pyrophosphate, condensed phosphates, phosphonates and other phosphate compounds on the dissolution of hydroxyapatitein vitro and on bone resorption induced by parathyroid hormone in tissue culture and in thyroparathyroidectomised rats. Calcif Tissue Res. 1970;6(1):183–96.

246. Rogers MJ. New insights into the molecular mechanisms of action of bisphosphonates. Curr Pharm Des. 2003;9(32):2643–58.

247. Landesberg R, Cozin M, Cremers S, Woo V, Kousteni S, Sinha S, et al. Inhibition of oral mucosal cell wound healing by bisphosphonates. J Oral Maxillofac Surg. 2008;66(5):839–47.

248. Vescovi P, Nammour S. Bisphosphonate-Related Osteonecrosis of the Jaw (BRONJ) therapy. A critical review. Minerva Stomatol. 2010;59(4):181–203, 4–13

249. Yoneda T, Hagino H, Sugimoto T, Ohta H, Takahashi S, Soen S, et al. Bisphosphonate-related osteonecrosis of the jaw: position paper from the allied task force committee of Japanese Society for Bone and Mineral Research, Japan Osteoporosis Society, Japanese Society of Periodontology, Japanese Society for Oral and Maxillofacial Radiology, and Japanese Society of Oral and Maxillofacial Surgeons. J Bone Miner Metab. 2010;28(4):365–83.

250. Lazarovici TS, Yahalom R, Taicher S, Schwartz-Arad D, Peleg O, Yarom N. Bisphosphonate-related osteonecrosis of the jaw associated with dental implants. J Oral Maxillofac Surg. 2010;68(4):790–6.

251. Van Bezooijen RL, Roelen BA, Visser A, Van Der Wee-pals L, De Wilt E, Karperien M, et al. Sclerostin is an osteocyte-expressed negative regulator of bone formation, but not a classical BMP antagonist. J Exp Med. 2004;199(6):805–14.

252. Li X, Zhang Y, Kang H, Liu W, Liu P, Zhang J, et al. Sclerostin binds to LRP5/6 and antagonizes canonical Wnt signaling. J Biol Chem. 2005;280(20):19883–7.

253. van Bezooijen RL, ten Dijke P, Papapoulos SE, Löwik CW. SOST/sclerostin, an osteocyte-derived negative regulator of bone formation. Cytokine Growth Factor Rev. 2005;16(3):319–27.

254. Durrington P. Dyslipidaemia. Lancet. 2003;362(9385):717–31.

255. Pedersen T. Randomised trial of cholesterol lowering in 4444 patients with coronary heart disease: the Scandinavian Simvastatin Survival Study (4S). Atheroscler Suppl. 2004;5(3):81–7.

256. Bagger Y, Rasmussen HB, Alexandersen P, Werge T, Christiansen C, Tanko L, et al. Links between cardiovascular disease and osteoporosis in postmenopausal women: serum lipids or atherosclerosis per se? Osteoporos Int. 2007;18(4):505–12.

257. Luisetto G, Camozzi V. Statins, fracture risk, and bone remodeling. J Endocrinol Investig. 2008;32(4 Suppl):32–7.

258. Tsartsalis AN, Dokos C, Kaiafa GD, Tsartsalis DN, Kattamis A, Hatzitolios AI, et al. Statins, bone formation and osteoporosis: hope or hype. Hormones (Athens). 2012;11(2):126–39.

259. van Staa T-P, Wegman S, de Vries F, Leufkens B, Cooper C. Use of statins and risk of fractures. JAMA. 2001;285(14):1850–5.

260. Mundy G, Garrett R, Harris S, Chan J, Chen D, Rossini G, et al. Stimulation of bone formation in vitro and in rodents by statins. Science. 1999;286(5446):1946–9.

261. Ayukawa Y, Okamura A, Koyano K. Simvastatin promotes osteogenesis around titanium implants. Clin Oral Implants Res. 2004;15(3):346–50.

262. Du Z, Chen J, Yan F, Xiao Y. Effects of Simvastatin on bone healing around titanium implants in osteoporotic rats. Clin Oral Implants Res. 2009;20(2):145–50.

263. Canonica GW, Blaiss M. Antihistaminic, antiinflammatory, and antiallergic properties of the nonsedating second-generation antihistamine desloratadine: a review of the evidence. World Allergy Organ J. 2011;4(2):47–53.

264. Gebhard JS, Johnston-Jones K, Kody MH, Kabo JM, Meals RA. Effects of antihistamines on joint stiffness and bone healing after periarticular fracture. J Hand Surg. 1993;18(6):1080–5.

265. Fitzpatrick L, Buzas E, Gagne T, Nagy A, Horvath C, Ferencz V, et al. Targeted deletion of histidine decarboxylase gene in mice increases bone formation and protects against ovariectomy-induced bone loss. Proc Natl Acad Sci. 2003;100(10):6027–32.

266. Kinjo M, Setoguchi S, Solomon DH. Antihistamine therapy and bone mineral density: analysis in a population-based US sample. Am J Med. 2008;121(12):1085–91.

267. Lesclous P, Guez D, Baroukh B, Vignery A, Saffar J. Histamine participates in the early phase of trabecular bone loss in ovariectomized rats. Bone. 2004;34(1):91–9.

268. Deyama Y, Kikuiri T, Ohnishi G-i, Feng Y-G, Takeyama S, Hatta M, et al. Histamine stimulates production of osteoclast differentiation factor/receptor activator of nuclear factor-κB ligand by osteoblasts. Biochem Biophys Res Commun. 2002;298(2):240–6.

269. Arnsten JH, Freeman R, Howard AA, Floris-Moore M, Lo Y, Klein RS. Decreased bone mineral density and increased fracture risk in aging men with or at risk for HIV infection. AIDS (London, England). 2007;21(5):617.

270. Carpenter CC, Cooper DA, Fischl MA, Gatell JM, Gazzard BG, Hammer SM, et al. Antiretroviral therapy in adults: updated recommendations of the International AIDS Society–USA Panel. JAMA. 2000;283(3):381–90.

271. Tebas P, Powderly WG, Claxton S, Marin D, Tantisiriwat W, Teitelbaum SL, et al. Accelerated bone mineral loss in HIV-infected patients receiving potent antiretroviral therapy. AIDS (London, England). 2000;14(4):F63.

272. Brown TT, McComsey GA, King MS, Qaqish RB, Bernstein BM, da Silva BA. Loss of bone mineral density after antiretroviral therapy initiation, independent of antiretroviral regimen. J Acquir Immune Defic Syndr. 2009;51(5):554–61.

273. Ofotokun I, Weitzmann MN. HIV-1 infection and antiretroviral therapies: risk factors for osteoporosis and bone fracture. Curr Opin Endocrinol Diabetes Obes. 2010;17(6):523.

274. Beard EL Jr. The American Society of Health System Pharmacists. JONAS Healthc Law Ethics Regul. 2001;3(3):78–9.

275. Simann M, Schneider V, Le Blanc S, Dotterweich J, Zehe V, Krug M, et al. Heparin affects human bone marrow stromal cell fate: promoting osteogenic and reducing adipogenic differentiation and conversion. Bone. 2015;78:102–13.

276. Irie A, Takami M, Kubo H, Sekino-Suzuki N, Kasahara K, Sanai Y. Heparin enhances osteoclastic bone resorption by inhibiting osteoprotegerin activity. Bone. 2007;41(2):165–74.

277. Barbour LA, Kick SD, Steiner JF, LoVerde ME, Heddleston LN, Lear JL, et al. A prospective study of heparin-induced osteoporosis in pregnancy using bone densitometry. Am J Obstet Gynecol. 1994;170(3):862–9.

278. Dahlman TC, Sjöberg HE, Ringertz H. Bone mineral density during long-term prophylaxis with heparin in pregnancy. Am J Obstet Gynecol. 1994;170(5):1315–20.

279. Douketis J, Ginsberg J, Burrows R, Duku E, Webber C, Brill-Edwards P. The effects of long-term heparin therapy during pregnancy on bone density. A prospective matched cohort study. Thromb Haemost. 1996;75(2):254–7.

280. Siegal D, Yudin J, Kaatz S, Douketis JD, Lim W, Spyropoulos AC. Periprocedural heparin bridging in patients receiving vitamin K antagonists: systematic review and meta-analysis of bleeding and thromboembolic rates. Circulation. 2012;126(13):1630–9.

281. Mukherjee S. Alcoholism and its effects on the central nervous system. Curr Neurovasc Res. 2013;10(3):256–62.
282. Klein RF, Fausti KA, Carlos AS. Ethanol inhibits human osteoblastic cell proliferation. Alcohol Clin Exp Res. 1996;20(3):572–8.
283. Dai J, Lin D, Zhang J, Habib P, Smith P, Murtha J, et al. Chronic alcohol ingestion induces osteoclastogenesis and bone loss through IL-6 in mice. J Clin Invest. 2000;106(7):887–95.
284. Koo S, Bruno König J, Mizusaki CI, Sérgio Allegrini J, Yoshimoto M, Carbonari MJ. Effects of alcohol consumption on osseointegration of titanium implants in rabbits. Implant Dent. 2004;13(3): 232–7.
285. Alissa R, Oliver RJ. Influence of prognostic risk indicators on osseointegrated dental implant failure: a matched case-control analysis. J Oral Implantol. 2012;38(1):51–61.
286. Friedlander AH, Marder SR, Pisegna JR, Yagiela JA. Alcohol abuse and dependence: psychopathology, medical management and dental implications. J Am Dent Assoc. 2003;134(6):731–40.

Preoperative Radiological Assessment

5

Matthieu Schmittbuhl

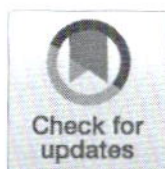

Abstract

An accurate radiographic presurgical assessment is required for planning implant placement in edentulous mandible. The radiographic evaluation helps the clinician to determine the quantity and quality of bone available in the alveolar ridge to support implants. Accurate information concerning the location of anatomical structures is of fundamental importance for preoperative planning. Damage to these structures or implant placement beyond the anatomical boundaries can cause considerable complications. This chapter provides thus information regarding the various imaging modalities available, their specific application and the potential information that each can provide concerning the anatomical appearance, location, dimensions and variations of critical structures that are routinely encountered during implant placement.

Careful gathering of clinical and radiological information results in high success rate for dental implant placement in edentulous mandible [1]. Important aspects in the planning of dental implants are consideration of the bone morphology and the relationship between the implant and the anatomical structures such as neurovascular bundles. An accurate radiographic presurgical assessment of bone quantity and quality is thus required to obtain this information and provides the opportunity to prevent complications during implant placement [2, 3]. The radiographs help the clinician to visualize the alveolar ridge and adjacent structures in all three dimensions and guide the choice of site, number, size and orientations of the implants [4, 5]. Imaging modalities also contribute information for intraoperative and postoperative assessment of the implants. The aim of this chapter is not only to provide information regarding the various imaging modalities available but also their specific application and the potential information that each can provide concerning the anatomical appearance, location, dimensions and variations of critical structures that are routinely encountered during implant placement.

Usually a combination of radiographic techniques is applied to dental implant case management, including panoramic radiography, intraoral radiography and cone beam CT. Each examination has specific indications, advantages and disadvantages, and the decision about ordering specific imaging is based on clinician judgment.

M. Schmittbuhl
Faculty of Dentistry, Université de Montréal, Montreal, QC, Canada
e-mail: matthieu.schmittbuhl@umontreal.ca

© Springer International Publishing AG, part of Springer Nature 2018
E. Emami, J. Feine (eds.), *Mandibular Implant Prostheses*,
https://doi.org/10.1007/978-3-319-71181-2_5

5.1 Panoramic Imaging

Panoramic radiography is considered as the imaging modality of choice for initial implant site assessment [3]. Although the resolution and sharpness of panoramic radiographs are less than those of intraoral radiographs, panoramic radiographic technique provides a single comprehensive image of jaws and related anatomical structures [6]. Its broad coverage of the maxillomandibular structures, low dose of radiation (Table 5.1) and simple and easy-to-use extraoral technique are some advantages of this imaging modality. It is particularly useful in making preliminary estimations of alveolar ridge and boundaries of the mandibular canal. However, measurements with panoramic radiograph are unreliable because of geometrical distortion such as unequal magnification [10]. Image size distortion varies significantly between images from different panoramic units and at different locations within the same radiograph. Patient's head positioning errors and discrepancies between the curvature of the dental arch and focal trough of the machine can also exacerbate distortions [6]. Compared with contact radiographs of dissected anatomic specimens, only 17% of panoramic measurements between the alveolar crest and superior wall of the mandibular canal were found to be accurate within 1 mm [11]. As other imaging techniques which are two-dimensional, panoramic radiographs are further limited by the lack of information on the buccolingual dimensions.

5.2 Intraoral Radiography

Periapical radiography can be used to supplement the preliminary information from panoramic radiography [3]. The paralleling technique provides an image with minimal distortion and can thus be used for determining vertical and mesiodistal dimensions of the edentulous mandibular area being examined [11]. Periapical radiographs provide also images of excellent resolution with fine bony details allowing determination of bone architecture and bone quality (bone density, amount of cortical and trabecular bone among other factors). But extra cautions should be applied while interpreting the images. Firstly, the technique is highly operator dependent and requires a moderate level of patient compliance to provide images with minimal geometrical distortions [3]. Even if paralleling technique is used, it is often difficult to achieve an optimal projection when dealing with a resorbed edentulous alveolar ridge. The position of the image receptor may thus not result in an accurate display of the height of the alveolar ridge, and the image receptor holder may dig into the lingual sulcus causing patient discomfort [12]. The technique presents also anatomic limitations. Although only a limited area of the dentoalveolar region is visualized, intraoral radiograph is subject to anatomic superimposition and misinterpretation. The lack of information in the third dimension may lead the clinician to use preoperative sectional imaging for planning of implant length/diameter [13]. However, periapical radiograph can be used to

Table 5.1 Effective dose from conventional dental radiography, cone beam CT and CT scan and equivalent background exposure

	Effective dose (µSv)	Equivalent background exposure (days)	References
Intraoral radiography	15[a]	1.5	Granlund et al. [7]
Panoramic radiography	4–30	0.5–3	Okano and Sur [8]
Cone beam CT	11–674 (small FOV)[b] 30–1073 (large FOV)	1–67 3–107	European Commission (EC) [9]
CT scan for dental implant	250–860	25–86	Okano and Sur [8]

[a]Full-mouth intraoral examination
[b]Height of field of view (FOV): small FOV <10 cm; large FOV >10 cm

confirm whether implant placement has been satisfactory in terms of angulation and depth. Periapical radiograph is also indicated in the postoperative follow-up, specifically to assess the bone-implant interface and marginal peri-implant bone height at regular intervals for depicting a possible lack of osseointegration or bone loss due to peri-implantitis [11].

5.3 Cone Beam CT Imaging

Cone beam CT (CBCT) is a fairly recent imaging modality as these devices were introduced in dentomaxillofacial imaging in the late 1990s [14]. CBCT imaging has progressed rapidly and is now a widely used imaging approach in dentomaxillofacial radiology [10]. This imaging modality offers a much reduced exposure to radiation [8], the production of images of higher resolution than medical CT scan and much lower capital investment in the purchase of equipment [10]. In comparison with conventional two-dimensional imaging modalities, CBCT imaging presents as main advantages the elimination of superimposition of adjacent structures and absence of image magnification. CBCT provides images of highly contrasting structures and is therefore particularly well suited for the imaging of osseous structures of the jaws. This imaging modality allows thus a complete 3D evaluation of alveolar ridge topography prior the implant insertion. Bone quantity is assessed by measuring the height and width of available alveolar bone and by the morphology of the alveolar ridge. Cross-sectional images at approximatively 1 mm intervals are very useful for determining buccolingual width and height of the ridge and angulations of bone [15, 16].

CBCT allows thus more than diagnosis; it facilitates image-guided surgery [17]. Planning software are available to facilitate virtual implant placement and to create surgical implant guidance templates. Among the various imaging modalities available, CBCT has been proved to have the greatest impact on the planning of dental implant placements [18]. Careful examination

and planning of the treatment result in a high success rates of 97% for dental implants [1]. The CBCT is therefore considered as the imaging modality of choice for preoperative cross-sectional imaging of potential implant sites [3]. This technology also provides the practitioner with a modality extending maxillofacial imaging from diagnosis to image guidance of operative and surgical implant placement procedures.

Nevertheless, artefacts can seriously degrade the quality of CBCT images. Among the many different types of artefacts encountered in CBCT, patient motion can be a major cause of misregistration of data [10], particularly in edentulous patient. These artefacts can be attributed to improper stabilization or fixation of the patient's head during acquisition. In CBCT, any movement of the patient affects the quality of the entire volume of data, causing image blurring or double images. Since the resolution in CBCT is very high, ranging from 0.070 to 0.300 mm, even small motion can impair image quality [19]. Motion artefacts can be minimized by stabilizing edentulous mandible with positioning aids and using as short a scan time as possible [18].

5.4 Radiation Dose

Because a certain amount of radiation is inevitably delivered to patients, the main objective is to produce images of optimal quality with the least amount of radiation exposure, a principle known as ALARA (as low as reasonably achievable). The radiation exposure from CBCT is generally higher than in conventional radiography (intraoral and panoramic radiographs) but considerably lower than in CT scan [10]. Reported effective doses for intraoral radiography, panoramic radiography and cone beam CT are listed in Table 5.1.

The radiation dose from any CBCT device largely depends on the type of machine and scan settings including field of view (FOV), number of basis image projections or exposure time (s) and scan modes, among other factors [20, 21]. As dose received being strongly related to field size, patient radiation dose can be significantly lowered by adequately collimating the primary X-ray beam to the minimum size needed to image the structures of interest [22, 23]. On the other hand, the radiation dose is depending on the voxel size, i.e. higher radiation doses are needed when decreasing voxel size [24]. Radiation dose is also depending on the region being scanned because radiosensitive organs as salivary glands or thyroid gland can be exposed to scattered radiation or primary beam during acquisition [10]. Accordingly, the use of lead shielding is appropriate to protect the thyroid gland during radiographic examination [25]. Thyroid skin exposure can indeed be reduced by 33–84% in adults and 63–92% in children by using thyroid shield [26].

5.5 Preoperative Implant Imaging

As recommended by evidence-based guidelines [3], initial implant imaging is best achieve with panoramic radiography. Periapical radiography may supplement the preliminary information from panoramic radiography in obtaining images of excellent resolution for demonstrating fine details of bone architecture and quality. For the preoperative diagnosis phase, CBCT imaging is recommended for cross-sectional imaging of potential implant sites [3].

Candidates for dental implants are preoperatively evaluated to determine the quantity and quality of bone available in the alveolar ridge to support implants. In addition to evaluation of internal anatomy, consideration should be given to jaw shape, orientation and boundaries [27]. The amount of bone varies considerably because the edentulous regions undergo bone resorption. This can considerably diminish the height and thickness of the alveolar ridge. Patients must also be evaluated to determine the precise location of the mandibular anatomical structures. A meticulous radiographic examination is required to obtain all this information. Violation or damage

to these structures or implant placement beyond the anatomical boundaries can cause considerable complications [2, 28–31]. Some of the anatomical structures that are routinely encountered during implant placement are discussed below.

5.5.1 Posterior Mandible

Depiction of the mandibular canal is of fundamental importance for preoperative planning of implant placement involving the posterior mandible [32]. This canal travels within the mandible and houses a neurovascular bundle consisting of the inferior alveolar nerve, the inferior alveolar artery and the inferior alveolar vein. This neurovascular bundle enters the mandibular canal through the mandibular foramen on the medial surface of the ramus and exits through the mental foramen. The average diameter of the canal in its horizontal part is approximatively 3.4 mm wide [33]. As the nerve and vessels proceed in the mandibular canal, the canal follows usually (70%) the lingual cortical plate at the mandibular ramus and body [34]. The mental nerve and vessels exit the mental foramen, and the canal continues anteriorly as the mandibular incisive canal. Damage to the inferior alveolar bundle is one of the major complications in dental implant surgery in the mandible and results in most cases from poor characterization of the location of the mandibular canal [30]. The identification of the mandibular canal is therefore a requirement for planning implant placement particularly in case of ridge atrophy of the posterior part of the mandible [35]. The radiographic appearance usually involves a radiolucent channel lined by two more or less sclerotic borders. Indeed the cortication of walls of the canal is quite variable which may explain why in some cases the delineation of the mandibular canal course is not always so evident. The visibility of the canal decreases towards the mental foramen (Fig. 5.1), and when only one border of the canal is seen, it is typically the inferior border [35]. In severe atrophic mandible, the man-

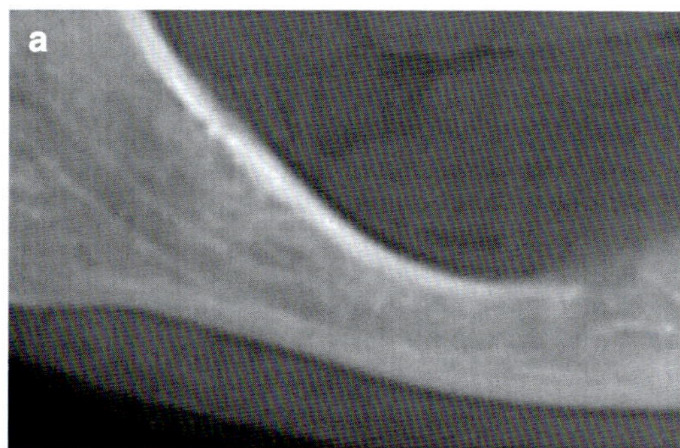

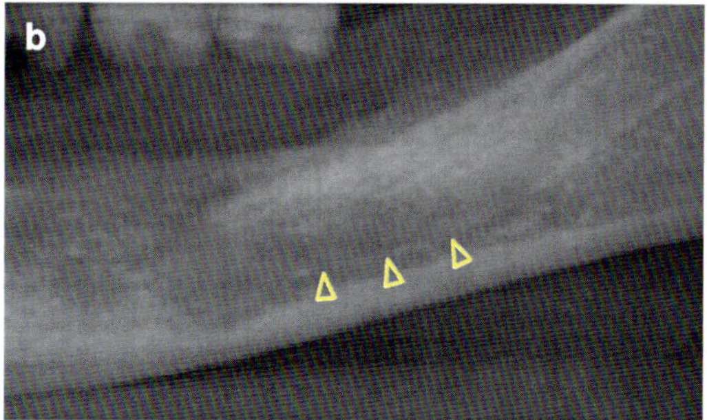

Fig. 5.1 Panoramic images showing the mandibular canal. (**a**) The posterior segment of the mandibular canal is more identifiable than the portion of the canal near to mental foramen. (**b**) The inferior border of the canal (empty yellow arrowheads) is usually easier to identify than the superior border on panoramic radiograph

dibular canal can be adjacent to the crest of the alveolar ridge [36] (Fig. 5.2). Moreover, the edentulous mandibular regions may present a reduction in size of the neurovascular bundle influencing the visibility of the mandibular canal [37]. However, CBCT shows significantly better visualization of the mandibular canal than panoramic radiograph [35, 38, 39], and depiction of the canal clearly increases when the assessment is performed from every sequential cross-sectional image available [40].

Although panoramic radiographs allow the detection of the mental foramen in 94% [41], the conventional two-dimensional presurgical radiological assessment often fails to reflect the actual position of the foramen [42]. Accurate information concerning the location of the mental foramen is generally provided by cone beam CT [29, 43]. This foramen is located on the buccal side of the anterior mandible (Fig. 5.3) and transmits the mental nerve in conjunction with blood vessels. The mental foramen is typically found halfway between the alveolar crest and the inferior border of the mandible [44]. Nevertheless, the location of the mental foramen in edentulous patient

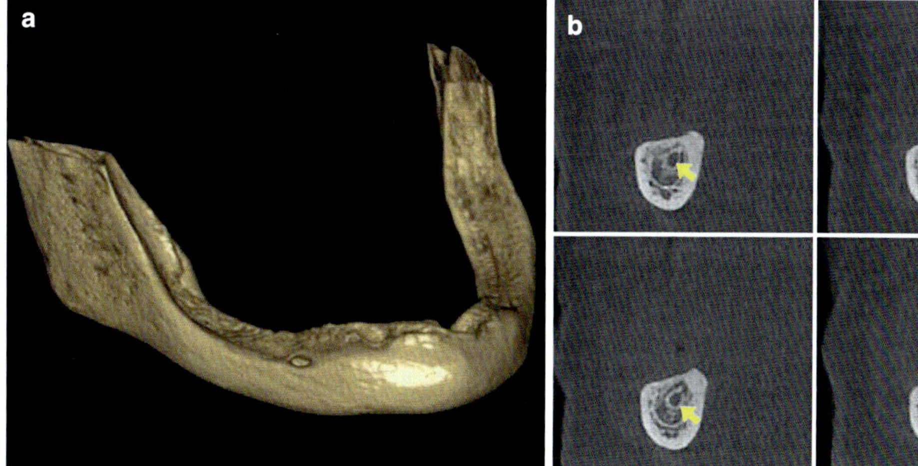

Fig. 5.2 Cone beam CT imaging of severe atrophy of the alveolar ridge. (**a**) 3D volumetric rendering of the edentulous mandible. (**b**) Series of cross-sectional images in the mandibular premolar and molar areas showing the close proximity between the roof of the mandibular canal (yellow arrows) and the alveolar crest. The bone resorption associated with the presence of the mandibular canal limits the available remaining bone for implant placement

can be influenced by the amount of crestal bone loss. After resorption of alveolar bone, the mental foramen is closer to the alveolar crest

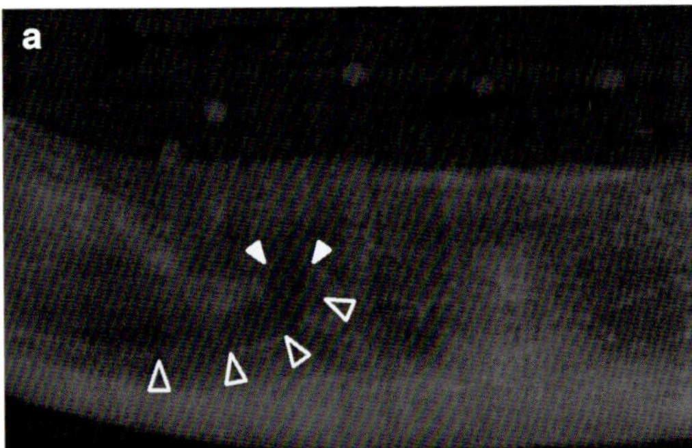

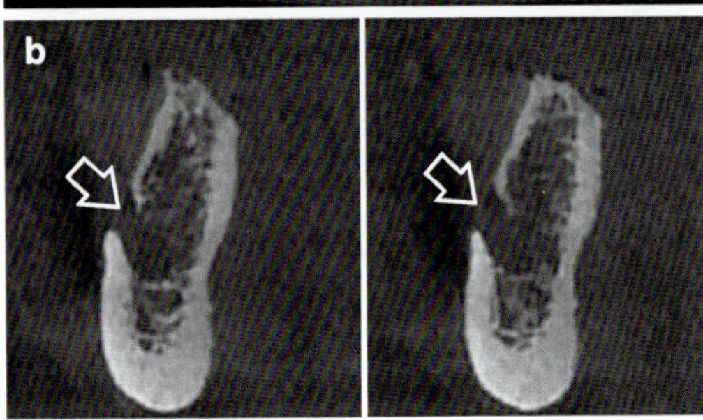

Fig. 5.3 Detection of the mental foramen for preimplant assessment. (**a**) Panoramic radiograph showing the course of mandibular canal and its anterior loop (empty white arrowheads) towards the mental foramen (filled white arrowheads). (**b**) Cone beam CT cross-sections. Emergence of the mental neurovascular bundle into the buccal surface of the mandibular bone. Typically, the mental foramen (white arrows) is located halfway between the alveolar crest and the lower border of the mandible

(Fig. 5.4). In severely atrophic mandible, the loss in bone height extends down to the roof of the mandibular canal and causes an eventual exposure of the mental foramen. Radiographs or cone beam CT demonstrating therefore close proximity of the foramen to the alveolar crest dictate that the foramen should be surgically located to avoid nerve damage prior surgical procedure as implant placement.

Lingual undercuts are common in the posterior region of the mandible and pose the risk of perforating the lingual cortical plate during placement of implants. Panoramic radiograph does not provide information on buccolingual dimensions and thus fails to predict not only the presence of any concavities in the posterior part of the mandible but also the extent and depth of such concavity. As reported by Nickenig et al. [27], the prevalence of lingual undercut is significantly higher in the second molar region than in the first molar region. Compared to conventional two-dimensional radiological assessment (panoramic radiographs, periapical radiographs), cross-sectional analysis using CBCT provides the opportunity to determine the presence of a lingual undercut (Fig. 5.5), and the virtual implant planning avoids complications by perforation of the lingual cortical bone.

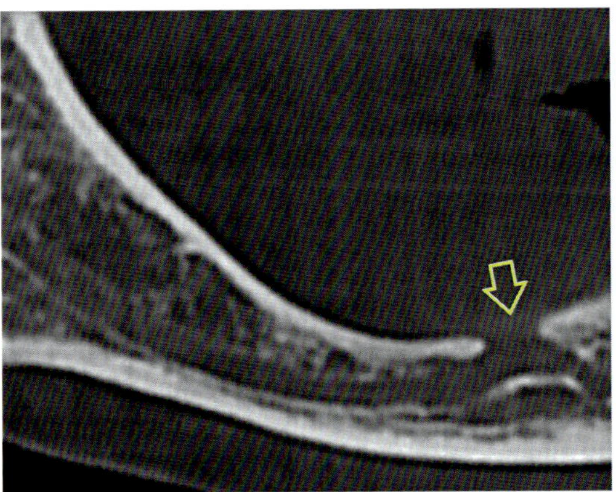

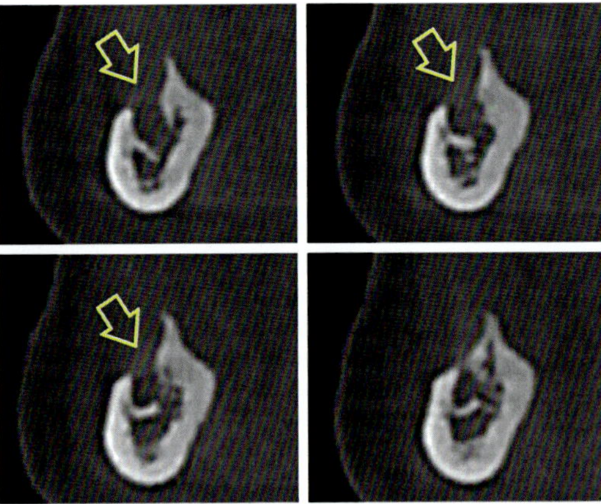

Fig. 5.4 Location of the mental foramen in severe atrophic mandible. Panoramic and cross-sectional images of edentulous patient. Atrophic loss of ridge height causes an opening of the mental foramen (yellow arrows) near the crest of the ridge and an eventual exposure of the mental neurovascular bundle

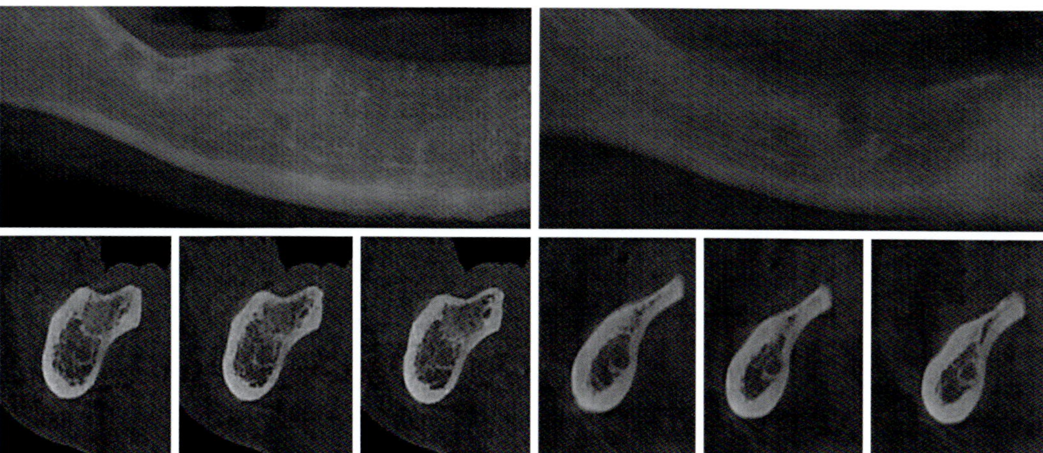

Fig. 5.5 Detection of lingual undercuts and prevention of lingual cortical perforation. In these two patients, panoramic radiograph fails to predict the presence of lingual concavities in the premolar and molar areas. Cross-sectional analysis of the posterior mandibular region not only demonstrates the lingual undercut but also shows the marked lingual inclination of the tooth-bearing part of the alveolar bone (see right lower cross-sections)

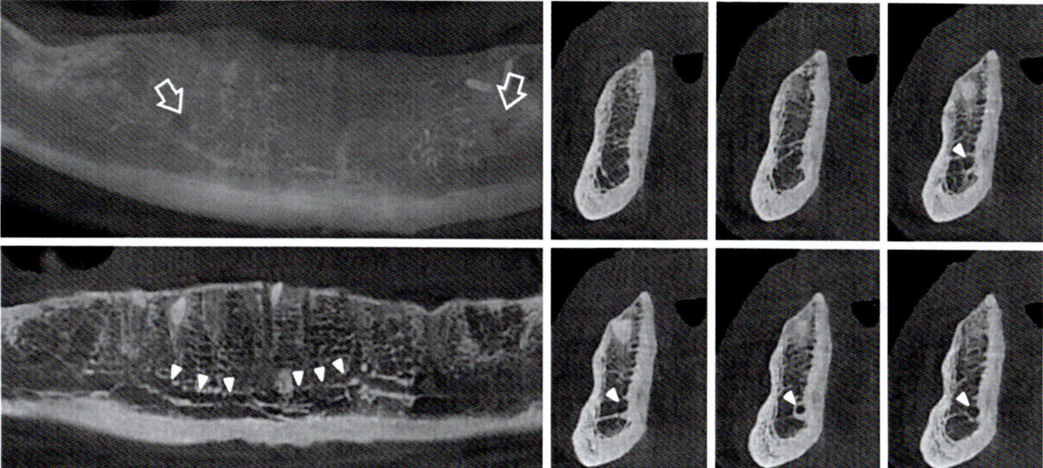

Fig. 5.6 Assessment of the mandibular incisive canal. Cone beam CT examination has definitive advantage over panoramic radiograph for identification of the course of the mandibular incisive canal. The depiction of the canal clearly increases using a combination of panoramic and cross-sectional cuts. (Mandibular incisive canal, white arrowheads; mental foramen, white arrows)

5.5.2 Interforaminal Region

The interforaminal region of the mandible contains the mandibular incisive canal. This canal continues the mandibular canal mesially to the mental foramen and contains one of the terminal branches of the inferior alveolar nerve, the mandibular incisive nerve (Fig. 5.6). Radiographically, the mean diameter of the incisive canal is 1.8 mm; the mean distance from the inferior border of the mandible is 11.5 mm, and its course is closer to the buccal border of the mandible [45]. Panoramic radiograph can detect only 2.7% of mandibular incisive canal, whereas its occurrence has been shown in 95% of cases [46]. In contrast cross-sectional imaging using CBCT allows the delineation of the incisive canal in more than 90% of the case [45, 47, 48]. A significant anatomical

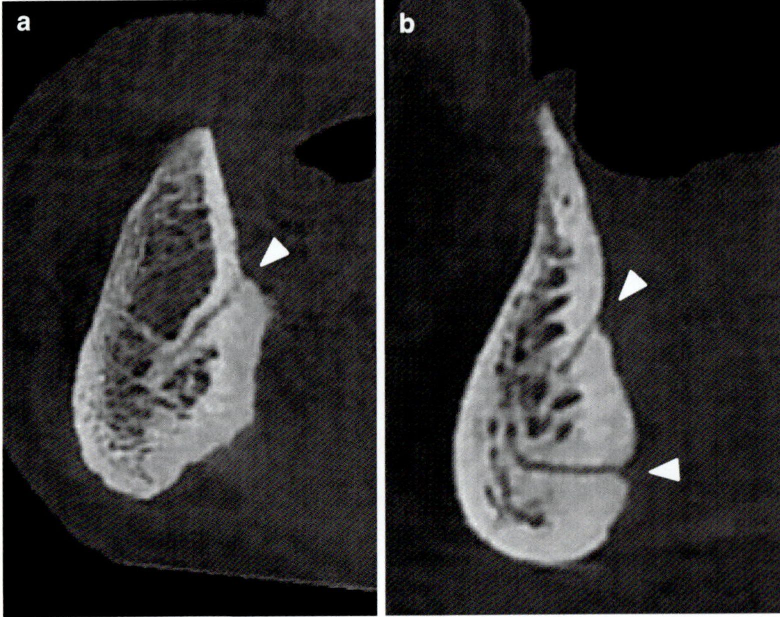

Fig. 5.7 Median lingual foramen. (**a**) The canal perforating the lingual cortex superior to the genial tubercles corresponds to the lingual foramen (white arrowhead). (**b**) Example of multiple accessory canals along the midline of the mandible

structure in the internal region of the mandible, at the level of the genial tubercles, is the lingual foramen or foramina, which contains an artery that develops from the anastomosis of the two sublingual arteries. These foramina are located at the midline and are oriented at an upper-lingual direction (Fig. 5.7). They are identified fairly inferior, unless severe bone resorption is noted. Lingual foramina can be identified in 83.5% of CBCT cross sections [45]. The radiological assessment of the accurate location of these anatomical structures is of significant importance before implant placement in the interforaminal region [32, 44]. Intraoperative or postoperative complications in this region may be in fact attributed to a direct trauma of these structures [49].

Significant variation exists concerning the shape of the anterior mandible in cross sections. In canine and first premolar region, a lingual undercut is observed in 5–18% [50]. Nevertheless the extent of the lingual concavity is less marked than in the molar region [27]. Bone loss can also cause progressive labiolingually thinning of the alveolar crest. The shape of the residual ridge may then alter into a thin and sharp knife edge (Fig. 5.8). Further resorption leads to a low well-rounded ridge reduced in height and width. In advanced cases, CBCT cross sections may reveal the lingual canal and the superior genial tubercle becoming exposed to the ridge crest.

5.5.3 Bone Quality Evaluation

Bone quality, besides the quantity of the surrounding bone, is another important factor influencing the success rate obtained with dental implants [51]. As mentioned in the literature, CBCT imaging can provide useful information on bone quality [52, 53], particularly the reformatted alveolar cross-sectional CBCT images which facilitate the assessment of both cortical plate and trabecular bone [17]. Lekholm and Zarb [54] classified bone quality into four groups (types I–IV) according to the ratio of compact bone to trabecular bone tissues. Anterior mandible generally presents the highest bone density (type I) and posterior maxilla has the lowest one (type IV). The trabecular bone is generally denser and more coarsely woven in the anterior region than in either the premolar region or molar part of the mandible (Fig. 5.9). These regional differences in

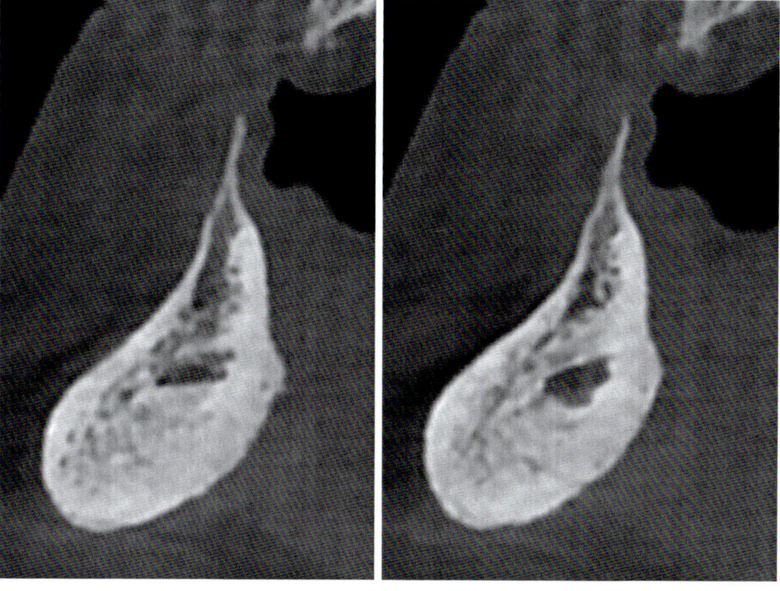

Fig. 5.8 Example of alveolar bone resorption leading to a thin and sharp knife edge (CBCT cross-sections of the anterior mandible)

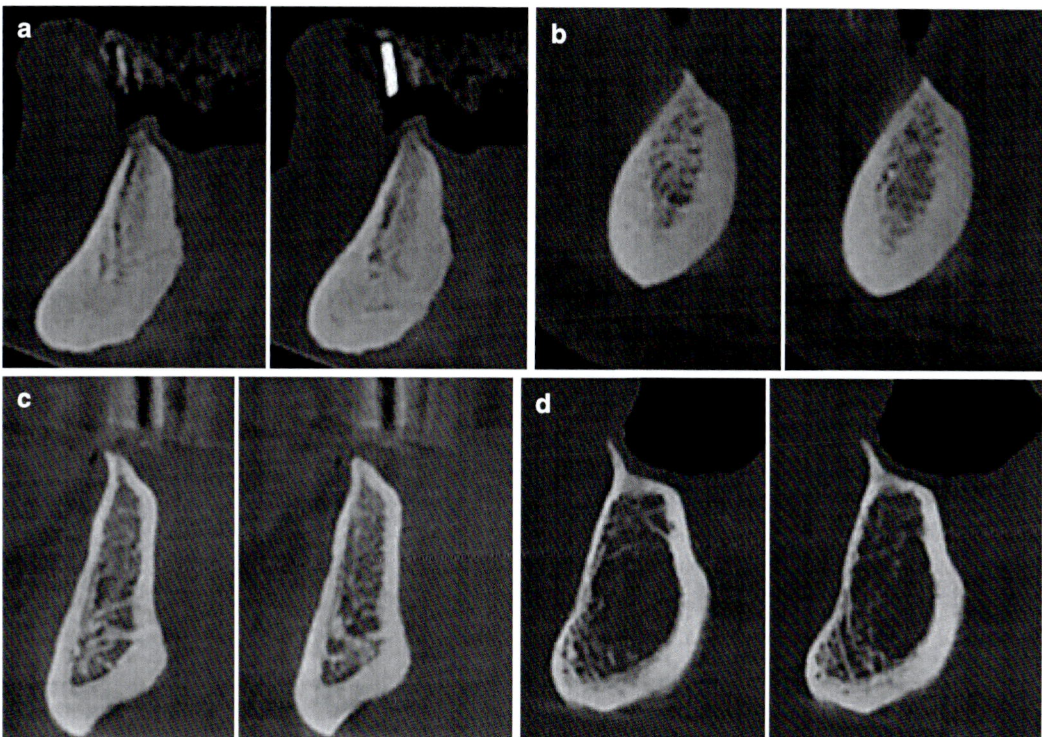

Fig. 5.9 Mandibular bone quality. Based on its radiographic appearance, bone quality is categorized into four groups (Zarb and Lekholm). (**a**) Type I: almost the entire bone is composed of homogenous compact bone. (**b**) Type II: thick cortical layer surrounding a dense medullar bone. (**c**) Type III: thin layer of cortical bone surrounding a core of dense trabecular bone. (**d**) Type IV: thin cortical layer surrounding a sparse medullar bone

bone density may explain some of the variation in clinical success rate of implant therapy. Indeed it has been demonstrated that the poorer quality of bone (type IV) is associated with higher failure rates [51, 55]. Preoperative evaluation of bone quality is thus crucial to assist the clinician when planning implant therapy [56]. The higher bone mineral density in the anterior region of the mandible may be one of the reasons for increased success rate of osteointegration [57].

Considering bone density assessment, high correlation between HU from CBCT and CT scan voxel grey values has been reported suggesting the potential of CBCT in estimation of bone mineral density [58–60]. Nevertheless the large amounts of scattered radiation and technology-specific artefacts produced by CBCT can significantly influence the grey-level values measurements [61]. Grey-level values are also largely dependent on the selected FOV and scan settings [62]. Furthermore, the lack of a technical standard for the development of CBCT systems has led to a wide disparity in physical parameters of each model, including, among others, grey value measurements [62]. Developing such standard as for CT scan may be very helpful for improving the robustness of the concordance between the grey value measurements in CBCT and the bone mineral densities.

References

1. Kopp KC, Koslow AH, Abdo OS. Predictable implant placement with a diagnostic/surgical template and advanced radiographic imaging. J Prosthet Dent. 2003;89:611–5.
2. Ardekian L, Dodson TB. Complications associated with the placement of dental implants. Oral Maxillofac Surg Clin North Am. 2003;15:243–9.
3. Tyndall DA, Price JB, Tetradis S, Ganz SD, Hildebolt C, Scarfe WC, American Academy of Oral and Maxillofacial Radiology. Position statement of the American Academy of Oral and Maxillofacial Radiology on selection criteria for the use of radiology in dental implantology with emphasis on cone beam computed tomography. Oral Surg Oral Med Oral Pathol Oral Radiol. 2012;113:817–26.
4. Hatcher DC, Dial C, Mayorga C. Cone beam CT for pre-surgical assessment of implant sites. J Calif Dent Assoc. 2003;31:825–34.
5. Kraut RA. Interactive CT diagnostics, planning and preparation for dental implants. Implant Dent. 1998;7:19–25.
6. Lurie AG. Panoramic imaging. In: White SC, Pharoah MJ, editors. Oral radiology principles and interpretation. 6th ed. St. Louis: Mosby; 2009. p. 175–90.
7. Granlund C, Thilander-Klang A, Ylhan B, Lofthag-Hansen S, Ekestubbe A. Absorbed organ and effective doses from digital intra-oral and panoramic radiography applying the ICRP 103 recommendations for effective dose estimations. Br J Radiol. 2016 Jul 25:20151052.
8. Okano T, Sur J. Radiation dose and protection in dentistry. Jpn Dent Sci Rev. 2010;46:112–21.
9. European Commission (EC). Radiation protection n°172: evidence based guidelines on cone beam CT for dental and maxillofacialradiology. Luxembourg: Office for Official Publications of the European Communities; 2014.
10. Suomalainen A, Pakbaznejad Esmaeili E, Robinson S. Dentomaxillofacial imaging with panoramic views and cone beam CT. Insights Imaging. 2015;6:1–16.
11. Benson BW, Shetty V. Dental implants. In: White SC, Pharoah MJ, editors. Oral radiology principles and interpretation. 6th ed. St. Louis: Mosby; 2009. p. 597–612.
12. White SC, Pharoah MJ. Oral radiology principles and interpretation. 6th ed. St. Louis: Mosby; 2009. p. 109–51.
13. Rathi S, Hatcher D. Radiologic evaluation of alveolar ridge in implant dentistry. CBCT technology. In: Tolstunov L, editor. Horizontal alveolar ridge augmentation in implant dentistry: a surgical manual. Hoboken, NJ: Wiley-Blackwell; 2016. p. 55–71.
14. Mozzo P, Procacci C, Tacconi A, Martini PT, Andreis IA. A new volumetric CT machine for dental imaging based on the cone-beam technique: preliminary results. Eur Radiol. 1998;8:1558–64.
15. Resnik RR, Kircos L, Misch CE. Diagnostic imaging and techniques. In: Misch CE, editor. Contemporary implant dentistry. 3rd ed. St. Louis: Mosby, Elsevier; 2008. p. 38–67.
16. Schropp L, Stavropoulos A, Gotfredsen E, Wenzel A. Comparison of panoramic and conventional cross-sectional tomography for preoperative selection of implant size. Clin Oral Implants Res. 2011;22:424–9.
17. Gulsahi A. Bone quality assessment for dental implants. In: Turkyilmaz I, editor. Implant dentistry—the most promising discipline of dentistry: Intech; 2011. p. 437–49.
18. Scarfe WC, Farman AG. Cone beam computed tomography. In: White SC, Pharoah MJ, editors. Oral radiology principles and interpretation. 6th ed. St. Louis: Mosby; 2009. p. 225–43.
19. Schulze R, Heil U, Gross D, Bruellmann DD, Dranischnikow E, Schwanecke U, Schoemer E. Artefacts in CBCT: a review. Dentomaxillofac Radiol. 2011;40:265–73.
20. Pauwels R, Beinsberger J, Collaert B, Theodorakou C, Rogers J, Walker A, Cockmartin L, Bosmans H,

Jacobs R, Bogaerts R, Horner K. Effective dose range for dental cone beam computed tomography scanners. Eur J Radiol. 2012;81:267–71.

21. Suomalainen A, Kiljunen T, Käser Y, Peltola J, Kortesniemi M. Dosimetry and image quality of four dental cone beam computed tomography scanners compared with multislice computed tomography scanners. Dentomaxillofac Radiol. 2009;38:367–78.

22. Horner K, Islam M, Flygare L, Tsiklakis K, Whaites E. Basic principles for use of dental cone beam computed tomography: consensus guidelines of the European Academy of Dental and Maxillofacial Radiology. Dentomaxillofac Radiol. 2009;38:187–95.

23. Pauwels R, Zhang G, Theodorakou C, Walker A, Bosmans H, Jacobs R, Bogaerts R, Horner K, SEDENTEXCT Project Consortium. Effective radiation dose and eye lens dose in dental cone beam CT: effect of field of view and angle of rotation. Br J Radiol. 2014;87:20130654.

24. Loubele M, Jacobs R, Maes F, Denis K, White S, Coudyzer W, Lambrichts I, van Steenberghe D, Suetens P. Image quality vs radiation dose of four cone beam computed tomography scanners. Dentomaxillofac Radiol. 2008;37:309–18.

25. Tsiklakis K, Donta C, Gavala S, Karayianni K, Kamenopoulou V, Hourdakis CJ. Dose reduction in maxillofacial imaging using low dose Cone Beam CT. Eur J Radiol. 2005;56:413–7.

26. Horner K. Radiation protection in dental radiology. Br J Radiol. 1994;67:1041–9.

27. Nickenig HJ, Wichmann M, Eitner S, Zöller JE, Kreppel M. Lingual concavities in the mandible: a morphological study using cross-sectional analysis determined by CBCT. J Craniomaxillofac Surg. 2015;43:254–9.

28. Dao TT, Mellor A. Sensory disturbances associated with implant surgery. Int J Prosthodont. 1998;11:462–9.

29. Greenstein G, Tarnow D. The mental foramen and nerve: clinical and anatomical factors related to dental implant placement: a literature review. J Periodontol. 2006;77:1933–43.

30. Klinge B, Petersson A, Maly P. Location of the mandibular canal: comparison of macroscopic findings, conventional radiography, and computed tomography. Int J Oral Maxillofac Implants. 1989;4:327–32.

31. Sharawy M, Misch CE. Anatomy for dental implants. In: Misch CE, editor. Contemporary implant dentistry. 3rd ed. St. Louis: Mosby, Elsevier; 2008. p. 217–24.

32. Greenstein G, Cavallaro J, Romanos G, Tarnow D. Clinical recommendations for avoiding and managing surgical complications associated with implant dentistry: a review. J Periodontol. 2008;79:1317–29.

33. Ikeda K, Ho KC, Nowicki BH, Haughton VM. Multiplanar MR and anatomic study of the mandibular canal. AJNR Am J Neuroradiol. 1996;17:579–84.

34. Kim ST, Hu KS, Song WC, Kang MK, Park HD, Kim HJ. Location of the mandibular canal and the topogra-phy of its neurovascular structures. J Craniofac Surg. 2009;20:936–9.

35. Kamrun N, Tetsumura A, Nomura Y, Yamaguchi S, Baba O, Nakurama S, Watanabe H, Kurabayashi T. Visualization of the superior and inferior borders of the mandibular canal: a comparative study using digital panoramic radiographs and cross-sectional computed tomography images. Oral Surg Oral Med Oral Pathol Oral Radiol. 2013;115:550–7.

36. Ulm CW, Solar P, Blahout R, Matejka M, Watzek G, Gruber H. Location of the mandibular canal within the atrophic mandible. Br J Oral Maxillofac Surg. 1993;31:370–5.

37. Wadu SC, Penhall B, Townsend GC. Morphological variability of the human inferior alveolar nerve. Clin Anat. 1997;10:82–7.

38. Angelopoulos C, Thomas SL, Hechler S, Parissis N, Hlavacek M. Comparison between digital panoramic radiography and cone-beam computed tomography for the identification of the mandibular canal as part of presurgical dental implant assessment. J Oral Maxillofac Surg. 2008;66:2130–5.

39. Oliveira Santos C, Cappelozza ALÁ, Dezzoti MSG, Fischer CM, Poleti ML, Rubira bullen IRF. Visibility of the mandibular canal on CBCT cross-sectional images. J Appl Oral Sci. 2011;19:240–3.

40. Lofthag-Hansen S, Gröndahl K, Ekestubbe A. Cone-beam CT for preoperative implant planning in the posterior mandible: visibility of anatomic landmarks. Clin Implant Dent Relat Res. 2009;11:246–55.

41. Jacobs R, Mraiwa N, Van Steenberghe D, Sanderink G, Quirynen M. Appearance of the mandibular incisive canal on panoramic radiographs. Surg Radiol Anat. 2004;26:329–33.

42. Yosue T, Brooks SL. The appearance of mental foramina on panoramic and periapical radiographs. II. Experimental evaluation. Oral Surg Oral Med Oral Pathol. 1989;68:488–92.

43. Sonick M, Abrahams J, Faiella RA. A comparison of the accuracy of periapical, panoramic, and computerized tomographic radiographs in locating the mandibular canal. Int J Oral Maxillofac Implants. 1994;9:455–60.

44. Mraiwa N, Jacobs R, van Steenberghe D, Quirynen M. Clinical assessment and surgical implications of anatomic challenges in the anterior mandible. Clin Implant Dent Relat Res. 2003;5:219–25.

45. Makris N, Stamatakis H, Syriopoulos K, Tsiklakis K, van der Stelt PF. Evaluation of the visibility and the course of the mandibular incisive canal and the lingual foramen using cone-beam computed tomography. Clin Oral Implants Res. 2010;(7):766–71.

46. Romanos GE, Papadimitriou DE, Royer K, Stefanova-Stephens N, Salwan R, Malmström H, Caton JG. The presence of the mandibular incisive canal: a panoramic radiographic examination. Implant Dent. 2012;21:202–6.

47. Jacobs R, Mraiwa N, vanSteenberghe D, Gijbels F, Quirynen M. Appearance, location, course, and morphology of the mandibular incisive canal: an

assessment on spiral CT scan. Dentomaxillofac Radiol. 2002;31:322–7.

48. Tepper G, Hofschneider UB, Gahleitner A, Ulm C. Computed tomographic diagnosis and localization of bone canals in the mandibular interforaminal region for prevention of bleeding complications during implant surgery. Int J Oral Maxillofac Implants. 2001;16:68–72.

49. Kalpidis CD, Setayesh RM. Hemorrhaging associated with endosseous implant placement in the anterior mandible: a review of the literature. J Periodontol. 2004;75:631–45.

50. Watanabe H, Mohammad Abdul M, Kurabayashi T, Aoki H. Mandible size and morphology determined with CT on a premise of dental implant operation. Surg Radiol Anat. 2010;32:343–9.

51. Jaffin RA, Berman CL. The excessive loss of Branemark fixtures in type IV bone: a 5-year analysis. J Periodontol. 1991;62:2–4.

52. Hao Y, Zhao W, Wang Y, Yu J, Zou D. Assessments of jaw bone density at implant sites using 3D cone-beam computed tomography. Eur Rev Med Pharmacol Sci. 2014;18:1398–403.

53. Parsa A, Ibrahim N, Hassan B, van der Stelt P, Wismeijer D. Bone quality evaluation at dental implant site using multislice CT, micro-CT, and cone beam CT. Clin Oral Implants Res. 2013b;26:1–7.

54. Lekholm U, Zarb GA. Patient selection and preparation. In: Branemark PI, Zarb GA, Albrektsson T, editors. Tissue-integrated prostheses: osseointegration in clinical dentistry. Chicago: Quintessence; 1985. p. 199–209.

55. Jemt T, Book K, Linden B, Urde G. Failures and complications in 92 consecutively inserted overdentures supported by Branemark implants in severely resorbed edentulous maxillae: a study from prosthetic treatment to first annual check-up. Int J Oral Maxillofac Implants. 1992;7:162–7.

56. Tolstunov L. Implant zones of the jaws: implant location and related success rate. J Oral Implantol. 2007;33:211–20.

57. Turkyilmaz I, McGlumphy EA. Influence of bone density on implant stability parameters and implant success: a retrospective clinical study. BMC Oral Health. 2008;8(32)

58. Naitoh M, Hirukawa A, Katsumata A, Ariji E. Evaluation of voxel values in mandibular cancellous bone: relationship between cone-beam computed tomography and multislice helical computed tomography. Clin Oral Implants Res. 2009;20:503–6.

59. Nomura Y, Watanabe H, Honda E, Kurabayashi T. Reliability of voxel values from cone-beam computed tomography for dental use in evaluating bone mineral density. Clin Oral Implants Res. 2010;21:558–62.

60. Parsa A, Ibrahim N, Hassan B, Motroni A, van der Stelt P, Wismeijer D. Reliability of voxel gray values in cone beam computed tomography for pre-operative implant planning assessment. Int J Oral Maxillofac Implants. 2012;27:1438–42.

61. Nackaerts O, Maes F, Yan H, Couto Souza P, Pauwels R, Jacobs R. Analysis of intensity variability in multislice and cone beam computed tomography. Clin Oral Implants Res. 2011;22:873–9.

62. Parsa A, Ibrahim N, Hassan B, Motroni A, van der Stelt P, Wismeijer D. Influence of cone beam CT scanning parameters on grey value measurements at an implant site. Dentomaxillofac Radiol. 2013a;42:79884780.

Clinical Assessment of Edentate Elders for Mandibular Implant Overdentures

6

Charlotte Stilwell

Abstract

A comprehensive clinical assessment is the basis of safe and predictable treatment planning. A systematic approach further ensures that all relevant aspects and factors are included and considered. With the specific focus on the elderly patient, the clinical assessment commences with the first approach for an appointment and the patient's ability and possible needs connected with attending the dental office. At the first visit, the clinical assessment is divided between obtaining a full patient history, performing a clinical examination and establishing the need for additional investigations. Specifically, for consideration of mandibular implant overdentures, investigations related to existing dentures and denture wearing history are important to establish clear indication for treatment. Similarly, a risk assessment in relation to implant therapy is recommended to ensure that the surgical aspect amongst other is appropriate and that no contraindications exist.

C. Stilwell
Specialist Dental Services, London, UK

6.1 Introduction

The aim of this chapter is to gather the clinical information that is required to safely and predictably plan and provide mandibular implant overdentures. Implant assistance for mandibular dentures is a therapy that is both scientifically and clinically validated, but it is not without risks [1]. Appropriate clinical assessment is therefore mentioned in recommendations for minimum standards of training for dentists who wish to undertake implant treatment (*UK Training Standards in Implant Dentistry*).

The focus on rehabilitation of the edentulous older patient adds a further important perspective to the clinical assessment. There is no age limit per se to provision of implant treatment [2], and the benefits of implant support for a mandibular denture are extensively documented [3–5]. Even so dental implants are still scarcely used in elderly patients and where indicated treatment should be encouraged, whilst patients are still in good health and able to live independently [6]. Barriers to implant treatment may be self-imposed by the patient. It could be through fear of the surgical aspect and it is important to discover this. The clinical assessment will also serve to determine if the implant therapy element is appropriate or whether there are risks and contra-indications against doing so. As outlined already in the previous chapters, specific treatment considerations may exist and careful assessment is

© Springer International Publishing AG, part of Springer Nature 2018
E. Emami, J. Feine (eds.), *Mandibular Implant Prostheses*,
https://doi.org/10.1007/978-3-319-71181-2_6

essential to identifying individual needs and challenges to provision of care.

This chapter sets out a systematic approach to clinical assessment to ensure that all relevant factors are considered. In turn this should assist the process of reaching the clinical diagnoses and indications that will guide the selection of the most appropriate treatment option.

6.1.1 Clinical Assessment

Clinical assessment includes a number of components. In a systematic approach, these are set out in a logical sequence as seen in Table 6.1. Assessment of the patient's general status commences from the moment of first contact and continues throughout the assessment. This part will reveal physical and cognitive considerations. Next it is important to establish the patient's reason for seeking treatment together with any other social, medical and dental information. This is followed by the actual clinical examination together with any additional investigations that may prove necessary or helpful to finally reaching diagnoses and summarising indications for treatment (the radiographic imaging under additional investigations has been covered as a separate topic by itself in the previous chapter). A risk assessment can also be undertaken, and an example of this is offered towards the end of the chapter. Through the chapter, factors that may impact on difficulty of treatment process and risk of complications are marked with ⬤.

6.2 General Status of the Patient: Observations

As already mentioned, age is in itself not a barrier to implant therapy. Equally age is not a prognostic factor for the outcome of denture treatment [7]. However, advancing age and presence of medical conditions are likely to be reflected in both the patient's physical and cognitive status [8]. In turn these may impact on the patient's access to dental care and ability to cope with dental procedures in a dental chair. As such it is necessary to consider the needs of the individual throughout the whole treatment process. Useful information can be gained from the moment of first contact. This could be when the patient makes an appointment with the dental office or through a request for a dental visit to the patient's abode.

6.2.1 Physical Status

The Seattle Care Pathway for securing oral health in older patients [9] is aimed at a structured, pragmatic and evidence-based approach to assessment, and it is designed to be globally applicable. It offers a helpful point of reference in this context through its Pathway categories which are based on level of dependency. The categories are 'no dependency', 'pre-dependency', 'low dependency', 'medium dependency' and 'high dependency'. These categories are also closely linked with the Canadian Study of Health and Aging (CSHA) frailty scores [10].

Table 6.1 Diagrammatic representation of the components in a clinical assessment set out in a logical sequence

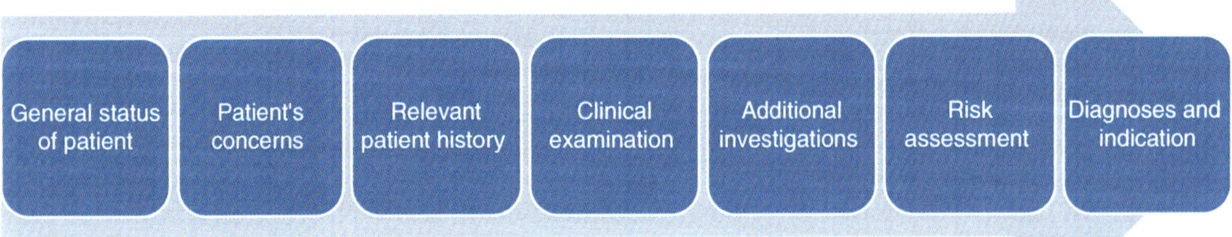

The general status of the no dependency patient presents no immediate impediment to implant therapy although there may be other risk factors to be explored as detailed later in this chapter. The pre-dependency/less dependency patients will need more detailed evaluation of their medical status and its potential impact on oral health and implant treatment. The medium dependency patient will need careful investigation of the medical factors that are impacting on oral health before implant therapy can be considered. The health of the high dependency patient together with the difficulties of moving the patient may preclude consideration of implant therapy.

Signs of reduced mobility and frailty may be immediately obvious. The patient may be accompanied as a means of overcoming both of these, and it is sensible to enquire from the outset what measures might be needed to make the patient comfortable in the dental setting. Frailty could further hint at concern about nutritional status and give rise to more detailed history taking on this point.

There may also be clear signs of medical conditions. Examples are shortness of breath associated with chronic obstructive pulmonary disease (COPD), bruising of the skin linked to anticoagulation or changes to hands caused by arthritis. It could also be reduced sight and or hearing which can both impact on effective communication with the patient.

From an oral perspective, it may be immediately obvious that the patient is edentulous. The patient may present with no dentures or only one denture in situ or with dentures that are not restoring the patient's physiognomy. The psychosocial impact of this is one concern, and the impact on nutritional status is very likely to be another [11].

Arthritic hands and details of the patient's dress appearance with Velcro bands on shoes instead of shoelaces may hint at diminished dexterity. This is likely to be directly relevant to the patient's ability to maintain oral hygiene around implants and associated prostheses. In turn, this has an important bearing on the complexity of the dental work that the patient will be able to manage.

The above are helpful in forming an initial if subjective impression of the patient. It should be backed up by more detailed assessment as outlined later in the chapter.

6.2.2 Personal Interest and Motivation

It is important to assess the patient's personal interest and motivation for treatment. Even if the patient is unaccompanied, the driving force behind seeking a professional consultation may be a significant other person or event in the background. 'My wife thinks I need new teeth' or 'my daughter is getting married'. The type and source of motivation is also likely to have a bearing on the expectations to outcome of the treatment.

The patient may also be attending at the behest of a relative or, as a decision of physician, care home or home carer. This may be a pointer to the cognitive status of the patient.

6.2.3 Signs of Anxiety

As for all dental patients, it is important to detect signs or suggestions of anxiety in the patient's manner. For the older patient, the anxiety could be centred on being able to hear what the dentist is saying or being able to sit comfortably in the dental chair. It is always sensible to listen out for concerns that are expressed at the time of the initial arrangement of the appointment and to enquire from the outset what measures might be needed to make the patient comfortable in the dental setting.

Anxiety could also be linked to the prospect of implant therapy. Many older patients are known to refuse dental implants because of their fear of surgical complications, their feelings of frailty and distrust of the dental profession [12].

It is also important to consider that signs of anxiety could be due to reasons not related to the dental situation. If there is suggestion that this could be the case, the dental practitioner should consider and explore alternative explanations including the possibility of elder abuse.

6.2.4 Cognitive Status

It may be tempting to see an accompanying person as an immediate help to communication with or about the patient. However, unless there is clear information to the contrary, it is wise to explore and where possible first and foremost maintain direct communication with the patient.

Where the accompanying person has an official role as a guardian, they should be involved in any treatment planning decisions. A carer should also be party to the oral health education that is provided.

A specific reason for involving an accompanying person may be the presence of dementia. A patient with mild cognitive impairment (MCI) may also feel happier if a person of trust is present during the assessment. It will assist recollection and discussion after the consultation. Cognitive considerations have been covered in an earlier chapter, but as a quick reference here, MCI is defined as 'cognitive decline greater than expected for an individual's age and education level but not interfering notably with activities of daily life' [13]. Epidemiological studies suggest a prevalence of 3–19% in adults older than 65 years. MCI can be stable or can even return to normal over time, but more than half progress to dementia within 5 years.

6.3 Reason for Attending

6.3.1 Patient's Concerns

As in all treatment planning, it is very important to be clear on why the patient is seeking dental attention. This may be quite different from the professional findings arising from the ensuing clinical examination [14], and it must feature prominently in the overall treatment considerations and documentation.

The reason for attending is an entry point to gauging the nature and the magnitude of patient's concerns. These may be specifically dental or more generally tied up with the physical impairment of tooth loss. The impact of tooth loss should not be underestimated [15].

The concerns may be linked to the patient's daily life and activities such as eating, smiling and speaking [16, 17]. They could also present an impediment to participating in sport or sexual activity. They could even be forcing the patient into avoiding social events altogether—'I don't accept dinner invitations for fear of not being able to chew the food that is served'; 'I don't trust my denture not to move when I laugh'; and 'the denture glue does not last long enough for me to go through an afternoon out with my friends'.

6.3.2 Expectations

The patient may have specific wishes that translate into expectations. Expectations to a new prosthesis can be very high. This has been shown in a study where patients were asked to indicate how satisfied they expected to be with their new prosthesis [18]. The patient may have specific hopes that implant therapy will resolve all of their concerns. This could to some extent be justified as there is evidence that implant-supported overdentures can have a positive impact on social and sexual activity by reducing the patient's uneasiness [18]. However, expectations may exceed what is realistic. An example is a husband who requests the same implant treatment as his wife. She is very happy with her implant-supported maxillary and mandibular overdentures. Unfortunately, her successful outcome does not mean that implant therapy is indicated or even possible for him. It is therefore important to identify the patient's expectations from the outset and address them individually to determine to which extent they are realistic and achievable.

Expectations can also be negative and based on apprehension about treatment. These could be due to past dental experiences or a result of fear of potential pain and complications associated with surgery [12]. For many the prospect of being without their denture(s) for even a short period is an immediate barrier to implant therapy. Older people may feel they are not strong enough to go through the surgical procedure. They are worried about infection, period of recovery and that their gum and jaw may be too thin and weak. As such they may feel the risks outweigh the potential benefits.

Studies show that only a limited number of elderly patients are as yet benefitting from the improvement that dental implants can offer for a mandibular denture. Time taken to present and discuss the advantages of implant therapy to older patients who are still in good health and able to live independently [6] is an important healthcare service both to the individual and for spreading the message to the age group in general. It is may also be essential to overcome a patient-imposed barrier to the most appropriate treatment.

6.4 Patient History

This part of the clinical assessment is intended to elicit any further information from the patient that may be relevant to the treatment planning. It can broadly be divided into three parts aimed at covering and exploring social, medical and dental information not already volunteered by the patient.

6.4.1 Social Factors

There may be a number of factors that could impact on a patient's ability and willingness to accept a treatment plan. For older patient who still have work commitments these will need to be considered in the execution of the treatment plan. The patient may also have pre-existing booked events, e.g. holidays that need to be factored in. The importance of support from family and friends is well recognised [12] as is the absence of same. There can also be restrictions on the patient's freedom if they are acting as a carer for a partner or significant other (Table 6.2).

6.4.2 Medical Factors

🟠 The patient's full medical history and current treatment need to be explored and discussed.

Table 6.2 Social factors that may impact on a patient's ability and willingness to undergo implant therapy

Socioeconomic status	Functional and aesthetic needs
Marital status and family support	Treatment expectations
Work or voluntary project responsibilities	Past dental experiences

Medical and pharmacological considerations have been covered in detail in a previous chapter. It should be noted that this point comes ahead of the clinical examination in the assessment sequence. This is to ensure that any medical impediment to the clinical or radiographic examination is picked up here.

The medical history should include details of current treatment, presence of systemic and local disease, list of prescription medicines and intake of any other over-the-counter or alternative therapy remedies. The medical history should also disclose any allergies and absolute or relative contraindications to dental treatment in general or implant therapy in particular as well as presence of known risk factors.

🟠 Smoking is a proven risk factor for implant therapy [19]. The impact of alcohol consumption is less clear but could play a contributory role in terms of malnutrition, poor oral hygiene and compliance in terms of risk [20]. Smoking is classified as heavy when the patient smokes more than ten cigarettes per day. The guidelines for maximum units of alcohol per week vary between countries, but the general trend is in favour of a reduction.

Where malnutrition is suspected or it forms the basis of a medical referral for dental treatment, further information is needed. This is to ascertain the specific limitations imposed by the dental status on diet and nutrition as well as the impact on the patient's health. Provision of an implant-supported mandibular overdenture does not in itself ensure a positive effect on nutrition compared to conventional complete dentures [21]. However, a customised diet advice may have a beneficial effect [22]. Through better chewing ability, the mandibular implant overdenture wearer is more likely to include fresh whole fruits and vegetables in their diet (Table 6.3).

Table 6.3 Medical factors that may influence implant therapy, bone healing or patient compliance

Pre-existing medical conditions	Tobacco and alcohol consumption
Medication	Patient's ability to comply with
Allergies	intra- and post-operative
	instructions

Table 6.4 Dental factors to consider when assessing patients for implant therapy

Age	Previous implant history
Reasons for tooth loss	Previous denture history
Bruxism	Oral hygiene and compliance

6.4.3 Dental Factors

The patient's dental history is relevant to throwing light on potential dental risk factors. It should also include enquiry about previous denture wearing experience. The dental risk factors include reason for tooth loss, history or present evidence of parafunctional habits and previous implant history or experience.

Amongst the reasons for tooth loss, a history of periodontal disease is particularly relevant. Patient susceptibility does not change simply because teeth have been removed [23]. A history of caries can also throw light on the patient's understanding of dental disease, its prevention and past compliance.

Bruxism is a documented risk factor for the durability of implant prostheses and components. It is also a factor to consider in choice of implant loading protocols. Confirmed presence would favour conventional loading and less ambitious surgical approaches.

Details of previous implant therapy may disclose a history of complications or failure.

Current oral medicine concerns or treatment also comes under dental factors. These would include diseases of the oral mucosa such as denture stomatitis and lichen planus.

Based on current dental status, the consideration of denture wearing experience can be divided into two categories:

- Partially edentulous looking at transition to edentulous
- These patients may have no previous experience. The current trend is that the older population will keep teeth longer. The prosthodontically accepted recommendation to reduce the dental burden of maintenance through shortened dental arch solutions (SDA) [24, 25] may have obviated need for partial dentures. The age at which the transition to edentulous becomes necessary may therefore be advanced and linked to sudden changes in the patient's circumstances. This could be due to changes in medical factors or in level of dependency that in turn leads to significant change in the patient's own ability to maintain the residual dentition.
- If the patient does have partial denture wearing experience, it is important to learn from both positive and negative comments. Positive comments could point to which implant configurations to explore in order to carry forward a hitherto successful partial denture design. From negative comments, there may be diagnostic measures to be considered under additional investigations to address any previously unsuccessful partial denture aspects.
- Already edentulous
- These patients can be divided into patients with short-term only experience versus long-term denture wearing. The short-term experience group may be patients who have recently made the transition to conventional complete dentures and are still struggling with coping with conventional dentures, in particular the mandibular denture. For the long-term group, the denture wearing experience as a whole may be favourable, but more recent changes due to advanced alveolar atrophy may have affected retention, stability or comfort of the denture(s) (Table 6.4).

6.5 Clinical Examination

The systematic approach to the assessment overall should also be developed and followed for the clinical examination. This ensures that a broader evaluation is undertaken even if the patient presents with a request for a specific focus for treatment. The aim is to record any and all clinical information that is relevant to reaching diagnosis and to detect any conditions outside of the normal range.

It is important to document what has been examined and what the findings are. A systematic clinical examination would include both an extraoral and an intraoral examination. In the context of mandibular overdentures, the examination would also include evaluation of the prosthodontic and surgical aspects. The categories to be considered are set out in Table 6.5.

6.5.1   Extraoral

6.5.1.1 Craniomandibular Examination

This involves the examination of the temporomandibular joints and muscles of mastication to detect any symptoms or signs of pain or dysfunction. If any are present, etiological factors should be evaluated together with their possible consequences for prosthodontic rehabilitation [26]. The range of opening of the mandible and range of lateral and protrusive movement should be checked together with deviations during the movements. Deviations and audible sounds such as click and crepitation suggest internal derangement in the joints. Limitations in the range of movement could be a sign of muscle tension, but it could also be a further sign of internal joint derangement.

⚠ Limited opening, for example, can interfere with access for treatment and lead to strain and further discomfort to the patient. Internal derangement in the joints can put a question mark against the most suitable joint position to use for jaw registration. It should be noted that the prevalence of signs and symptoms of temporomandibular disorders amongst edentulous patients has been reported to be low [27]. This prevalence applies to both denture and non-denture wearers.

The extraoral examination should also include palpation of the regional lymph nodes.

This palpation may detect a localised infection. It could also detect more serious underlying conditions.

Movement disorders associated with, for example, Parkinson's disease may also manifest themselves in the face and jaw. They could result in both an increase and a decrease of movement. This would be an important factor to take into consideration for the stability and retention of the prostheses.

6.5.1.2 Facial Examination

This involves the examination of facial proportions and symmetry, midline, lip support and vertical dimension. The lip support and vertical dimension of occlusion are particularly relevant to the partially and completely edentulous patient. Tooth loss and associated atrophy of the alveolar process will lead to a reduction in both. The assessment therefore centres on whether the existing prostheses are restoring both parameters correctly. Often the lip support and the vertical dimension are inadequate. This may be associated with the angular cheilitis or inflammation in the corners of the mouth caused by bacteria or fungal infections.

The lip support and vertical dimension may also be increased. To detect this error, patients with a removable dental prosthesis should be evaluated both with and without the existing prosthesis.

The facial examination should also note any other signs of pathology of the lips and face. This could be signs of paralysis, changes in colour or skin lesions that should be investigated further (Fig. 6.1).

Table 6.5 Clinical examination in overview

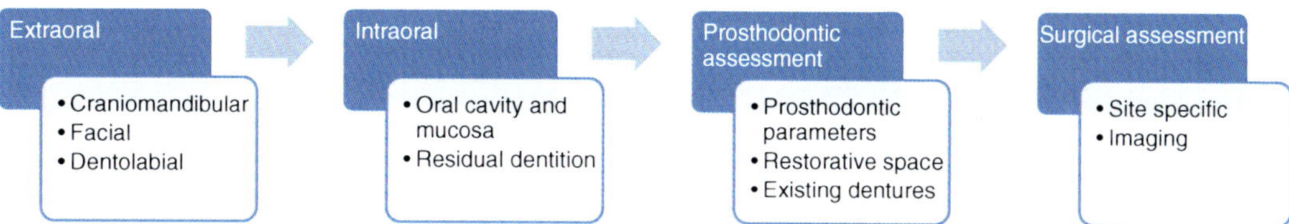

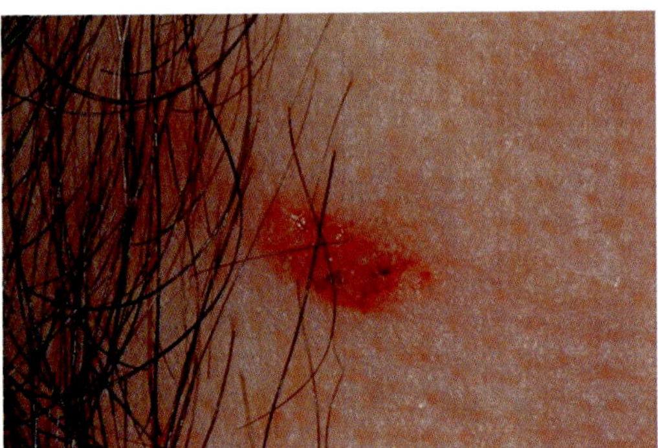

Fig. 6.1 Skin lesion that should be investigated further

6.5.1.3 Dentolabial Examination

This part centres on assessing facial proportions, upper and lower lip support, competency and lines at rest and in smile. It also includes assessment of position and relationship of upper and lower incisors. The position of the incisors is guided by aesthetics and functional requirements. It is helpful to observe the incisors during speech, and phonetics can provide a useful guide to incisal edge position. However, additional investigation via a diagnostic set-up may be needed to assess these parameters properly.

6.5.2 Intraoral Examination

6.5.2.1 Oral Cavity and Mucosa

Regardless of the patient's primary reason for seeking dental attention, regular screening for oral pathology is recognised as an important factor in early detection and diagnosis of oral cancer; early intervention is likely to result in less extensive and more effective treatment. Oral cancer is the largest group of head and neck cancers. It is more common in men than in women, and the vast majority of cases are in people over the age of 50 [28, 29].

In a specific report on the geriatric population, the non-neoplastic lesions outnumbered the neoplastic [30]. The five most prevalent oral lesions in descending order of frequency were squamous cell carcinoma, focal fibrous hyperplasia (irritation fibroma), radicular cyst, osteomyelitis and epithelial dysplasia. The site of predilection was the labial/buccal mucosa, followed by the gingiva, mandibular bone, tongue and maxillary bone, respectively. Figure 6.2a shows a sessile lump that could be related to an underlying saliva gland. It could also interfere with the positioning of a post-dam compression area just anterior to the hard/soft palate vibration line.

Diseases of the oral mucosa may be relevant to both the denture aspect of treatment and to implant therapy. High success rates have been demonstrated for implants in patients affected by these diseases, but the severity of the diseases and medical complications should be evaluated [31]. The diseases may also compromise the patient's ability to maintain adequate oral hygiene. Examples of diseases that affect the oral mucosa are lichen planus, epidermolysis bullosa and Sjögren's syndrome.

The subjective sensation of dry mouth is referred to as xerostomia. This disorder is part of Sjögren's syndrome, but it is also associated with medication, systemic diseases, other pathologies of the salivary glands and head and neck radiotherapy. Xerostomia is a side effect of a large number of drugs, and 70% of adults who take some kind of medication can suffer from it. Xerostomia has clear, negative effects on oral-dental tissue. Some of the best known side effects include demineralisation of tooth enamel, rampant caries, superinfections caused by fungal diseases (candidiasis), reactive gingival enlargement due to dehydration and loss of salivary antimicrobial properties. Xerostomia can also influence ingestion, swallowing and speech articulation, thus negatively affecting the quality of life of people suffering from it [32]. For documentation purposes, the extent of dry mouth should be described, for example, by referral to a dry mouth scale [33], and management should be considered as part of the subsequent treatment planning.

Mucosal findings may also be more specifically related to the existing dentures. The prevalence for at least one mucosal lesion has been reported as 54% [34]. The same study found the three most common lesions to be angular cheilitis (34%), traumatic ulcers (15%) and denture stomatitis (14%) amongst 84 elderly denture wear-

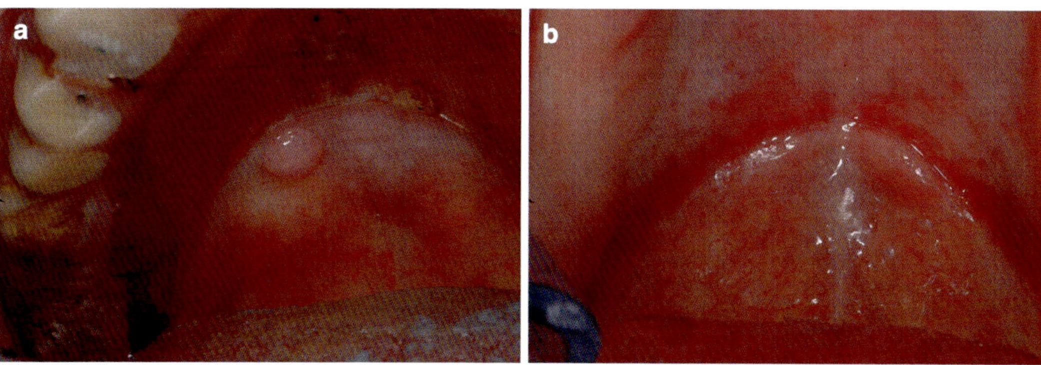

Fig. 6.2 (**a**) Sessile lump in palate in area of potential post-dam compression zone. (**b**) Denture-induced ulcer along post-dam compression area of maxillary denture

ers recruited from geriatric residences and day care centres. In some cases of long-standing mucosal issues, the changes can be so marked as to be sinister in appearance (Fig. 6.2b). As a first measure, further questioning of the patient together with examination of the denture hygiene as well as the dentures(s) in situ may confirm a denture-induced diagnosis [35]. If concern remains, however, appropriate further investigation is required and by referral if necessary. The changes may also require some form of surgical correction, but often the situation will improve through appropriate adjustment of the denture.

A white crest line in the cheek referred to as linea alba and scalloping along the lateral border of the tongue may indicate tooth contact during parafunction.

6.5.2.2 Residual Dentition

The presence of teeth can provide very useful information for the overall assessment and subsequent treatment planning. The patient's level of oral hygiene can be assessed together with evidence of present and past dental disease. Findings include caries, endodontic issues, periodontal disease and tooth surface loss through mechanical attrition or chemical erosion. Evaluation of whether disease is active or controlled is important for the subsequent treatment planning. The presence of localised acute or chronic infection should be noted.

Even a reduced dentition may offer helpful prosthodontic information about the facial pro-

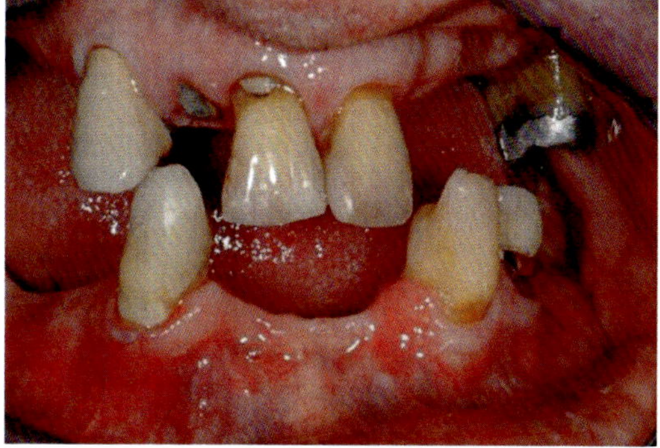

Fig. 6.3 A reduced dentition still offers helpful prosthodontic information

file, incisor relationship, occlusal classification and vertical dimension of occlusion (Fig. 6.3). It is important to document this information in order that it can be used for reference after the teeth have been removed.

It could also be important to determine whether natural teeth could serve as the overdenture abutments, thereby avoiding the need for implant therapy. This could be very relevant in patients who are at risk of medication-related osteonecrosis of the jaw (MRONJ). MRONJ in connection with implant placement is relatively rare, and the risk is considered similar to that of tooth extraction. However, in view of the potentially serious consequences of MRONJ, patients treated with antiresorptive drugs such as high-dose intravenous bisphosphonates are not candidates for implant therapy [36].

6.5.3 Prosthodontic Assessment

The anatomical situation of residual ridges has a bearing on the stability and retention than can be achieved particularly for the mandibular denture. Both the height and the shape of the residual ridge play a part, and continued loss of alveolar bone over time can cause previously stable dentures to become ill-fitting. It has been reported that more than 50% of those with mandibular complete dentures may have problems with stability and retention [4].

There are a number of descriptive classifications for the extent of atrophy of the alveolar ridges. One of these is the often cited Cawood and Howell classification [37] which describes five different stages of alveolar atrophy of the mandible classified as II to VI. A class II ridge is equivalent to the alveolar bone around a retained healthy root with a sound bone support. A mandibular class III retains a good, high and rounded ridge form, whereas class IV is the often seen knife-edge ridge shape. Class V is a flat ridge, and class VI is concave with atrophy extending beyond the original alveolar ridge into the basal bone of the mandible (Fig. 6.4).

In addition to the ridge classification, it is highly relevant to note encroachment by muscles and ligaments on the denture-supporting area. Equally, areas of flabby soft tissues with no underlying bony support will impact on both denture construction and performance and scope for implant placement (Fig. 6.5).

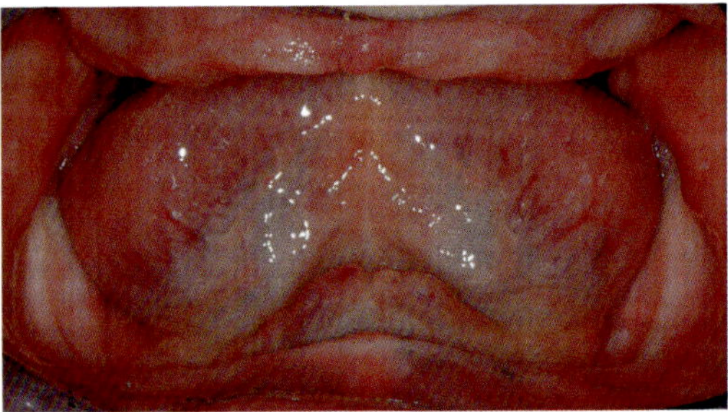

Fig. 6.4 Clinical representation of Cawood and Howell classification class V ridges in both the maxilla and mandible

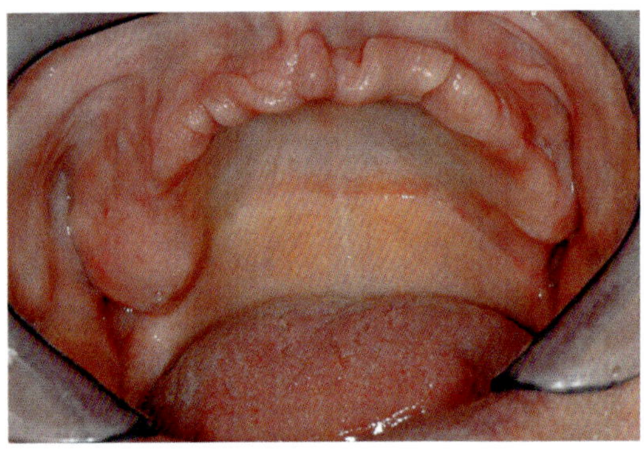

Fig. 6.5 Maxillary arch with prominent posterior ridge form on the right and a flabby anterior ridge

The mucosal status of denture-supporting areas changes in the older patient, and the tissues are likely to be thinner, less resilient and more friable. 🔶 Specifically for implant therapy, the evidence as to the true value of attached, keratinised mucosa in the formation of a stable peri-implant cuff is equivocal [38]. It is suggested, however, that the patient will find it easier to perform oral hygiene around the implant if it has a keratinised cuff. In turn, this may reduce susceptibility to inflammation, recession of the peri-implant mucosa and crestal bone loss.

6.5.3.1 Restorative Space

In a prosthodontically driven approach to implant therapy, the desired parameters of the definitive prostheses determine the appropriate implant configurations and individual implant positions. This ensures that the restorative dimensions are adequate to accommodate the spatial dimensions of both the implant and denture attachment components together with any internal denture reinforcement that may be required. Assessment and definition of the restorative space is therefore a very important consideration.

🔶 The interarch distance has a direct bearing on the vertical dimension of the prostheses and hence the volume for attachment components within. In a Cawood and Howell class III situation, the benefits of a good high ridge may be countered by limited restorative space in which to accommodate denture teeth, body and attachments (Fig. 6.5).

Conversely a class V or class VI ridges are likely to have a correspondingly greater restorative space. Construction of a stable denture in these situations can be challenging. Irrespective of whether implant assistance is planned, the prosthesis stability, comfort and function should be maximised through physiologically optimal denture contours and physiologically appropriate denture tooth arrangement [39].

6.5.3.2 Existing Dentures

The aim of any new dentures is to restore the patient to optimal aesthetics, function and quality of life. As such the evaluation of the patient's existing dentures, both previous and present, against established design principles can provide very helpful pointers to changes required or compromises to be accepted. For example, the patient may present with recent conventional complete dentures constructed in line with optimal design principles, but concerns persist regarding retention, stability and support of one or both dentures. At the other end of the spectrum, the dentures may be unsatisfactory from both a patient and professional point of view. It is also possible that the patient has previous dentures that used to be more successful than the present ones.

The denture evaluation can be divided into assessment of:

- Fit and extension of base
  - Both have a direct bearing on denture support and retention. The examination should determine whether the base has a retentive seal and (Fig. 6.6) the extent to which the existing denture base is making use of the support that is available. Scope for improvement should also be assessed.
- Facial support and position of incisors
  - Restoration of the patient's physiognomy requires correct facial support. This is achieved through a combination of upper and lower lip support. The position of the

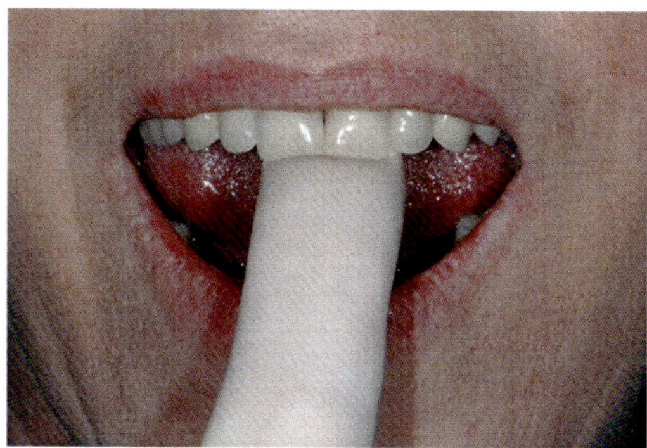

Fig. 6.6 Testing stability and retention of maxillary denture

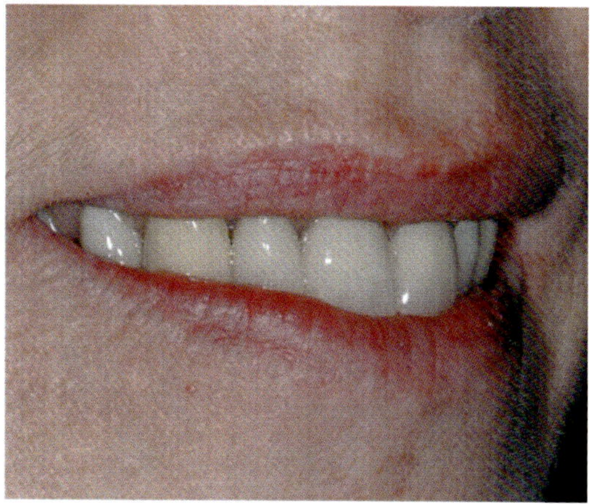

Fig. 6.7 Position of the incisors is guided by a combination of aesthetic and functional requirements

incisors is guided by a combination of aesthetic and functional requirements (Fig. 6.7).
- Jaw relationship
  - A comfortable three-dimensional relationship between the upper and lower jaws requires a correct lower face height and vertical dimension of occlusion as well as a comfortable jaw position.
- Denture occlusion
  - This should be stabilising the position of the mandible against the maxilla. This is important during both static and dynamic occlusion. The posterior teeth should transfer the occlusal load as effectively as possible

to the underlying ridges to aid stability of the dentures and thereby enhance chewing efficiency.

- Features and contours of denture body
  - These should restore the missing tissue volume and assist the patient with muscular control of the denture. They should avoid contours and crevices that may encourage retention of food and buildup of extrinsic stains and complicate oral hygiene removal of bacterial biofilm (Fig. 6.8). Obvious signs of wear and damage should be noted.

The patient's bite force should be assessed (Fig. 6.9). As a rule of thumb, the greater the bite force, the more implant support is indicated for the mandibular overdenture.

Patient satisfaction with a well-constructed maxillary denture can be equal to satisfaction after implant therapy [40]. Even so in an assessment for MI OVD, the potential impact on the performance and satisfaction, positive or negative, of the opposing conventional maxillary denture should be considered.

6.5.4 Surgical Assessment

Where the restorative assessment involves the entire prostheses, the surgical assessment for implant therapy is more site specific. The aim is to relate the prosthodontically preferred implant positions to the anatomical situation of soft and hard tissues at the prospective sites. In addition to the aforementioned presence or absence of keratinised mucosa, the 🟠 evaluation includes assessment of bone volume and proximity to vital structures such the mental foramen and mandibular canal. This assessment has already been covered in detail in the previous chapter in connection with additional investigations via radiographic imaging.

6.6 Radiographic Imaging (See Previous Chapter)

6.7 Additional Investigations

The need for and value of additional investigations have been mentioned throughout the chapter.

6.7.1 Diet-Related Investigations

- Testing masticatory efficiency
  - It is suggested that masticatory efficiency decreases over time regardless of the denture quality [41]. An almond and an artificial food made from a moulding material are the most constantly employed test foods and could also be used as a guide in the dental office as well as in studies [42].

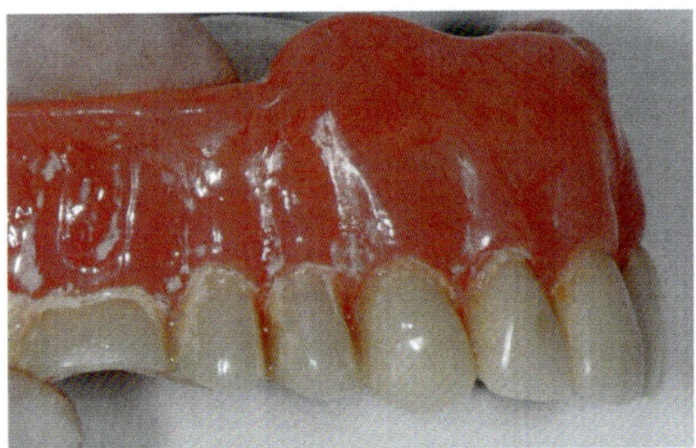

Fig. 6.8 Contours and crevices that encourage calculus formation and food retention

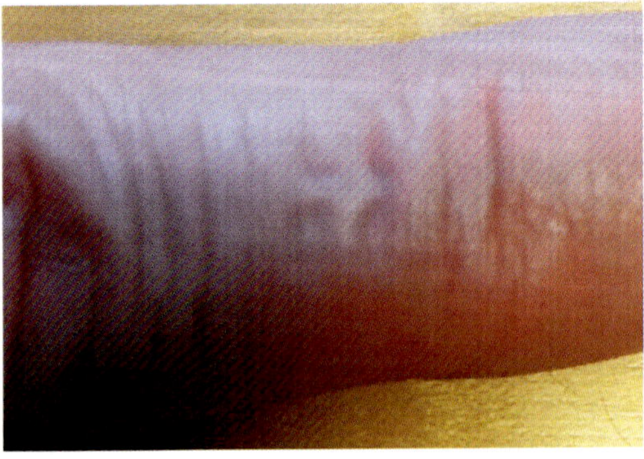

Fig. 6.9 Visible tooth imprint on finger as indication of good bite force

- Diet investigation and analyses [43]
  - Diminished masticatory efficiency may lead to a change in diet. Equally, the restoration of masticatory function via mandibular implant overdenture will not in itself necessarily lead to an improved diet. A diet analysis at the assessment stage can therefore disclose valuable information regarding the need for both functional denture improvement and professional diet advice [44].

6.7.2 Denture-Related Investigations

Diagnostic approach to new dentures:
Can be based on:

- Testing possible changes for improvements by reversible measures
  - This could be by addition of wax to existing dentures to test scope for improvement of denture base extension, lip support and vertical dimension of occlusion (Fig. 6.10).
- Use of photos from the patient's dentate past
  - Useful information about the shape and size of the patient's natural teeth, incisal relationship and facial contours can be gleaned from photos.

- Dental information from dentate relatives
  - Guidance to tooth size, shape and arrangement can in some cases be gained from relatives.

Can lead to:

- Trial/training bases
  - For patients who have a history of difficulty in accepting the presence of dentures, a gradual training process via training base can be very helpful.
- Diagnostic set-up
  - This is essential in a prosthodontically driven approach to implant planning to ensure that the implant placement is determined by and compatible with the planned denture.

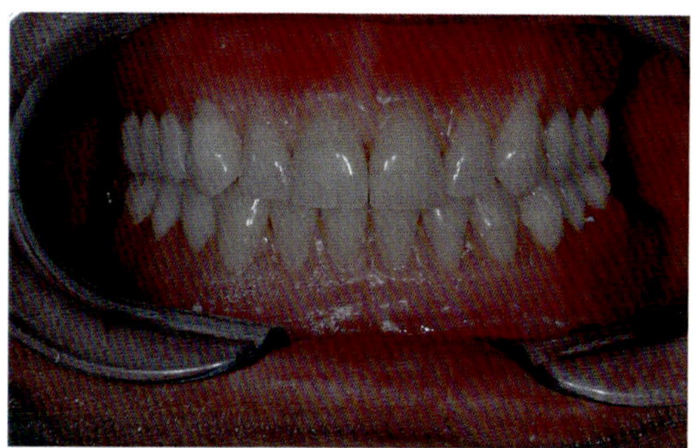

- Radiographic/surgical templates
  - A diagnostic set-up or a successful existing denture can also be the basis for both radiographic and surgical templates to be used in implant planning and to guide placement.

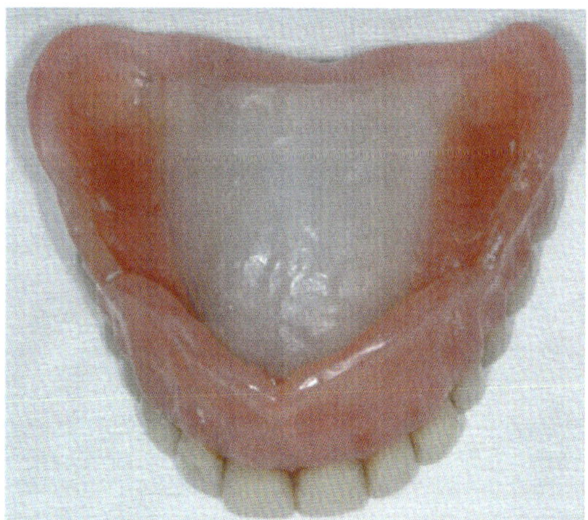

Fig. 6.10 Diagnostic addition of wax to form a post-dam compression area

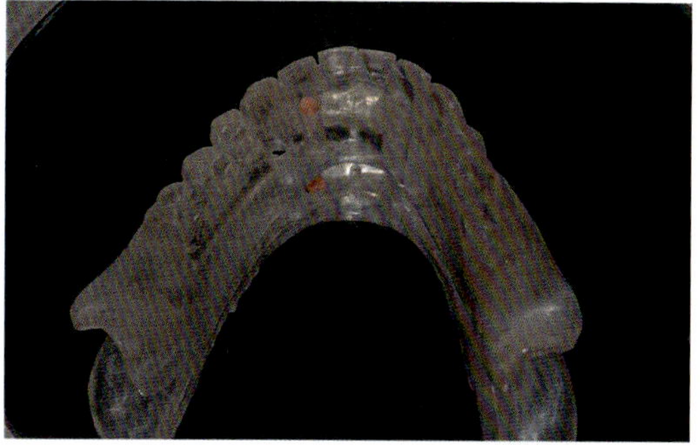

6.8 Diagnoses and Specific Indications for Implant Therapy

Once the clinical assessment is completed, the information is synthesised into diagnoses. In addition to determining the need and scope for treatment, the diagnoses will also be the basis of defining indications for prosthodontic treatment and specific indications for implant therapy. With the potential risks of implant therapy in mind, it is a good idea at this point to consider some form of risk assessment.

6.9 Risk Assessment

It is important to remember that implant therapy is an elective treatment modality with the purpose of facilitating prosthodontic rehabilitation. By its nature, implant placement is also an invasive treatment. Whilst implant therapy is now considered routine, it is clear that implant therapy also presents with differing levels of difficulty and differing degrees of risk for prosthodontic and surgical complications. To ensure that the patient or a legal guardian is able to give full informed consent to treatment, it is important to document that both degree of treatment difficulty and potential risks have been assessed and discussed.

Amongst the information collected during the clinical assessment, there are findings that could influence/impact on treatment complexity and risk modifiers. These have been marked by the symbol . These factors can be used to assess difficulty of the treatment process and risk of complication involved in prospective implant therapy.

The International Team for Implantology (www. iti.org) offers a free online risk assessment tool (https://academy.iti.org) for this purpose. The tool is based on a book entitled *The SAC Classification in Implant Dentistry* [45], and it offers a systematic assessment to identify and document modifying factors and risks, thereby allowing contingency planning to be undertaken to minimise risks and undesirable outcomes (Fig. 6.11).

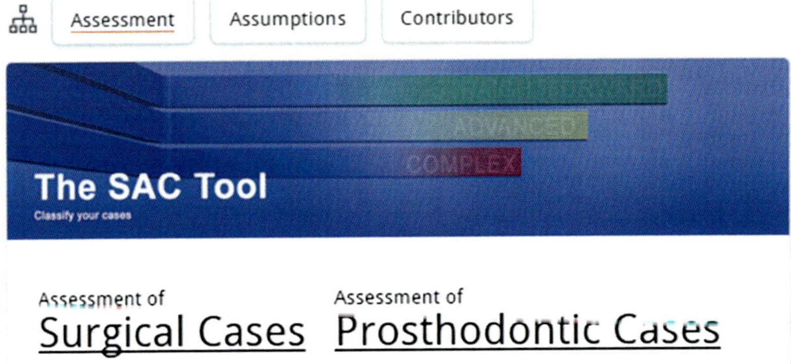

Fig. 6.11 ITI SAC tool

Table 6.6 Examples of patient-modifying factors in an implant therapy risk assessment

Patient expectations
Medical status
Medication
Periodontal status
General oral health
Oral hygiene and compliance
Smoking habit
Access to treatment site
Reasons for tooth loss
Bruxism
Anatomic risk
Bone volume
Keratinised mucosa
Interarch distance
Interim prosthesis needs
Previous implant history

The tool poses a series of questions, and the user selects the most appropriate answer from a number of options. The patient factors highlighted by 🟠 through this clinical assessment chapter (summarised in Table 6.6) will provide the patient-specific information to guide which answer option to select. Depending on the selected answer, the underlying algorithm of the tool will pose further questions until a classification of the case as straightforward, advanced or complex can be offered. The tool also lists modifying factors that should be considered in the further treatment planning.

Conclusion

The clinical assessment is a process of information gathering. It is a comprehensive undertaking, and a systematic approach is helpful to ensure that all relevant aspects have been included. With the particular focus on the older patient and the possibility of implant therapy, this includes consideration of specific factors as well as a risk assessment. A complete clinical assessment forms an important precursor to effective treatment planning and also to ensuring a safe and predictable outcome of the ensuing treatment.

References

1. Doundoulakis JH, Eckert SE, Lindquist CC, Jeffcoat MK. The implant-supported overdenture as an alternative to the complete mandibular denture. J Am Dent Assoc. 2003;134:1455–8.
2. Park JC, Baek WS, Choi SH, Cho KS, Jung UW. Long-term outcomes of dental implants placed in elderly patients: a retrospective clinical and radiographic analysis. Clin Oral Implants Res. 2017;28(2):186–91.
3. Feine JS, Carlsson GE, Awad MA, Chehade A, Duncan WJ, Gizani S, et al. The McGill Consensus Statement on Overdentures. Montreal, Quebec, Canada. May 24-25, 2002. Int J Prosthodont. 2002;15:413–4.
4. Thomason JM, Kelly SA, Bendkowski A, Ellis JS. Two implant retained overdentures—a review of the literature supporting the McGill and York consensus statements. J Dent. 2012;40:22–34.
5. British Society for the Study of Prosthetic Dentistry. The York consensus statement on implant-supported overdentures. Eur J Prosthodont Restor Dent. 2009;17:164–5.
6. Muller F, Salem K, Barbezat C, Herrmann FR, Schimmel M. Knowledge and attitude of elderly persons towards dental implants. Gerodontology. 2012;29:e914–23.
7. Critchlow SB, Ellis JS. Prognostic indicators for conventional complete denture therapy: a review of the literature. J Dent. 2010;38:2–9.
8. Katsoulis J, Schimmel M, Avrampou M, Stuck AE, Mericske-Stern R. Oral and general health status in patients treated in a dental consultation clinic of a geriatric ward in Bern, Switzerland. Gerodontology. 2012;29:e602–10.
9. Pretty IA, Ellwood RP, Lo EC, MacEntee MI, Muller F, Rooney E, et al. The Seattle Care Pathway for securing oral health in older patients. Gerodontology. 2014;31(Suppl 1):77–87.
10. Rockwood K, Song X, MacKnight C, Bergman H, Hogan DB, McDowell I, et al. A global clinical measure of fitness and frailty in elderly people. Can Med Assoc J. 2005;173:489–95.
11. Gil-Montoya JA, Ponce G, Sanchez Lara I, Barrios R, Llodra JC, Bravo M. Association of the oral health impact profile with malnutrition risk in Spanish elders. Arch Gerontol Geriatr. 2013;57(3):398–402.
12. Ellis JS, Levine A, Bedos C, Mojon P, Rosberger Z, Feine J, et al. Refusal of implant supported mandibular overdentures by elderly patients. Gerodontology. 2011;28:62–8.
13. Gauthier S, Reisberg B, Zaudig M, Petersen RC, Ritchie K, Broich K, et al. Mild cognitive impairment. Lancet. 2006;367:1262–70.
14. Awad MA, Feine JS. Measuring patient satisfaction with mandibular prostheses. Community Dent Oral Epidemiol. 1998;26:400–5.
15. Davis DM, Fiske J, Scott B, Radford DR. The emotional effects of tooth loss: a preliminary quantitative study. Br Dent J. 2000;188:503–6.

16. Hyland R, Ellis J, Thomason M, El-Feky A, Moynihan P. A qualitative study on patient perspectives of how conventional and implant-supported dentures affect eating. J Dent. 2009;37:718–23.

17. Trulsson U, Engstrand P, Berggren U, Nannmark U, Branemark PI. Edentulousness and oral rehabilitation: experiences from the patients' perspective. Eur J Oral Sci. 2002;110:417–24.

18. Heydecke G, Thomason JM, Awad MA, Lund JP, Feine JS. Do mandibular implant overdentures and conventional complete dentures meet the expectations of edentulous patients? Quintessence Int. 2008;39:803–9.

19. Heitz-Mayfield LJ, Huynh-Ba G. History of treated periodontitis and smoking as risks for implant therapy. Int J Oral Maxillofac Implants. 2009;24(Suppl):39–68.

20. Ekfeldt A, Christiansson U, Eriksson T, Linden U, Lundqvist S, Rundcrantz T, et al. A retrospective analysis of factors associated with multiple implant failures in maxillae. Clin Oral Implants Res. 2001;12:462–7.

21. Awad MA, Morais JA, Wollin S, Khalil A, Gray-Donald K, Feine JS. Implant overdentures and nutrition: a randomized controlled trial. J Dent Res. 2012;91:39–46.

22. Ellis JS, Elfeky AF, Moynihan PJ, Seal C, Hyland RM, Thomason M. The impact of dietary advice on edentulous adults' denture satisfaction and oral health-related quality of life 6 months after intervention. Clin Oral Implants Res. 2010;21:386–91.

23. Quirynen M, Van Assche N. Microbial changes after full-mouth tooth extraction, followed by 2-stage implant placement. J Clin Periodontol. 2011;38:581–9.

24. Kayser AF. Shortened dental arches and oral function. J Oral Rehabil. 1981;8:457–62.

25. Gerritsen AE, Witter DJ, Bronkhorst EM, Creugers NH. An observational cohort study on shortened dental arches—clinical course during a period of 27-35 years. Clin Oral Investig. 2013;17:859–66.

26. Chisnoiu AM, Picos AM, Popa S, Chisnoiu PD, Lascu L, Picos A, et al. Factors involved in the etiology of temporomandibular disorders—a literature review. Clujul Med. 2015;88:473–8.

27. Dervis E. Changes in temporomandibular disorders after treatment with new complete dentures. J Oral Rehabil. 2004;31:320–6.

28. Scully C, Kirby J. Statement on mouth cancer diagnosis and prevention. Br Dent J. 2014;216:37–8.

29. Petersen PE. Oral cancer prevention and control—the approach of the World Health Organization. Oral Oncol. 2009;45:454–60.

30. Dhanuthai K, Rojanawatsirivej S, Somkotra T, Shin HI, Hong SP, Darling M, et al. Geriatric oral lesions: a multicentric study. Geriatr Gerontol Int. 2016;16(2):237–43.

31. Candel-Marti ME, Ata-Ali J, Penarrocha-Oltra D, Penarrocha-Diago M, Bagan JV. Dental implants in patients with oral mucosal alterations: an update. Med Oral Patol Oral Cir Bucal. 2011;16:e787–93.

32. Miranda-Rius J, Brunet-Llobet L, Lahor-Soler E, Farre M. Salivary secretory disorders, inducing drugs, and clinical management. Int J Med Sci. 2015;12:811–24.

33. Challacombe SJ, Proctor GB. Clinical assessment. Br Dent J. 2014;217:486.

34. Martori E, Ayuso-Montero R, Martinez-Gomis J, Vinas M, Peraire M. Risk factors for denture-related oral mucosal lesions in a geriatric population. J Prosthet Dent. 2014;111:273–9.

35. Freitas JB, Gomez RS, De Abreu MH, Ferreira EFE. Relationship between the use of full dentures and mucosal alterations among elderly Brazilians. J Oral Rehabil. 2008;35:370–4.

36. Ruggiero SL, Dodson TB, Fantasia J, Goodday R, Aghaloo T, Mehrotra B, et al. American Association of Oral and Maxillofacial Surgeons position paper on medication-related osteonecrosis of the jaw—2014 update. J Oral Maxillofac Surg. 2014;72:1938–56.

37. Cawood JI, Howell RA. A classification of the edentulous jaws. Int J Oral Maxillofac Surg. 1988;17:232–6.

38. Wennstrom JL, Derks J. Is there a need for keratinized mucosa around implants to maintain health and tissue stability? Clin Oral Implants Res. 2012;23(Suppl 6):136–46.

39. Cagna DR, Massad JJ, Schiesser FJ. The neutral zone revisited: from historical concepts to modern application. J Prosthet Dent. 2009;101:405–12.

40. Thomason JM, Heydecke G, Feine JS, Ellis JS. How do patients perceive the benefit of reconstructive dentistry with regard to oral health-related quality of life and patient satisfaction? A systematic review. Clin Oral Implants Res. 2007;18:168–88.

41. Ribeiro JA, de Resende CM, Lopes AL, Mestriner W Jr, Roncalli AG, Farias-Neto A, et al. Evaluation of complete denture quality and masticatory efficiency in denture wearers. Int J Prosthodont. 2012;25:625–30.

42. Oliveira NM, Shaddox LM, Toda C, Paleari AG, Pero AC, Compagnoni MA. Methods for evaluation of masticatory efficiency in conventional complete denture wearers: a systematized review. Oral Health Dent Manag. 2014;13:757–62.

43. Moynihan PJ, Bradbury J, Müller F. Dietary consequences of oral health in frail elders. In: MI ME, Müller F, Wyatt C, editors. Oral healthcare and the frail elder: a clinical perspective. Ames: Wiley-Blackwell; 2011. p. 73–95.

44. Müller F, Nitschke I. Oral health, dental state and nutrition in older adults. Zeitschrift für Gerontologie und Geriatrie. 2005;38:334–41.

45. Dawson A, Chen S. The SAC Classification in implant dentistry. Berlin: Quintessence Publishing Co. Ltd. 2009.

Further Reading

The *SAC Classification in Implant Dentistry* jointly published by the ITI and the Quintessence Publishing Group (Dawson and Chen 2009)

Training standards in implant dentistry: Faculty of General Dental Practice, The Royal College of Surgeons of England. Available from: http://www.fgdp.org.uk/pdf/training_stds_imp_dent_guide_2008.pdf; 2008

Elham Emami and Pierre-Luc Michaud

Abstract

Many individuals are exposed to worse oral and general health when they transition from dentate to edentate status. In fact, edentulism is associated with high levels of physical and psychological disability, which are only partially reduced with the use of conventional prostheses as replacement for the missing natural teeth. The implant-assisted overdenture has thus become a viable option to replace denture because of the accumulating evidence on its advantages from both clinical and patient perspectives.

Various types of implant-assisted prostheses are available to treat partially or completely edentate patients. The functional capacity, time needed to treat, maintenance, complications and cost vary amongst the different types of implant prostheses and may address patients' physical, psychological and social needs in different ways. To ensure the delivery of high-quality implant care within the available options, clinicians need to consult the literature and become aware of scientific evidence, exchange this knowledge with their patients and consider the level of their clinical expertise, as well as patients' needs and preferences, to make a shared treatment decision and arrive at an agreement on the treatment to implement.

In this chapter, the authors distinguish between fixed and removable options for mandibular implant-assisted prostheses and provide a summary on different factors that should be considered in the choice between these two prosthetic designs.

E. Emami, D.D.S., M.Sc., Ph.D. (✉)
Department of Restorative Dentistry, Faculty of Dentistry, Université de Montréal,
Montreal, QC, Canada
e-mail: Elham.emami@mcgill.ca

P.-L. Michaud, D.M.D., M.Sc., F.R.C.D.(C)
Department of Dental Clinical Sciences, Faculty of Dentistry, Dalhousie University, Halifax, NS, Canada
e-mail: PL.Michaud@dal.ca

7.1 Mandibular Implant-Assisted Prostheses: Classification

In general, classification of prostheses depends on arch coverage (complete or partial) and anchorage (fixed or removable). Regarding implant-assisted prostheses, other subcategorizations may include the type of support, type of superstructure and infrastructure design (number and position of implants) and prosthetic materials.

© Springer International Publishing AG, part of Springer Nature 2018
E. Emami, J. Feine (eds.), *Mandibular Implant Prostheses*,
https://doi.org/10.1007/978-3-319-71181-2_7

7.1.1 Implant-Assisted Fixed Prostheses

The terms *implant-assisted fixed complete prosthesis*, *implant fixed complete denture* or *implant fixed complete prosthesis* all describe a prosthesis that is entirely supported by implants and covers the entire arch (Fig. 7.1a–e) [1, 2]. This type of prosthesis (previously known as a hybrid prosthesis) is directly connected to its superstructure using screws and, therefore, can only be removed by the clinician. Implant-fixed prostheses can be made of a substructure of metal or zirconia layered with porcelain, a metallic substructure layered with

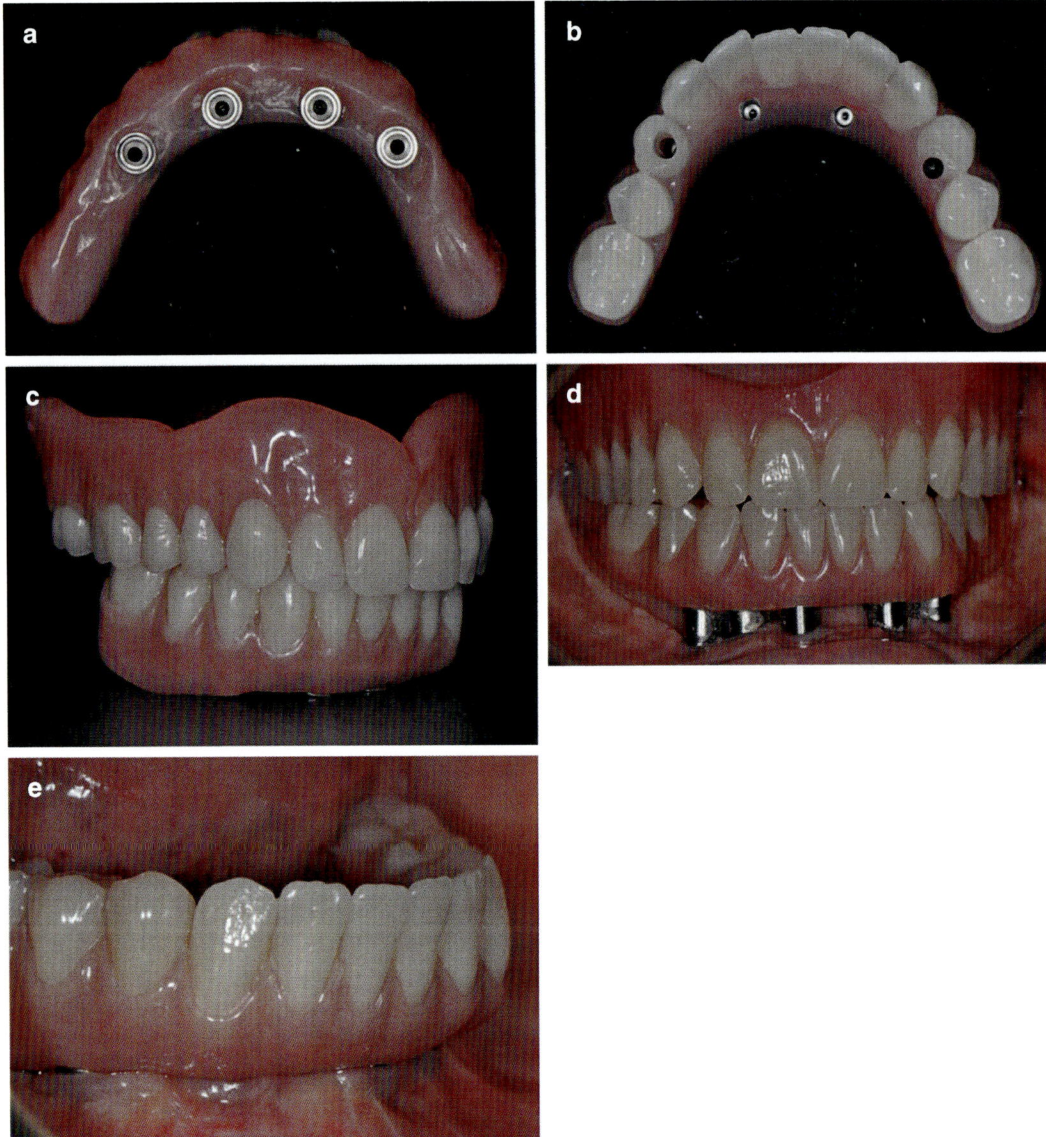

Fig. 7.1 Implant-assisted fixed prosthesis (Courtesy of Dr. Samer Abi-Nader). (**a**) View from under the prosthesis. (**b**) Occlusal view. (**c**) Lateral view. (**d**) Implant-fixed metal-acrylic mandibular prosthesis with long abutments to create space between the prosthesis and the gingiva to help better oral hygiene. (**e**) Implant-fixed metal-acrylic mandibular prosthesis without space between the gingiva and prosthesis, making it harder to clean but causing less food trapping and phonetic problems

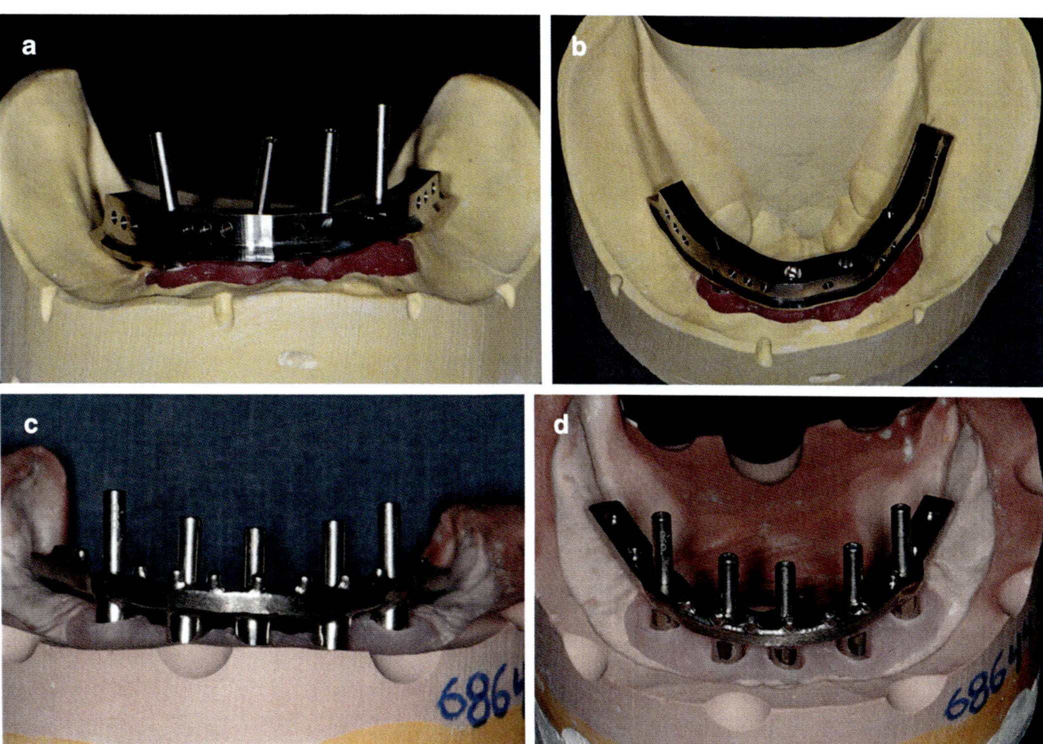

Fig. 7.2 (**a**, **b**) Metal structure used in implant-assisted fixed prosthesis with metal polished surface underneath. (**c**, **d**) Metal structure used in implant-assisted fixed prosthesis with a wrap-around acrylic design (Courtesy of Dr. Samer Abi-Nader and Dr. Pierre-Luc Michaud)

acrylic, or monolithic zirconia [2]. Metal-acrylic implant-assisted fixed prostheses could be fabricated with a metallic gingival surface underneath (Fig. 7.2a, b) or with a wrap-around acrylic design (Figs. 7.1 and 7.2c, d). A metallic smooth surface is usually easier to clean and more hygienic compared to an acrylic surface, which is more porous. However, a wrap-around acrylic design offers more adjustment possibilities since acrylic resin may be added to fill spaces, for example, in situations when patients complain of air escaping through the space, with associated phonetic problems [2].

7.1.2 Implant-Assisted Removable Prostheses

The terms *implant-assisted removable prosthesis*, *implant-assisted removable complete prosthesis* or *implant overdenture* refer to a prosthesis that is connected to implants via various types of attachment and that can be removed by the patient (Fig. 7.3a, b) [1, 2]. Implant-assisted removable prostheses can be supported by implants alone (*implant-supported overdenture*) via a rigid bar with posterior extensions (Figs. 7.3b and 7.4c) or by implant attachments and soft tissues (*tissue-implant-supported overdenture*) (Fig. 7.4b) [2, 3]. While the implant-supported overdenture gets both its support and retention across the entire arch via a bar with cantilevers, the tissue-implant-supported overdenture gets its retention and anterior support from the implant superstructure, such as a cantilever-free ovoid/round bar, and its posterior support from mucosal tissues. Finally, implant overdentures are called tissue-supported overdentures or implant-retained overdentures when their support is solely through the soft tissue, but their retention is obtained by individual abutments with vertical relief such as stud abutments (e.g., Locator) (Figs. 7.3a and 7.4a). Figure 7.4 shows different types of superstructure used within removable overdenture.

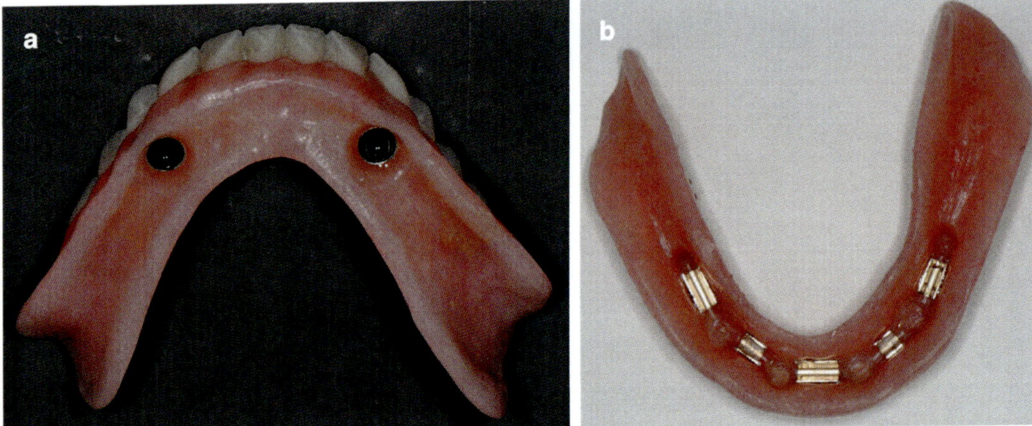

Fig. 7.3 Implant-assisted removable prostheses (Courtesy of Dr. Samer Abi-Nader and Dr. Pierre-Luc Michaud). (**a**) Two locator attachments provide retention and anterior support for the prosthesis. (**b**) A long Dolder bar with cantilevers provides retention and most of the anterior and posterior support for the prosthesis

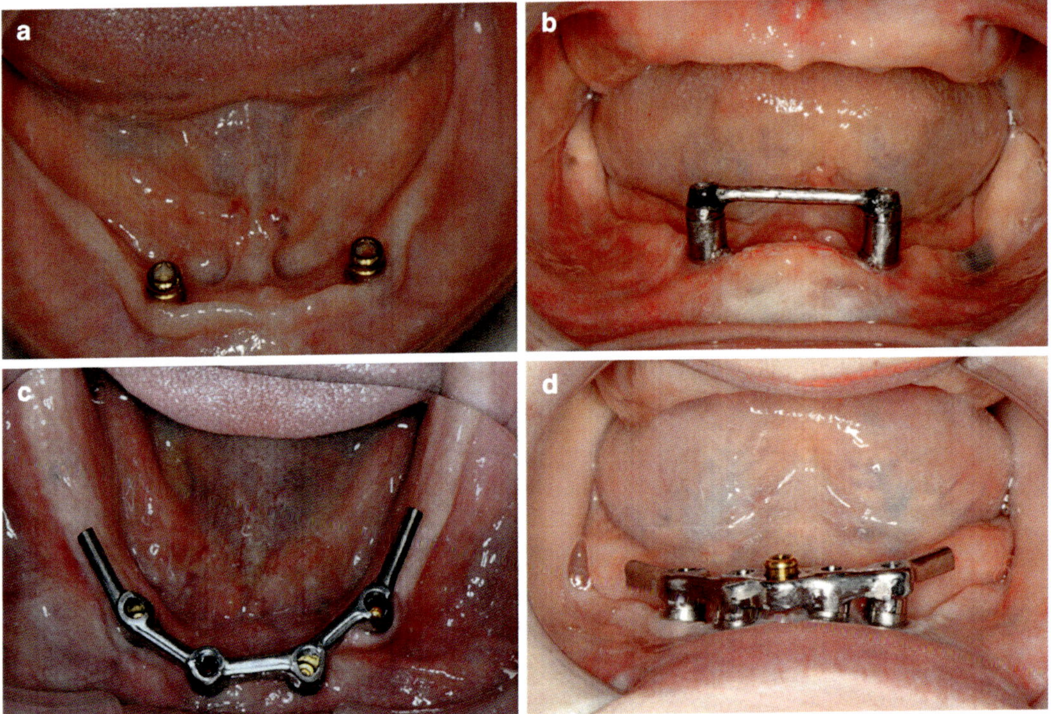

Fig. 7.4 Types of superstructure used in removable implant overdenture (Courtesy of Dr. Samer Abi-Nader and Dr. Pierre-Luc Michaud). (**a**) Locator abutments. (**b**) Dolder bar without cantilever. (**c**) Long Dolder bar with bilateral cantilevers. (**d**) Long Dolder bar with bilateral cantilevers and a Locator abutment on its surface

7.2 Towards the Favourable Choice of Treatment for Edentate Mandible

7.2.1 Clinical Considerations

A successful prosthetic treatment depends upon an ideal treatment planning that is comprehensive and evidence-based. A complete assessment of various factors will indicate which of the different treatment modalities available will be the most appropriate choice for a particular patient.

The consideration of implant-assisted prostheses as a treatment choice for the edentate mandible should start with a discussion with the patient explaining the prosthetic choices, their advantages and limitations as well as the anatomical constraints, and asking them their needs and preferences. To inform patients on the evidence-based advantages of implant prostheses, the clinician can explain how implants prevent bone resorption, improve denture stability and retention, increase chewing capacity and masticatory efficacy, decrease soft tissue trauma and associated ulceration and pain, as well as enhance satisfaction and quality of life [4–21]. According to the latest meta-analysis on this subject, including 11 randomized controlled trials published since 1995, other factors such as health status, oral condition and patient characteristics should also be discussed and considered in treatment planning [21]. During this process of shared decision-making, clinicians may notice that, for some of their patients, conventional dentures will remain their first choice because of satisfaction with the current conventional denture, fear of surgical risk and cost of treatment [22, 23]. The factors influencing their refusal of implant-assisted prostheses should then be considered by the clinician to tailor the best treatment choice for the patient. Since cost is one of the most important limiting factors for a large part of the population, offering a prosthesis with a minimum number of implants may impact on the decision of prosthesis type. For these patients, a prosthesis requiring only a single mandibular implant could make implant-assisted treatment possible [24]. Since with fixed prostheses, a minimum of four implants are required [25], this option should be automatically eliminated from the treatment plan when patients cannot afford high treatment costs. Similarly, for patients requiring surgical bone augmentation, if fear of surgery and cost restrain their choice of treatment, implant-assisted removable prostheses could be considered to reduce both morbidity and cost [26–28].

Other conditions may also steer the decision towards removable rather than fixed prostheses. For instance, in anatomical conditions where there are moderate to severe vertical and horizontal atrophy, a concave and prognathic profile, inadequate lip support and phonetic problems, implant-assisted removable prostheses are preferable [29, 30] because they allow the construction of labial acrylic flanges and help to provide aesthetic lip support. Implant-fixed prostheses are usually not recommended if lip support needs to be enhanced. Nevertheless, in such cases, implant-fixed mandibular prostheses produce fewer aesthetic complications than their maxillary counterparts because of reduced vertical lip movement and lesser need for lip support.

People with acquired or congenital oral and maxillofacial defects could also greatly benefit from implant-assisted removable prostheses, which can be easily removed for check-up appointments and when complications occur [26]. Removable designs may also be preferable in elders who may lack dexterity and have limited visual acuity and in general for patients with poor oral hygiene [28, 31, 32], because these prostheses are much easier to clean. It is more difficult to clean under fixed prostheses because floss has to be threaded between the implants, but depending on the design of the fixed prosthesis, ease of hygiene can vary greatly (Fig. 7.1d, e). Patients whose tongues cannot reach the palate (tongue hypomobility) could also benefit from the shortened distance offered by the acrylic thickness of overdentures, and the use of a fixed prosthesis in these cases could cause speech problems. Furthermore, when the opposing arch is dentate or restored with an implant-fixed prosthesis and the potential for parafunctional activity is present, an implant-assisted removable prosthesis is recommended because it can be removed at night which may help decrease the rate of biomechanical complications [33]. However, a larger denture-bearing area is covered, and more attached soft tissue is necessary with removable prostheses. Thus, patients with high muscle attachments, sensitive mandibular ridges or tori or knife-edge ridges may be more satisfied with fixed prostheses [26].

Fixed prostheses are also often recommended for younger edentate patients, those who psychologically could not tolerate the sense of tooth loss, those suffering from prosthetic-related recurrent sores and patients with an excessive gag reflex [26].

If the vertical space is limited and there is no need to replace soft or hard tissues, a fixed prosthesis is usually the best option, as there would otherwise be no space to accommodate acrylic flanges associated with removable prostheses. When only 8–10 mm of vertical space is available between the soft tissue and the occlusal plane, the treatment of choice is to use an implant-fixed porcelain fused to metal restoration [25]. With less than 8 mm, the outcome could have poor aesthetics due to very short crowns, and soft and/or hard tissue remodelling should be considered [25]. If more soft or hard tissues have to be replaced vertically by the prosthesis, a fixed restoration consisting of acrylic supported by a metallic bar (Figs. 7.1 and 7.2) could be used instead of a porcelain fused to metal prosthesis. The advantages of this type of prosthesis are the absence of dark triangles, lower cost and easier maintenance and repairs. The optimal vertical space for this type of implant-fixed restoration is 15 mm [25]. With a vertical space of more than 15 mm, a horizontal defect will usually also be present due to the angulation of the alveolar bone. Using implant-fixed prostheses in such defects could lead to aesthetic problems, such as long and/or flared teeth, black triangles and visible abutments [34, 35] and may also cause excessive air space and additional speech problems [26]. In these cases, in order to enhance the aesthetic outcome, it is suggested to use implant-assisted removable prostheses to fill the defects by using acrylic flanges.

Removable prostheses are indicated when the anteroposterior bone resorption exceeds 10 mm [36]. If implant-assisted removable prostheses are chosen for the treatment of edentate patients, it is important to ensure having sufficient inter-arch space for the substructure and to consider recontouring the bone to obtain enough space for the substructure when needed [37]. Individual attachments such as Locator abutments, ball attachments and magnets could be used with an interarch space of 12 mm [25, 38]. More space is required to accommodate the space below the bar, the bar itself, the clips, the acrylic and the teeth. Usually, for a standard Dolder bar, 15 mm is necessary [25, 38]. In certain situations where not enough inter-implant space exists, it might not be possible to use clips. Locator abutments could be placed on top of the bar (Fig. 7.4d), but with this design, up to 20 mm of vertical space might be necessary.

Summary Table: Comparison between fixed and removable implant-assisted prostheses (Adapted from: Implant-assisted complete prostheses, Emami E, Michaud PL, Sallaleh I, Feine JS. Periodontol 2000. 2014 Oct;66(1):119–31. doi: https://doi.org/10.1111/prd.12041) [2]

| | Mandibular implant-assisted prosthesis | |
	Removable	Fixed
Indications	• Severe bone loss	• Mild/moderate bone loss
	• Vertical space required: – Locator abutments: ~12 mm – Dolder bar: ~15 mm – Dolder bar with locator attachments: ~20 mm	• Vertical space required: – PFM: ~8–10 mm – Metal-acrylic: ~15 mm
	• Oral/maxillofacial defects	• No horizontal bone loss
	• Patients lacking dexterity	• Psychological needs
	• Malpositioned implants	• Younger patients
	• High nocturnal parafunction	
	• Financial limitation	

	Mandibular implant-assisted prosthesis	
	Removable	Fixed
Advantages	• Easier to clean	• Can be made of acrylic or porcelain
	• No air trap during speech	• Aesthetics
	• Provides lip support	• Higher bite force
	• Technically easier to make and repair	• Better stability/retention
Disadvantages	• More mucosal problems	• More implants required
	• Wear of components	• Accumulation of food posteriorly
		• More difficult and expensive to make, adjust and redo

7.3 Research Evidence

The results of the studies and systematic reviews reporting on disease-oriented and patient-centred outcomes in regard to mandibular implant-assisted prostheses demonstrated favourable outcomes regardless of the prosthetic design (fixed or removable) or the type of attachments [39–42]. Biological complications such as peri-implantitis, peri-mucositis, tissue hyperplasia, peri-implant bone loss and residual ridge resorption have been reported for both types of treatment.

According to the systematic review conducted by Bryant et al. [42] in 2007, there is no difference in implant survival, success rate and peri-implant bone loss between these two types of treatment. The pooled implant survival for mandibular fixed and removable prostheses was more than 90% at 10 years. The success rate ranged from 71 to 95.7%. The peri-implant bone loss was 1.2 mm after the first year of prosthesis function and up to 0.4 mm per subsequent year. In regard to mandibular two-implant removable prostheses, a cumulative success rate of 97% and 96% was reported after 12 years and 20 years of follow-up, respectively [43]. Numerous studies reported non-significant marginal bone loss with the use of implant-assisted removable prostheses [44–46]. Failures caused by peri-implant infection were rarely reported. Most failures occurred before loading and were mostly due to bone quality and quantity rather than the type of prosthesis [47]. Wright et al. [48] compared the effect of two-implant overdenture and fixed prostheses on bone resorption over a period of 7 years and showed a low rate of residual ridge resorption with removable prostheses and bone apposition with implant-fixed prostheses.

Also, according to longitudinal studies, fixed prostheses showed less soft tissue complications than their removable counterparts. The most prevalent soft tissue complication, especially with the use of bars, was hyperplasia [45, 49]. Wear or fracture of prosthetic components, loosening and wear of retentive mechanisms, as well as maintenance needs (remakes, relines and adjustments), have been reported for both types of prosthesis and seem to be more prevalent for removable prostheses than for fixed prostheses [50–55]. Loosening of the overdenture retention mechanism was the most prevalent complication (33%), followed by relines (19%) and clip/attachment fracture (16%) [54]. Higher maintenance rate have been reported for those implant-fixed prostheses that are opposed by fixed prostheses, compared to those opposed by natural teeth or conventional complete prostheses [50, 52].

Study findings also showed that using implant-assisted prostheses leads to greater improvement in patient satisfaction and oral health-related quality of life compared to conventional prostheses. According to these studies, equal numbers of patients expressed preference for each of the two types of implant-assisted prosthesis (fixed or removable) [27]. Research has also shown that elders' preference is towards removable implant prostheses, with the ease of cleaning being the most important factor in their decision-making. Those who prefer fixed prostheses usually rank stability as the most important factor [56]. Research evidence suggests that the fixed option better addresses the needs of patients in regard to chewing ability [27, 28].

Although there is a paucity in terms of economic analyses, evidence shows that, in the long term, mandibular implant-assisted removable prostheses are more cost effective than implant-fixed prostheses [57–60].

References

1. Simon H, Yanase RT. Terminology for implant prostheses. Int J Oral Maxillofac Implants. 2003;18(4):539–43.
2. Emami E, Michaud PL, Sallaleh I, Feine JS. Implant-assisted complete prostheses. Periodontol. 2014;66(1):119–31. https://doi.org/10.1111/prd.12041.
3. Zitzmann NU, Marinello CP. A review of clinical and technical considerations for fixed and removable implant prostheses in the edentulous mandible. Int J Prosthodont. 2002;15(1):65–72.
4. Wyatt CC. The effect of prosthodontic treatment on alveolar bone loss: a review of the literature. J Prosthet Dent. 1998;80(3):362–6.
5. Carlsson GE. Responses of jawbone to pressure. Gerodontology. 2004;21(2):65–70.
6. Emami E, de Grandmont P, Rompre PH, Barbeau J, Pan S, Feine JS. Favoring trauma as an etiological factor in denture stomatitis. J Dent Res. 2008;87(5):440–4.
7. Raghoebar GM, Meijer HJ, Stegenga B, van't Hof MA, van Oort RP, Vissink A. Effectiveness of three treatment modalities for the edentulous mandible. A five-year randomized clinical trial. Clin Oral Implants Res. 2000;11(3):195–201.
8. Pan S, Dagenais M, Thomason JM, Awad M, Emami E, Kimoto S, et al. Does mandibular edentulous bone height affect prosthetic treatment success? J Dent. 2010;38(11):899–907.
9. Awad MA, Lund JP, Dufresne E, Feine JS. Comparing the efficacy of mandibular implant-retained overdentures and conventional dentures among middle-aged edentulous patients: satisfaction and functional assessment. Int J Prosthodont. 2003;16(2):117–22.
10. Heydecke G, Locker D, Awad MA, Lund JP, Feine JS. Oral and general health-related quality of life with conventional and implant dentures. Community Dent Oral Epidemiol. 2003;31(3):161–8.
11. Allen PF, McMillan AS. A longitudinal study of quality of life outcomes in older adults requesting implant prostheses and complete removable dentures. Clin Oral Implants Res. 2003;14(2):173–9.
12. Wismeijer D, Van Waas MA, Vermeeren JI, Mulder J, Kalk W. Patient satisfaction with implant-supported mandibular overdentures. A comparison of three treatment strategies with ITI-dental implants. Int J Oral Maxillofac Surg. 1997;26(4):263–7.
13. Boerrigter EM, Geertman ME, Van Oort RP, Bouma J, Raghoebar GM, van Waas MA, et al. Patient satisfaction with implant-retained mandibular overdentures. A comparison with new complete dentures not retained by implants—a multicentre randomized clinical trial. Br J Oral Maxillofac Surg. 1995;33(5):282–8.
14. Raghoebar GM, Meijer HJ, van't Hof M, Stegenga B, Vissink A. A randomized prospective clinical trial on the effectiveness of three treatment modalities for patients with lower denture problems. A 10 year follow-up study on patient satisfaction. Int J Oral Maxillofac Surg. 2003;32(5):498–503.
15. Watson RM, Jemt T, Chai J, Harnett J, Heath MR, Hutton JE, et al. Prosthodontic treatment, patient response, and the need for maintenance of complete implant-supported overdentures: an appraisal of 5 years of prospective study. Int J Prosthodont. 1997;10(4):345–54.
16. Emami E, Heydecke G, Rompre PH, de Grandmont P, Feine JS. Impact of implant support for mandibular dentures on satisfaction, oral and general health-related quality of life: a meta-analysis of randomized-controlled trials. Clin Oral Implants Res. 2009;20(6):533–44.
17. Ellis JS, Burawi G, Walls A, Thomason JM. Patient satisfaction with two designs of implant supported removable overdentures; ball attachment and magnets. Clin Oral Implants Res. 2009;20(11):1293–8.
18. Bouma J, Boerrigter LM, Van Oort RP, van Sonderen E, Boering G. Psychosocial effects of implant-retained overdentures. Int J Oral Maxillofac Implants. 1997;12(4):515–22.
19. Meijer HJ, Raghoebar GM, Van 't Hof MA, Visser A, Geertman ME, Van Oort RP. A controlled clinical trial of implant-retained mandibular overdentures; five-years' results of clinical aspects and aftercare of IMZ implants and Branemark implants. Clin Oral Implants Res. 2000;11(5):441–7.
20. de Albuquerque Junior RF, Lund JP, Tang L, Larivee J, de Grandmont P, Gauthier G, et al. Within-subject comparison of maxillary long-bar implant-retained prostheses with and without palatal coverage: patient-based outcomes. Clin Oral Implants Res. 2000;11(6):555–65.
21. Kodama N, Singh BP, Cerutti-Kopplin D, Feine J, Emami E. Efficacy of mandibular 2-implant overdenture: an updated meta-analysis on patient-based outcomes. Clin Trans Res. 2016;01(01):20–30.
22. Palmqvist S, Soderfeldt B, Arnbjerg D. Subjective need for implant dentistry in a Swedish population aged 45-69 years. Clin Oral Implants Res. 1991;2(3):99–102.
23. Walton JN, MacEntee MI. Choosing or refusing oral implants: a prospective study of edentulous volunteers for a clinical trial. Int J Prosthodont. 2005;18(6):483–8.
24. Walton JN, Glick N, Macentee MI. A randomized clinical trial comparing patient satisfaction and prosthetic outcomes with mandibular overdentures retained by one or two implants. Int J Prosthodont. 2009;22(4):331–9.
25. Misch CE. Contemporary implant dentistry. 3rd ed. St. Louis, MI: Mosby-Elsevier; 2008. 1102 p.
26. DeBoer J. Edentulous implants: overdenture versus fixed. J Prosthet Dent. 1993;69(4):386–90.
27. de Grandmont P, Feine JS, Tache R, Boudrias P, Donohue WB, Tanguay R, et al. Within-subject

comparisons of implant-supported mandibular prostheses: psychometric evaluation. J Dent Res. 1994;73(5):1096–104.

28. Feine JS, de Grandmont P, Boudrias P, Brien N, LaMarche C, Tache R, et al. Within-subject comparisons of implant-supported mandibular prostheses: choice of prosthesis. J Dent Res. 1994;73(5):1105–11.

29. Zitzmann NU, Marinello CP. Treatment outcomes of fixed or removable implant-supported prostheses in the edentulous maxilla. Part I: patients' assessments. J Prosthet Dent. 2000;83(4):424–33.

30. Zitzmann NU, Marinello CP. Treatment plan for restoring the edentulous maxilla with implant-supported restorations: removable overdenture versus fixed partial denture design. J Prosthet Dent. 1999;82(2):188–96.

31. Heydecke G, Boudrias P, Awad MA, De Albuquerque RF, Lund JP, Feine JS. Within-subject comparisons of maxillary fixed and removable implant prostheses: patient satisfaction and choice of prosthesis. Clin Oral Implants Res. 2003;14(1):125–30.

32. Brennan M, Houston F, O'Sullivan M, O'Connell B. Patient satisfaction and oral health-related quality of life outcomes of implant overdentures and fixed complete dentures. Int J Oral Maxillofac Implants. 2010;25(4):791–800.

33. Misch CE. In: Rudolph P, editor. Dental implant prosthetics. St. Louis, MI: Mosby-Elsevier; 2005. 626 p.

34. Mericske-Stern RD, Taylor TD, Belser U. Management of the edentulous patient. Clin Oral Implants Res. 2000;11(Suppl 1):108–25.

35. Mertens C, Steveling HG. Implant-supported fixed prostheses in the edentulous maxilla: 8-year prospective results. Clin Oral Implants Res. 2011;22(5):464–72.

36. Drago C, Carpentieri J. Treatment of maxillary jaws with dental implants: guidelines for treatment. J Prosthodont. 2011;20(5):336–47.

37. Michaud PL, Patel A. Hereditary gingival fibromatosis with extreme ridge thickness and insufficient interarch distance: a clinical report of surgical and prosthetic management. J Prosthet Dent. 2016;116(1):15–20.

38. Trakas T, Michalakis K, Kang K, Hirayama H. Attachment systems for implant retained overdentures: a literature review. Implant Dent. 2006;15(1):24–34.

39. Quirynen M, Alsaadi G, Pauwels M, Haffajee A, van Steenberghe D, Naert I. Microbiological and clinical outcomes and patient satisfaction for two treatment options in the edentulous lower jaw after 10 years of function. Clin Oral Implants Res. 2005;16(3):277–87.

40. Cehreli MC, Karasoy D, Kokat AM, Akca K, Eckert S. A systematic review of marginal bone loss around implants retaining or supporting overdentures. Int J Oral Maxillofac Implants. 2010;25(2):266–77.

41. SH O, Kim Y, Park JY, Jung YJ, Kim SK, Park SY. Comparison of fixed implant-supported prostheses, removable implant-supported prostheses, and complete dentures: patient satisfaction and oral health-related quality of life. Clin Oral Implants Res. 2016;27(2):e31–7.

42. Bryant SR, MacDonald-Jankowski D, Kim K. Does the type of implant prosthesis affect outcomes for the completely edentulous arch? Int J Oral Maxillofac Implants. 2007;22(Suppl):117–39.

43. Vercruyssen M, Marcelis K, Coucke W, Naert I, Quirynen M. Long-term, retrospective evaluation (implant and patient-centred outcome) of the two-implants-supported overdenture in the mandible. Part 1: survival rate. Clin Oral Implants Res. 2010;21(4):357–65.

44. Meijer HJ, Raghoebar GM, Batenburg RH, Visser A, Vissink A. Mandibular overdentures supported by two or four endosseous implants: a 10-year clinical trial. Clin Oral Implants Res. 2009;20(7):722–8.

45. Jemt T, Chai J, Harnett J, Heath MR, Hutton JE, Johns RB, et al. A 5-year prospective multicenter follow-up report on overdentures supported by osseointegrated implants. Int J Oral Maxillofac Implants. 1996;11(3):291–8.

46. van Steenberghe D, Quirynen M, Naert I, Maffei G, Jacobs R. Marginal bone loss around implants retaining hinging mandibular overdentures, at 4-, 8- and 12-years follow-up. J Clin Periodontol. 2001;28(7):628–33.

47. Montes CC, Pereira FA, Thome G, Alves ED, Acedo RV, de Souza JR, et al. Failing factors associated with osseointegrated dental implant loss. Implant Dent. 2007;16(4):404–12.

48. Wright PS, Glantz PO, Randow K, Watson RM. The effects of fixed and removable implant-stabilised prostheses on posterior mandibular residual ridge resorption. Clin Oral Implants Res. 2002;13(2):169–74.

49. Bressan E, Tomasi C, Stellini E, Sivolella S, Favero G, Berglundh T. Implant-supported mandibular overdentures: a cross-sectional study. Clin Oral Implants Res. 2012;23(7):814–9.

50. Davis DM, Packer ME, Watson RM. Maintenance requirements of implant-supported fixed prostheses opposed by implant-supported fixed prostheses, natural teeth, or complete dentures: a 5-year retrospective study. Int J Prosthodont. 2003;16(5):521–3.

51. Attard NJ, Zarb GA. Long-term treatment outcomes in edentulous patients with implant overdentures: the Toronto study. Int J Prosthodont. 2004;17(4):425–33.

52. Davis DM, Rogers JO, Packer ME. The extent of maintenance required by implant-retained mandibular overdentures: a 3-year report. Int J Oral Maxillofac Implants. 1996;11(6):767–74.

53. Tinsley D, Watson CJ, Russell JL. A comparison of hydroxylapatite coated implant retained fixed and removable mandibular prostheses over 4 to 6 years. Clin Oral Implants Res. 2001;12(2):159–66.

54. Goodacre CJ, Bernal G, Rungcharassaeng K, Kan JY. Clinical complications with implants and implant prostheses. J Prosthet Dent. 2003;90(2):121–32.

55. Naert IE, Hooghe M, Quirynen M, van Steenberghe D. The reliability of implant-retained hinging over-

dentures for the fully edentulous mandible. An up to 9-year longitudinal study. Clin Oral Investig. 1997;1(3):119–24.

56. Akoglu B, Ucankale M, Ozkan Y, Kulak-Ozkan Y. Five-year treatment outcomes with three brands of implants supporting mandibular overdentures. Int J Oral Maxillofac Implants. 2011;26(1):188–94.

57. Heydecke G, Penrod JR, Takanashi Y, Lund JP, Feine JS, Thomason JM. Cost-effectiveness of mandibular two-implant overdentures and conventional dentures in the edentulous elderly. J Dent Res. 2005;84(9):794–9.

58. Zitzmann NU, Marinello CP, Sendi P. A cost-effectiveness analysis of implant overdentures. J Dent Res. 2006;85(8):717–21.

59. Zitzmann NU, Sendi P, Marinello CP. An economic evaluation of implant treatment in edentulous patients-preliminary results. Int J Prosthodont. 2005;18(1):20–7.

60. Attard NJ, Zarb GA, Laporte A. Long-term treatment costs associated with implant-supported mandibular prostheses in edentulous patients. Int J Prosthodont. 2005;18(2):117–23.

Part II

Surgical Phase

Step-by-Step Surgical Considerations and Techniques

Robert Durand and René Voyer

Abstract

The management of the edentulous patient may represent a challenge in implantology for most surgeons. Careful planning using evidence-based methods will not only facilitate the surgical intervention but might also greatly improve the long-term prognosis of implant-supported prostheses. In this chapter, the anatomy of the mandible with a surgical perspective is reviewed in detail. The pre-, intra-, and postoperative elderly patient management including strategies to reduce anxiety, risk, and morbidity is reviewed. Mucogingival considerations, keratinized gingiva augmentation procedures, and steps for optimal implant placement are illustrated with clinical cases. Detailed pre- and postoperative instructions are presented as well as management of common surgical and postsurgical complications.

R. Durand, D.M.D., M.Sc., F.R.C.D.(C) (✉)
R. Voyer, B.Sc., D.M.D., M.Sc., F.R.C.D.(C)
Faculty of Dental Medicine, Université de Montréal, Montreal, QC, Canada
e-mail: robert.durand@umontreal.ca

8.1 Introduction

With newer implant surfaces, dental implants demonstrate high success rates in completely and partially edentulous patients. With life expectancy that will most likely continue to increase in coming decades, implants should be part of the treatment plan presented to elderly patients who are completely edentulous in the mandible [1]. Like their younger counterparts, they are seeking durable treatments that will enhance their physical appearance and quality of life. Consequently, implant-assisted mandibular complete dentures have gained popularity in recent years among the geriatric population. It has been established in the mid-1990s that the gold standard of care for rehabilitation of edentulous patients in the mandible includes a minimum amount of two implants to assist a complete removable denture [2, 3]. In addition, a recent meta-analysis evaluated the quality of life for patients with implant-supported mandibular overdentures compared to conventional dentures. The authors concluded that the implant overdenture group performed better in terms of functional limitation, psychological discomfort, physical disability, psychological disability, and social disability and for handicap [4]. Since age is not a contraindication for dental implants, implants should be part of the treatment plan presented to elderly patients who are completely edentulous in the mandible.

© Springer International Publishing AG, part of Springer Nature 2018
E. Emami, J. Feine (eds.), *Mandibular Implant Prostheses*,
https://doi.org/10.1007/978-3-319-71181-2_8

Indications for dental implants in elderly patients often do not differ from the rest of the population. The main differences between the geriatric population and younger individuals are that they are often affected by systemic and mental illnesses, take multiple medications, and can suffer from physical disabilities, which may diminish their ability to comply with instructions [5]. Therefore, a thorough dental and medical history, an assessment of patient's expectations, complete extra- and intraoral examinations including radiographs, and a cost-benefit analysis are necessary in order to establish an individualized treatment plan. Additional investigations may be required such as blood tests (e.g., HbA1c, INR, CBC), a complete physical examination, and cone beam computerized tomography (CBCT) of the mandible. Once the patient has shown motivation and is willing to put efforts in the execution of the treatment plan, it is important to discuss each single step of the treatment plan with the patient and, often, with at least one accompanying person to ensure that finances and logistics are well understood and, most importantly, to optimize clinical outcomes.

8.2   Patient Preparation

It is important to determine the patient's chief complaint at the initial visit. An edentulous patient is very likely to report issues related to the stability of the mandibular removable complete denture such as discomfort, reduced chewing ability to eat certain food, and trauma to the soft tissues.

When electing for a mandibular implant-retained removable prosthesis in individuals who are edentate in the upper maxilla, the dentist needs to determine if the maxillary prosthesis provides satisfaction for the patient primarily in terms of stability, retention, support, and comfort. Indeed, the implant-retained mandibular prosthesis will provide no advantages to the maxillary prosthesis if the latter is not stable and retentive.

Different treatment options need to be presented to the patient in terms of the desired stability, function, and esthetics. This will also give patients a sense of control and promote trust between the surgeon and the patient. For a completely edentulous patient, the anterior mandible provides the most favorable site for the placement of dental implants in terms of bone height and density. A few options are available and each one offers advantages:

- The fixed mandibular prosthesis requires four, five, or six implants and offers the best option in terms of stability, chewing capacity, and psychological advantages.
- The removable mandibular prosthesis requires from two to five implants depending on the desired stability.

The removable option presents two main retaining systems for the mandibular overdenture: individual ball or Locator™ (Zest Anchors LLC, Escondido, CA, USA) system and the bar with clip attachment. Attachment systems are comparable in terms of overdenture maintenance, implant survival rate, and patient's satisfaction [6].

An informed consent needs to be presented and obtained from the patient. It serves multiple purposes including preparing the patient both psychologically and financially, reminding the patient and the surgeon of the possible complications that could occur at implant placement or postoperatively, and a written proof that pertinent information related to the treatment plan were transmitted to the patient. This form must be used for complex treatments such as implant-retained prostheses in order to prevent miscommunication between the patient and the surgeon as well as potential legal issues.

Several items should be included in the informed consent form:

- Treatment option selected by the patient (fixed or removable prosthesis, the number of implants, and the type of attachment that will be used on the implant-retained prosthesis: ball, Locator™, or bar attachment).
- The cost of treatment and of the maintenance of the prosthesis including the replacement of some parts that will be replaced in the following years due to mechanical wear. Ball, Locator™, and bar attachments as well as prosthetic screws must be eventually replaced

when they have lost their retention. Also, denture teeth may wear faster, especially if the opposing dentition consists of natural teeth or porcelain restorations, having a higher degree of hardness compared to acrylic.

- The estimated prognosis of the prosthesis.
- Complications related to the implants and the attachment apparatus, e.g., peri-implantitis, fracture of an implant, fracture of an attachment component, fracture or loosening of the retaining screws, and loss of osseointegration.
- Surgical complications, e.g., infection, loss of sutures and healing by secondary intention, bruising, swelling, paresthesia, bleeding, difficulties when eating and talking, and trismus.
- The duration of the healing phase, e.g., the patient will not be able to wear the lower prosthesis for 1–2 weeks following the placement of the implants. Thereafter, a soft reline will be added to the denture once or at several occasions before the delivery of the final prosthesis.

There are several considerations regarding the hard and soft tissues to evaluate when evaluating the patient and planning the treatment:

- The number of implants and their location.
- The height and width of bone available for the placement of the implants.
- The quality of bone density.
- The surgical approach: one- or two-stage surgery.
- The anatomy of the edentulous mandible including the location of the mental foramina and the extent of the lingual undercuts in the anterior and posterior regions.
- The presence of residual roots, impacted teeth, or any bone pathology.
- The alveolar ridge morphology and the need for osseous recontouring.
- The presence of soft tissue pathologies (e.g., lichen planus, candidiasis).
- The depth of the vestibule and the width of keratinized gingiva on the edentulous ridge.
- The anterior interocclusal space: a minimum of 12 mm of space between the soft tissue

ridge and the occlusal plane of opposing maxillary dentition is generally required for a removable implant-supported prosthesis. With a smaller vertical space available, a fixed implant prosthesis must be contemplated.

8.3 Surgical Anatomy

Depending on the type of prosthetic rehabilitation in the mandible, fixed or removable, the recommended number of implants may vary. For a fixed prosthesis, a minimum of four implants is generally required to withstand the occlusal forces. For a removable prosthesis, the number of implants may vary between two and five, depending on the planned prosthetic system (individual attachments vs. bar with clips). Risks to damage vital structures increase with the number of implants to insert and the severity of bone resorption. Hence, several anatomical landmarks must be taken into consideration for the surgical placement of dental implants in the mandible.

A panoramic radiograph will provide an overview of the vital structures and provides an estimate of the bone height. A more precise measurement of bone width and height of the anterior mandibular region can be obtained with a cephalometric film. However, with the development of newer three-dimensional imaging techniques with minimal radiation exposure to the patient, a CBCT is recommended using a radiographic guide with radiopaque markers to diminish the risks of causing irreversible damages to vital structures (Figs. 8.1a, b). For example, if the mandibular canal or mental foramina are not easily visualized on a panoramic film or the distance between the crest and the canal seems to be somewhat limited, a CBCT analysis is essential. A radiographic guide is often fabricated from a duplicate of the old or a new denture and can be converted into a surgical guide after the radiographic examination is completed. Markers made with barium sulfate or gutta-percha are located at the ideal position of the implants. This information will facilitate the surgical planning for implant placement. The initial intraoral examination enables the surgeon to assess the mandibular

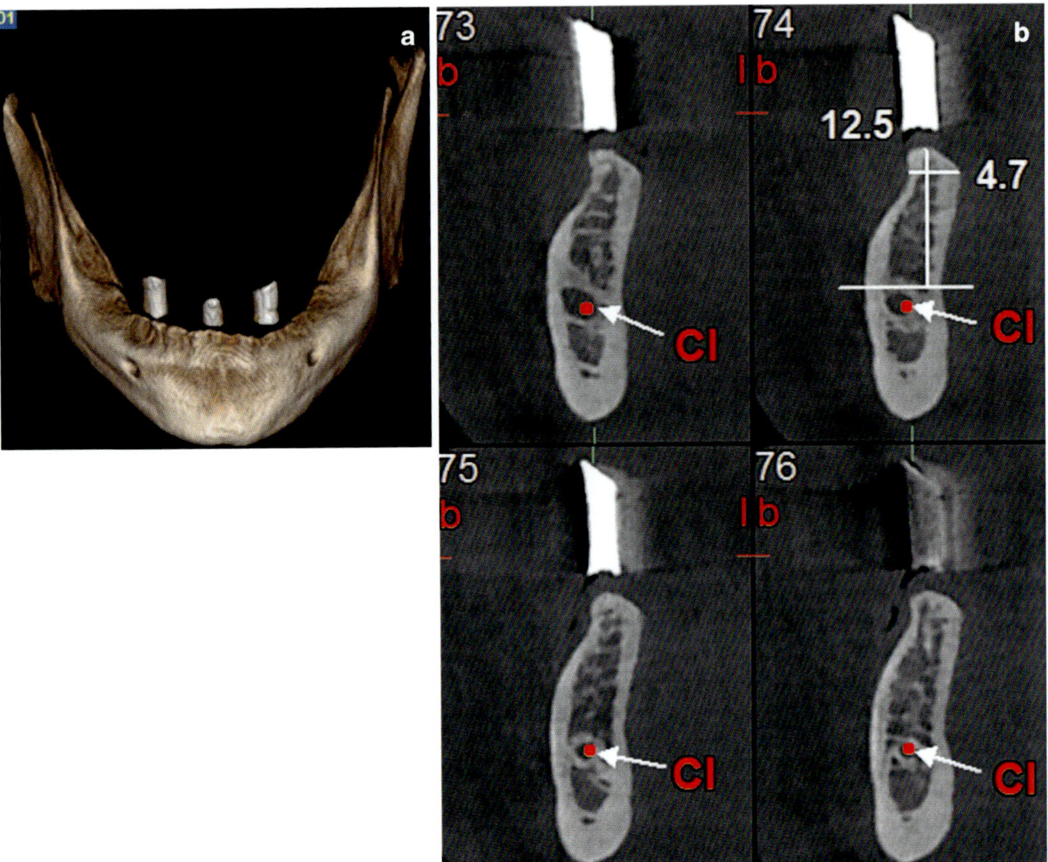

Fig. 8.1 (**a**) Three-dimensional reconstruction of an edentulous mandible using a CBCT technology with radiological guide in place. Photo courtesy of Dr. M. Schmittbuhl, Faculty of Dental Medicine, Université de Montréal, Canada. (**b**) Radiopaque marker with cross-sectional view of implant site #43: buccolingual width and bone height are measured in mm. The incisive canal is visible and marked. Photo courtesy of Dr. M. Schmittbuhl, Faculty of Dental Medicine, Université de Montréal, Canada

ridge anatomy and, often, the position of mental foramina through a visual examination and palpation. Once the restorative dentist and the surgeon have confirmed the implant positions on the surgical guide, the surgery may be scheduled. Extra care during the surgery needs to be taken in order to prevent severing of principal nerves or their branches as well as major blood vessels. Hence, the surgeon needs to be knowledgeable in oral and maxillofacial anatomy and be able to recognize and locate mandibular vital structures to reduce the incidence of intra- or postoperative complications.

8.3.1 Inferior Alveolar Canal

The mandibular nerve represents one of the three branches of the trigeminal nerve. One of its divisions is the inferior alveolar nerve, which enters the mandible through the mandibular canal on the medial surface of the ramus by the lingula. It extends anteriorly to the premolar region, where it divides into the mental and incisive canals [7, 8]. The mandibular canal contains the inferior alveolar neurovascular (IAN) bundle that provides a major part of the blood supply and innervation to the mandible. The IAN runs posteriorly from the lingual aspect of the mandible, is usually located midway between the lingual and buccal cortical plate in the molar region [9], and progressively shifts toward the buccal plate to finally exit the mental foramen. The IAN contains a large nerve trunk, a small artery, and a smaller vein [10]. Since an injury to the IAN caused by the implant osteotomy preparation can lead to temporary or permanent neuropathy or intraoperative excessive bleeding [11], it is important to locate the mandibular canal prior to the surgery. It has been suggested to keep a minimal safety distance of ≈2 mm from the mandibular canal [12]. If a panoramic radiograph is used to estimate vertical bone height, it is essential to take into consideration the magnification factor (≈25–30%) [13, 14]. One solution is to use a small metal bearing of known diameter on the film to calculate the magnification factor. If the mandibular canal is not visible on the panoramic radiograph or the bone height seems limited as often observed in the posterior area of the mandible of edentulous patients, a CBCT is recommended. In no circumstances the surgeon should rely on tactile feedback to locate the superior cortical plate of the mandibular canal while preparing the osteotomy, since the bone density may vary and the cortical plate might not always prevent penetration of the drill into the mandibular canal.

8.3.2 Mental Foramen

The inferior alveolar nerve emerges from the mental foramen in the premolar region to innervate the gingiva from the midline to the second premolar area, the mucosa, the lower lip, the skin in the interforaminal area, and the chin. At this point, an incisive branch of the inferior alveolar nerve continues mesially to provide innervation to the incisor teeth. It is believed that it goes either through an incisal canal or through medullary spaces of the trabecular bone [15–17]. The mental foramen is located 38% of the time between the first and second mandibular premo-

lars and 27.5% in line with the long axis of the second premolar [18], but it may be found in the canine or first molar area [19, 20] (Fig. 8.2). In rare cases, the mental nerve might be bifurcated (Fig. 8.3). There is a significant variation in the vertical position of the mental foramen [21], and therefore, its position must be precisely located using CBCT technology if implants are to be placed in its vicinity. With bone resorption that occurs in edentulous patients, it is common to find the mental foramen closer to the alveolar

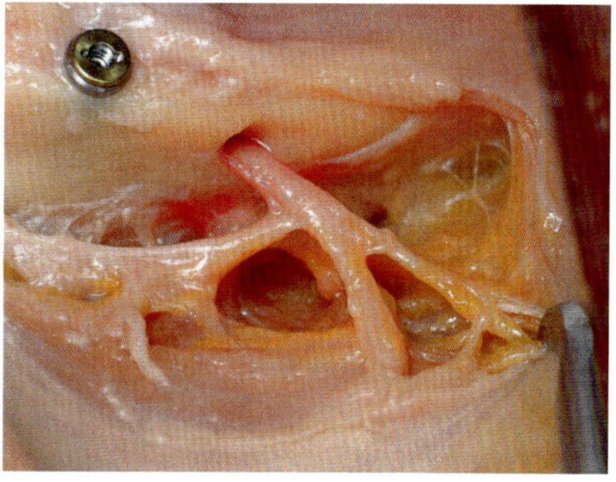

Fig. 8.2 Mental foramen exposed during dissection on cadaver. Photo courtesy of Drs. A. Boukari & M. Schmittbuhl, Faculty of Dental Medicine, University of Strasbourg, France

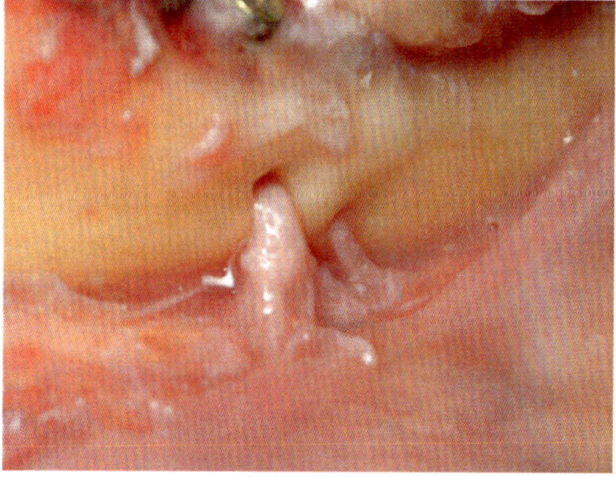

Fig. 8.3 Bifurcated mental foramen exposed during dissection on cadaver. Photo courtesy of Drs. A. Boukari & M. Schmittbuhl, Faculty of Dental Medicine, University of Strasbourg, France

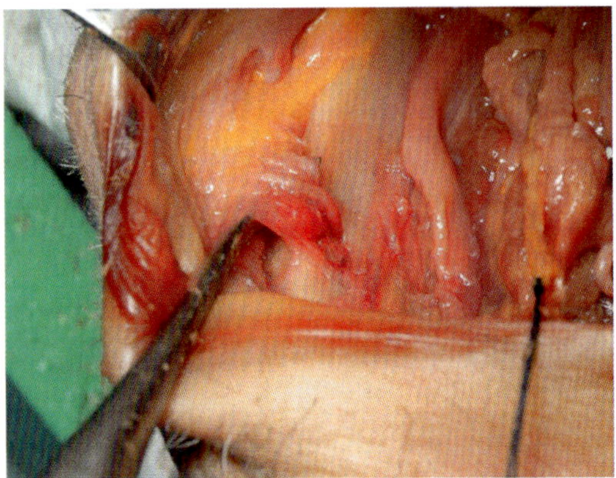

Fig. 8.4 Mental foramen located on top of the mandibular ridge exposed during dissection on cadaver. Photo courtesy of Drs. A. Boukari & M. Schmittbuhl, Faculty of Dental Medicine, University of Strasbourg, France

crest. In some severely resorbed mandibles, it may be located on the crest, and this may cause a chronic discomfort, and even in some cases, intermittent paresthesia can be triggered by compression of the mental nerve by a removable complete denture [22] (Fig. 8.4). The addition of implants to support the prosthesis will relieve the pressure on the mental foramen and prevent neurosensory complications.

The anterior loop of the inferior alveolar canal is an anterior extension exiting through the mental foramen. Conventional two-dimensional radiographs may underestimate or overestimate the anterior loop length [23]. From the foramen, it is located anteriorly and inferiorly, and its prevalence (31–97%) and length (0–7 mm) both vary greatly, depending on the methodology used (conventional radiographs vs. CBCT) [24–29]. Cadaver studies have shown similar prevalence (0–63%) and length (0–6 mm) [30–32]. It has been suggested that a safe distance of 6 mm between the distal aspect of the most distal implant and the mental foramen should be kept [33]. During the surgery, locating the mental foramen using a full-thickness mucoperiosteal flap will allow the surgeon to avoid any injury to its content. There is a bony prominence coronal to the entrance of the mental foramen that protects its content. This anatomical feature, once exposed during flap elevation, will hint the surgeon that the mental nerve is close by and light

pressure with blunt dissection must be used to expose the coronal part of the mental foramen to avoid severing one or multiple nerve branches of the mental nerve.

8.3.3 Lingual Foramen

In the midline area of the mandible, the sublingual and submental arteries form arterial anastomosis entering the lingual aspect of the mandible through one or multiple foramen [34] that may not be detected on two-dimensional radiographs. The lingual foramen was found in 99% of cadaver dissections [35]. There is also a possible anastomosis between sublingual and incisive arteries. Trauma with an implant drill of the lingual foramen/foramina may cause a hemorrhage resulting in a severe life-threatening hematoma of the floor of the mouth [36–38]. Through a CBCT study of 639 partially or completely edentulous patients from 5 different countries, it was found that the lingual foramen was 18.33 ± 5.45 mm apical to the alveolar crest, was 17.40 ± 7.52 mm coronal to the border of the mandible, and had a mean diameter of 0.89 ± 0.40 mm [39]. Most canal types were mono (76.8%) and 24.4% had a diameter >1 mm, which has the potential to cause excessive bleeding if damaged [40]. Therefore, implant placement in the midline exhibits potential risks, especially in elderly edentulous patients, where significant bone height might have been lost in the interforaminal area.

8.3.4 Incisive Canal

The incisive canal was found in 96% of cadavers and is a mesial extension of the inferior alveolar canal with a mean diameter of 1.8 ± 0.5 mm and reaching the mandible midline only 18% of the time [41]. It has been detected in 2.7–51% of panoramic radiographs [42, 43] but can be detected on CBCT images more than 90% of the time [43, 44]. It has been a common practice to ignore the presence of the incisive canal as long as the mental foramen is avoided during implant placement in the anterior region of the mandible. However, the wider the diameter of the canal is, the higher is the risk for neurosensory complications or intra-operative bleeding [45, 46]. Consequently, if long implants (>10 mm) are planned in the anterior region of the mandible, it is recommended to obtain a CBCT of the interforaminal area to prevent potential neurosensory complications.

8.3.5 Ridge Morphology

The alveolar mandibular ridge may vary significantly in shape. In the premolar and molar regions, the ridge can have either a parallel shape where its coronal part has a similar width to the apical part (type P) or have a coronal part narrower than its base (type C). Moreover, the posterior area of the mandible may exhibit a lingual undercut (type U) where lies the submandibular fossa, which may or may not limit the available bone height for implant placement [47, 48]. The submandibular fossa, located below the mylohyoid line where the mylohyoid muscle is attached, contains the submandibular gland and sublingual and submental arteries that run intimately with the lingual plate [49]. The sublingual fossa is located anteriorly and coronally to the submandibular fossa, above the mylohyoid line, in the premolar/canine region. It was found to be present 49% of the time, and the presence of lateral lingual foramen located in close proximity had a prevalence of 53% where branches of the submental artery entered the lingual plate of the mandible [50]. Therefore, maximum care is needed to prevent perforation of the lingual plate and trauma to these vital structures. In a CBCT study of edentulous first premolar/canine areas and first and second molar areas, it was found that an undercut was present in 90% of the second molar areas, 56% at the first molar, and 14% in the first premolar/canine regions [51]. The mean undercut depth was 3.7 mm in the molar region and 0.8 mm in the first premolar/canine region. The authors found that the closer the mandibular canal was to the basal bone, the higher was the prevalence of a lingual undercut. In the anterior region, an undercut may be observed. It was found that the lingual alveolar

process has an angle with the occlusal plane that may vary between 37° and 125° [52]. While palpation might be useful preoperatively and intra-operatively, a CBCT is recommended to detect lingual undercuts. Following a three-dimensional analysis, the angulation of the implant might have to be revised to keep the implant within bone during insertion and prevent perforation of the lingual plate. Failure to do so may put the patient at a greater risk for a life-threatening hemorrhage related to trauma to blood vessels located close to the lingual plate [53–55].

8.3.6 Mylohyoid Muscle

Several muscles attached to the mandible are involved during flap elevation procedures when an adequate access to the alveolar ridge is needed for implant placement. Of these muscles, the mylohyoid, mentalis, genioglossus, and geniohyoid muscles are of particular concern to the surgeon. Extending from the symphysis to the third molar region, the mylohyoid muscles originate from the mylohyoid line, insert the hyoid bone, and support the floor of the mouth by passing inferiorly to the tongue [56]. They represent an important barrier between the sublingual and submandibular fossae. They must be reflected using a sharp periosteal elevator since they are located in close proximity to the sublingual and submental arteries.

8.3.7 Mentalis Muscle

In the mandibular anterior region, part of the mentalis muscles must be reflected on the buccal aspect of the alveolar ridge with a full-thickness mucoperiosteal flap in order to expose the underlying bone. These paired muscles originate in the incisive fossae and insert into the skin of the chin [57]. Care must be taken not to fully reflect the mentalis muscles since the muscles may fail to reattach well on the alveolar bone and lower lip ptosis may result from this outcome [58]. Only partial reflection of the mentalis muscle is necessary to allow good visualization of the bone morphology of the coronal aspect of the alveolar ridge for implant placement (Fig. 8.5).

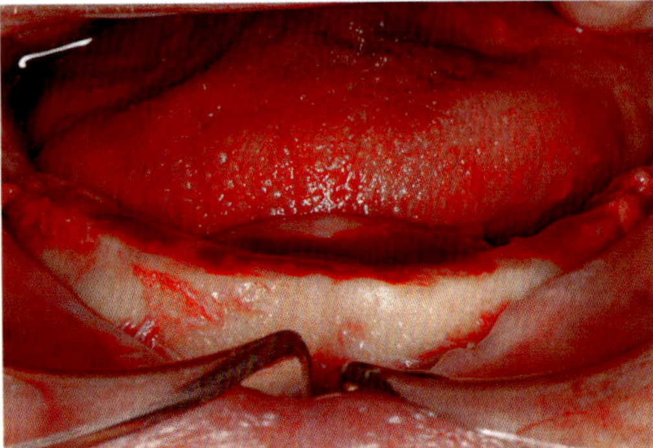

Fig. 8.5 Mentalis muscles reflected in the anterior mandible

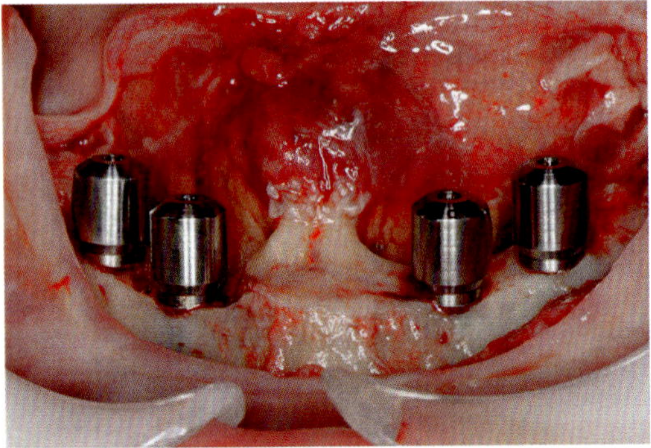

Fig. 8.6 Exposed genial tubercles in the severely resorbed patient

8.3.8 Genial Tubercles, Genioglossus, and Geniohyoid Muscles

Genial tubercles are small bony elevations located at the midline of the mandible on the lingual aspect of the alveolar ridge and close to the inferior border of the mandible [59]. The genioglossus and geniohyoid muscles originate from the superior and inferior tubercles, respectively. The lingual foramen/foramina may be located either between superior and inferior tubercles, apically or laterally to the tubercles [60]. Using CBCT images, the genial tubercle was found to be about 8–9 mm wide and 7–9 mm tall [61]. It is commonly exposed in severely resorbed mandibles and might be slightly modified by osteoplasty to allow placement of healing abutments immediately after implant placement (Fig. 8.6).

However, the genioglossus muscle should not be fully reflected to prevent retraction of the tongue and potential obstruction of the airway [62].

8.4 Strategies in Elderly Patients to Reduce Anxiety, Risk, and Morbidity

8.4.1 Surgical Planning and Time Management

Elderly individuals may become tired easily during long surgical procedures. Hence, a morning appointment is ideal for implant placement. When the patient has had a good night sleep and has a full reserve of energy, he/she might be able to cooperate more easily during the surgery. Also, it is imperative that the implant surgeon plans as much as possible the surgery before the patient enters the surgical room. This will optimize the use of time with the patient and will shorten the duration of the intervention. Shorter implant surgeries have been associated with lower visual analog scores (VAS) in patient-reported outcomes such as pain, swelling, bleeding, and bruising [63]. When indicated, all the necessary arrangements with the physician, i.e., medication holiday, physical examination, or blood tests, should have been made prior to the surgical appointment. For example, failure to obtain an INR within therapeutic range in a patient taking warfarin could significantly lengthen the surgery and increase the risk of postoperative bleeding-related complications. Obtaining appropriate radiographic images of the region of interest will allow the surgeon to evaluate potential anatomical obstacles during the surgery and anticipate practical solutions. By identifying vital structures as well as the available bone volume and alveolar ridge morphology, the surgeon will have a clearer idea of the surgical steps to accomplish. Also, training and keeping up with newer surgical techniques and technologies will enhance the surgeon's skills and efficiency. The surgical guide indicating the desired implant locations should be available at the time of surgery, as this will also contribute to reduce the duration of the appointment.

Since elderly individuals often have functional limitations, it is important to allow adequate time at the beginning and the end of the surgical appointment for pre- and postoperative instructions. Having an escort to assist and help the patient who has lost autonomy will save time for both the patient and the surgeon. The surgical room should be kept available for additional time at the end of surgery. If this is not possible, the other option is using a recovery room. Some patients might request to be in a semi-sitting position during the surgery or pause during the surgery. The surgical team should grant this request and adapt the room and schedule accordingly. Additional cushions and blankets should be readily available for elderly patients to enhance their comfort in the dental chair.

8.4.2　Communication Between the Surgeon and the Geriatric Patient

The prevalence of hearing and vision impairment was estimated to be 11.3% among 80 years and older individuals in the United States, among which only 19% were free of any sensory impairment [64]. Moreover, it is estimated that 40 million individuals worldwide have dementia, this condition affecting mostly individuals older than 60 years, and the numbers are expected to double every 20 years until 2050 [65]. Individuals who suffer from dementia may have memory loss and have difficulty to reason and think. This condition will interfere with their daily activities. Alzheimer's disease is the most common cause of dementia [66]. As a result, elderly individuals might not always hear, understand, or remember instructions given by the surgeon and the staff. In addition, introversion, conformity, rigidity, caution, and depression are personality traits that are frequently found in older individuals [67]. Consequently, the initial contact between the surgeon and the geriatric patient is extremely important.

Since some individuals might easily forget the instructions given at the time of surgery, someone who is knowledgeable about their condition should accompany these individuals to ensure the patient's comprehension of the treatment plan and compliance to postoperative care and follow-ups. The accompanying person should be present at the treatment planning and preoperative consultations as well as before and after the surgical appointment to ensure that the instructions, treatment steps, and related costs have been clearly understood by the patient. Psychological preparation of elderly patients is very important, as they might be very anxious about the implant surgery. The accompanying person should also be well prepared and should understand the different clinical steps involved in the confection of an implant-assisted complete mandibular prosthesis. Explanatory leaflets, illustrations, and short videos may assist the surgeon and restorative dentist to achieve this task. Short and clear explanations are therefore necessary to ensure that geriatric patients understand procedures and have realistic expectations related to the postoperative outcomes. The surgeon has to adapt several aspects of his verbal and nonverbal communication skills for the elderly patient who is affected with cognitive impairment [68]. For example, he should use short words and simple sentences, speak slowly and clearly, and wait for a response before going to the next question. He should be willing to repeat instructions and should assume that the elderly understands more than he/she may be able to express. Also, in conjunction with verbal communication, nonverbal skills are important to instill confidence and reduce the patient's anxiety such as maintaining eye contact, moving calmly, smiling, and using gentle gestures.

8.4.3　Anxiety Management

As with the younger population, elderly patients might exhibit fear or anxiety toward treatments involving surgical procedures such as implant placement. Dental anxiety or phobia in the geriatric population was estimated to be between 8 and 12% [69, 70]. Although it was found that the prevalence of dental-related anxiety is decreasing with age in individuals 50 years or older, it was found to be higher in edentulous patients [70]. One or multiple psychological strategies to manage anxiety should always be offered to the patient whether it is the sole option to reduce anxiety or is given in adjunct to sedative agents. It should always be used with compassion, patience, and respect toward the geriatric patient. Good communication between the surgeon and the patient must be maintained at every appointment. This will allow the surgeon to understand the patient's fears in order to find the best approach to reduce his/her anxiety. This will facilitate communication with the patient and will most likely contribute to improve the surgeon's efficiency during the execution of the clinical steps. A psychological approach might be sufficient for the less anxious patient, while a combination of both psychological approach and sedation might be required for the fearful patient. Regardless of the selected approach, a quiet and caring environment will play an important role in reducing the patient's anxiety and fears during the surgery.

For patients with mild anxiety, a trusting relationship and the transmission of specific and simple information about the treatment will generally allow the surgeon to manage and reduce the patient's anxiety [71]. The key is to provide the patient with the feeling that he/she is in control and that the treatment proceeds uneventfully. For patients with moderate to severe anxiety, anxiety management may require the use of sedative agents such as nitrous oxide and oral or intravenous (IV) sedation with additional strategies such as distraction, relaxation, or developing better coping methods [72]. When higher levels of anxiety are encountered, intravenous sedation and/or more complex psychological approaches may be necessary such as systematic desensitization, hypnosis, and cognitive restructuring. These approaches require additional training or the assistance of a psychotherapist knowledgeable in the field. In the most extreme cases, general anesthesia might be recommended although one might question if such patient should receive complex treatments such as the implant-assisted mandibular prosthesis.

The surgeon has to master several skills related to patient care and communication to provide a safe environment to reduce the patient's anxiety level:

- Allowing patient's control
- Demonstrating empathy
- Being receptive to patient's concerns
- Active listening (involves reflecting what the patient says)
- Providing information
- Creating a bond of trust and confidence

It may also involve using, although not exclusively, the following practical strategies:

- Allowing breaks between procedures
- Creating a signaling code so the patient can communicate easily with the surgeon
- Using visual or auditory distractions
- Using positive reinforcement
- Breathing techniques to induce relaxation

8.4.4 Sedation Techniques

The aging process often affects tissue and organ functions, which may have an impact on the patient's ability to respond to drugs. These changes cause a higher peak concentration and longer duration of drug effect after intake in the elderly individual. Aging does not affect all individuals in the same way, and some may be more prone than others to develop age-related diseases. For example, as age increases, elasticity in pulmonary tissues is reduced and the intercostal muscles become atrophied. Also, cardiac output and renal and hepatic blood flows are reduced with age [73]. Therefore, care must be taken when prescribing and giving sedatives to the geriatric population to prevent overdosing and undesired complications related to the respiratory and cardiovascular systems. At the first appointment, lower doses of local anesthetic agents, analgesics, or sedative agents should be given before being titrated at further appointments if necessary. Prior to recommend sedation to an elderly individual, the patient's physiological status and presence of coexisting diseases should be established with the collaboration of the physician. The American Society of Anesthesiologists (ASA) published a classification system for preoperative preparation of the patient (Table 1; [74]). Only ASA class I and II geriatric patients should be offered oral or intravenous sedation to reduce the risk of potentially lethal cardiovascular or respiratory complications. It is important to note that oral and IV sedation dosages will need to be lowered for elders having an impaired kidney or liver function. Routine medications should be taken as usual without any modification of their dosage, and liquids may be taken prior to any sedation procedure.

It is important to give precise and clear instructions prior to any sedation procedure should the patient choose that option to reduce his/her anxiety. It is important that he/she does not eat after midnight the night before the surgery to prevent nausea and allow the medication to be metabolized in a timely manner so its effect is felt as quickly as possible after sedative intake. No alcohol or other recreational drugs should be consumed while taking oral or IV sedatives. Since it is suggested to take oral sedatives 1 h preoperatively, a designated person should escort the patient to the clinic. For both oral and IV sedation procedures, the patient should be accompanied after the surgical appointment back to his/her home, and a designated person should stay with the patient for a period of 24 h to prevent any injuries that could result from an accidental fall. To minimize any misunderstanding, written instructions should be given to the patient and his/her escort.

Inhalation sedation with nitrous oxide (N_2O-O_2) is the safest method of sedation for the anxious geriatric patient. Nitrous oxide is a colorless, odorless, nonflammable, nonirritating, inorganic gas providing light to moderate sedation [75]. In addition, it provides oxygenation to the patient with light sedation and does not induce respiratory depression. It is rapidly eliminated by the patient and does not affect significantly the cardiovascular system. It is quickly reversible and usually does not impinge the surgeon's movements while operating on the mandible.

It can be difficult to use oral sedation in the elderly since they often take multiple medications that may interact with commonly used sedatives. In addition, titration tends to be more complicated in these individuals [76]. Benzodiazepines such as triazolam (0.0625–0.125 mg) and the newer nonbarbiturate sedative-hypnotic, zolpidem (5–10 mg), are indicated for the geriatric patient with mild anxiety since they do not have long half-lives (5.7–11 h and 1.4–4.5 h, respectively) [75]. Moreover, benzodiazepines possess anticonvulsant and muscle relaxant properties. The gastrointestinal tract absorbs them rapidly, and the liver metabolizes them, hence the importance of not taking any food prior intake. They should be given in lower doses for the elderly because of their decreased metabolism. Contraindications to benzodiazepines include history of an allergic reaction, psychoses, and acute narrow-angle glaucoma. Antihistamines like diphenhydramine (25–50 mg) and hydroxyzine (50–100 mg) may also be used and are considered safe for the elderly individual, although they do not have an anxiolytic effect [76]. Geriatric patients taking antihistamines might have hyposalivation that can exacerbate their current xerostomia induced by polypharmacy. Complications that may occur include hypotension, apnea, and loss of consciousness resulting from cardiovascular compromise or respiratory depression [76].

IV sedation is generally safe in the geriatric population. Continuous monitoring of vital signs including pulse oximetry, echocardiography, and blood pressure as well as oxygen delivery through nasal tubing is highly recommended during IV sedation procedures. It may be difficult to locate and access a patent vein in the elderly individual since their skin is thin and often has lost elasticity and their veins are generally more fragile. Midazolam (0.5–4 mg; max = 10 mg), a short-acting benzodiazepine, is the IV sedative of choice for the geriatric patient since it is short acting and can be reversed with flumazenil, its antagonist. Titration in the elderly should be done slowly and by an experienced professional. Postoperative monitoring is imperative due to the risk of delirium and increased risk of falls.

Discharge of the patient should not occur unless vital signs have returned to normal and his/her escort is present.

8.4.5 Minimally Invasive Surgical Approaches

The healthier the elder is, the more complex the treatment can be, including a higher number of implants. For ASA type II or III geriatric patients, surgeries of shorter duration with a minimal amount of local anesthetics are recommended. Therefore, in these individuals, minimally traumatic surgeries will enable the surgeon to attain these two goals. Two ways are suggested to achieve this goal: placing fewer implants or using computer-assisted guided surgery (CAGS) with a flapless surgery.

Two-implant-retained mandibular overdentures have shown to provide significantly greater improvements in satisfaction compared to conventional lower dentures [77]. This treatment option is therefore an excellent option for individuals who want to improve their quality of life while minimizing the cost of treatment and has been considered the minimum standard of care [78]. The placement of two implants in the interforaminal area is less complex than the placement of four or five implants since the mental foramen does not need to be exposed and identified, as long as its position has been clearly located. An incision located in the middle of the keratinized gingiva extending from the first premolar to the contralateral premolar will generally be sufficient to elevate a full-thickness flap to expose the buccal and lingual aspects of the alveolar ridge. If adequate visualization of the ridge is not obtained, short (3–4 mm long) vertical releasing incisions may be performed mesially to the mental foramen bilaterally. Thereafter, the surgical guide may be used for implant site preparation. With this approach, the flap is less extensive, and a smaller area of alveolar bone is exposed during surgery compared to the molar-to-molar crestal incision needed to locate the mental foramen with the standard approach. Consequently, it will reduce the duration of surgery and postoperative morbidity.

Another approach that has gained popularity in recent years is the computer-assisted guided surgery (CAGS) due to its minimal invasiveness. After a mean follow-up of 22.6 months, a recent systematic review has shown minimal postoperative morbidity and a survival rate of 97.2% in fully edentulous patients undergoing complete prosthetic rehabilitation with CAGS, which is similar to reported outcomes after freehanded flap surgeries [79]. This method requires several steps prior to surgery. First, a three-dimensional image (CT or CBCT) of the mandible with a radiological guide in place is taken. The radiological guide can be either a duplicate of the current denture or a new denture in clear acrylic. The resin has to be mixed with barium sulfate when fabricating the radiological guide to ensure its radiopacity on the images obtained. Once stored, the image is transferred to a computer software that will allow the surgeon to virtually place the implants in the ideal position, taking into account surrounding anatomical structures and the future prosthesis. Once the implant positions have been determined, the data is registered in the software and sent to the laboratory. There, the technician fabricates a virtual model of the mandible and creates a surgical guide using the computer-assisted manufacturing (CAM) technology. At the time of surgery, the CAM surgical guide can be maintained in place with fixation screws that are inserted in the underlying bone through the gingiva or the mucosa. On the surgical guide, sequential slots will allow drills of increasing diameter to be inserted at a precise angle and depth at each implant location. Therefore, there is no need to raise a flap with this technique. However, linear and angular deviations may occur with CAGS, especially with longer implants [80, 81]. Bony fenestrations caused by deviations may affect surgical and prosthetic results. Importantly, very few studies have evaluated the long-term (>5 years) success rate of prostheses placed using CAGS [82]. The high cost of this procedure may also influence patient's preferences. Furthermore, a flapless approach will not allow the surgeon to preserve the amount of KG and proceed with ridge recontouring if needed.

In recent years, efforts have been deployed to reduce the number of surgeries in medicine and dentistry. For the implant rehabilitation of the patient's mandible, one commonly used solution is to place the healing abutment at the time of implant placement. It was demonstrated in the edentulous mandible that there were no differences in success rate and crestal bone changes between one-stage implant surgeries with the healing abutment placed at time of placement and implants that were submerged and then exposed 8 weeks later [83]. Nowadays, it is a common practice to place the healing abutment at the time of implant placement to avoid an additional surgical procedure for the patient, unless simultaneous bone grafting at implant placement is required. In this case, a cover screw is placed on the implant platform, and a primary closure is obtained with sutures.

8.5 Mucogingival Considerations

8.5.1 Importance and Advantages of Keratinized Gingiva

Keratinized gingiva (KG) is defined as the gingiva located between the mucogingival junction and the gingival margin around the natural dentition and dental implants. It is pink, firm, and keratinized and is attached to the underlying alveolar bone, except for the zone adjacent to the gingival sulcus. Investigators initially found in a cross-sectional study that all sites with <2 mm of KG around natural teeth exhibited signs of inflammation, while 80% of sites with ≥2 mm of KG were clinically healthy [84]. According to their results, they recommended to keep a minimal width of KG of 2 mm around teeth to maintain a healthy periodontium. However, further studies have shown that periodontal health can be maintained through adequate oral hygiene and inflammation control with less than 2 mm of KG [85–87].

Like in the periodontium around teeth, implants have a biologic zone that includes connective tissue and epithelial attachments as well as a gingival sulcus. However, peri-implant tissues display fundamental differences with periodontal tissues around the natural teeth. From animal studies, it was demonstrated that the peri-implant epithelium has a lower sealing capacity compared to the junctional epithelium in the natural dentition [88, 89], although the explanation for this weaker bond between the implant surface and the epithelium remains unclear. Clinically, a mean additional probing depth of 1 mm on healthy peri-implant tissues was found compared to healthy periodontium around teeth when using a standardized pressure periodontal probe [90]. This was explained by the reduced resistance of peri-implant tissues to probing. Compared to the dentition, implants do not have cementum and a periodontal ligament. This might explain, in part, the reason why connective tissue fibers around implants have a more parallel orientation compared to a perpendicular direction around the natural dentition [91]. It has been suggested that this weaker peri-implant seal might predispose to gingival recessions [92] and to peri-implantitis, a chronic inflammatory disease of peri-implant tissues that is caused by the plaque biofilm and which is the equivalent of periodontitis in the natural dentition. Indeed, it was demonstrated in a split-mouth longitudinal animal study that peri-implantitis lesions extended deeper into the alveolar bone, while in periodontitis lesions, there was a connective tissue layer between the inflammatory lesion and the alveolar bone [93]. Several recent systematic reviews have shown that implant sites with presence of KG ≥1–2 mm were associated with lower values for plaque accumulation, signs of inflammation, recessions, and attachment loss compared to implant sites with minimal or no KG [94–96].

In individuals rehabilitated with implant-assisted complete dentures, an insufficient width of KG was associated with discomfort, and oral hygiene measures were reported to be painful in sites where there was no KG present [97]. The discomfort reported may be explained by the mobility of the nonkeratinized mucosa causing irritation during mastication [97, 98]. By its nature, keratinized gingiva is easier to handle surgically than mucosa since it is firmer. In the edentulous patient, where several muscle attachments need to be detached and elevated in order to access the underlying bone, it is technically less demanding to raise a mucoperiosteal flap that has been initiated through incisions in KG. Therefore, it is suggested that a minimal band of KG of 2 mm should be present preoperatively to facilitate soft tissue handling during implant placement surgery in edentulous patients. If it is not the case, several surgical procedures to increase the band of KG can be done before, at the second-stage surgery, or once the implant-assisted prosthesis is completed.

8.5.2 Keratinized Gingiva Augmentation Procedures in the Mandible

In the edentulous patients with moderate to severe mandibular resorption, it is not uncommon to observe a narrow band (<2 mm) of keratinized gingiva covering the alveolar ridge. Two surgical approaches can increase significantly the width of keratinized gingiva in the edentulous ridge [99]. The free gingival graft was initially described by Bjorn to correct mucogingival problems such as gingival recession and lack of KG [100]. The first case to illustrate this concept is a 67-year-old male patient who is a for-

mer smoker and had partial resection of the tongue due to the presence of a tongue neoplasm and had subsequently a skin graft four years ago. The band of KG is less than 2 mm (Fig. 8.7a, b). The patient has teeth #3.7 and 3.8 present in the mandible and most of his teeth in the maxilla that are heavily restored. The patient desired an implant-assisted and tooth-supported hybrid overdenture supported by two implants and Locator™ attachments to stabilize his future prosthesis. After local anesthesia through buccal and lingual infiltrations with lidocaine 2% 1:100,000 (or 1:50,000) epinephrine, an envelope flap is elevated in partial thickness in order to preserve the periosteum on the alveolar crest (Fig. 8.8a, b). Care must be taken to place the incision in the middle of the remaining KG in order to facilitate suturing. The surgeon harvests one or two 1.5-mm-thick gingival grafts of desired length and width in order to include the epithelium and a layer of connective tissue to ensure adequate revascularization. A band made with oxidized regenerated cellulose (Surgicel®, Ethicon Inc., Somerville, NJ, USA) stabilized with a cyanoacrylate oral adhesive (Periacryl®, GluStitch Inc., Delta, BC, Canada) was used to cover the donor sites in the palate (Fig. 8.9). The most common donor sites are the palate, the edentulous ridge, or the maxillary tuberosity. Two free gingival grafts were sutured in place

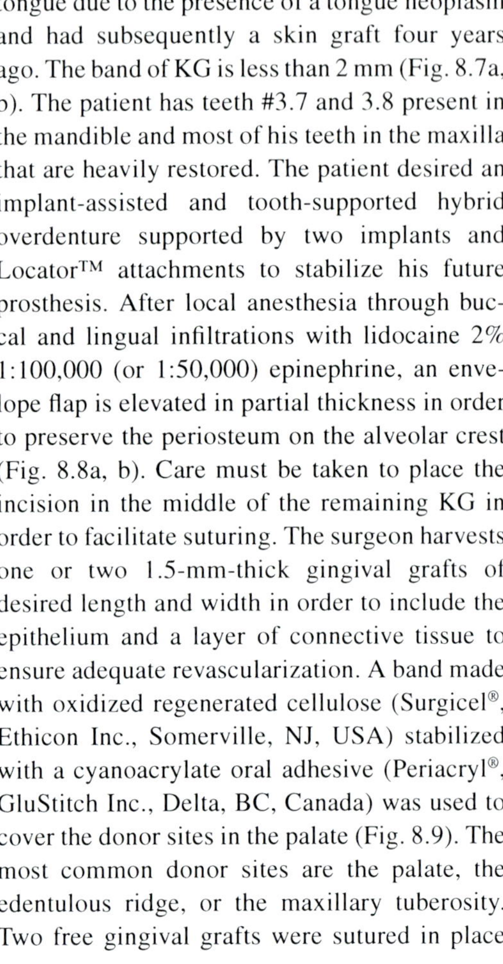

Fig. 8.7 (**a**, **b**) Buccal and occlusal views of the partially edentulous mandible of a patient that had a partial resection of the tongue

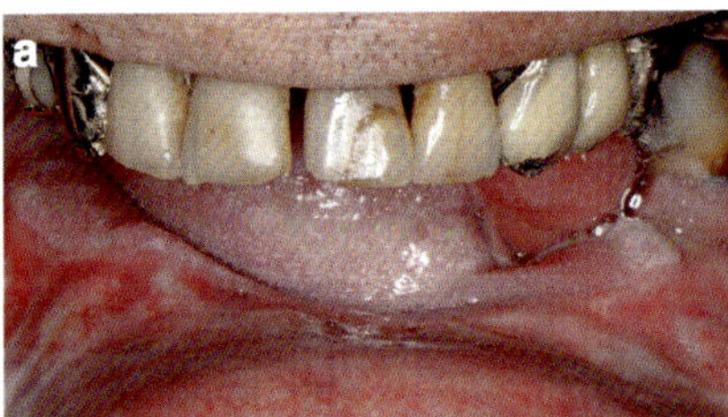
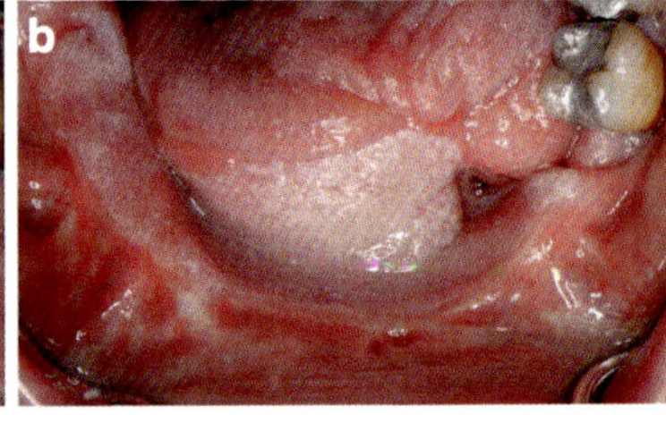

Fig. 8.8 (**a**, **b**) Buccal and occlusal views showing the buccal and lingual partial-thickness flaps exposing the periosteum on the alveolar crest

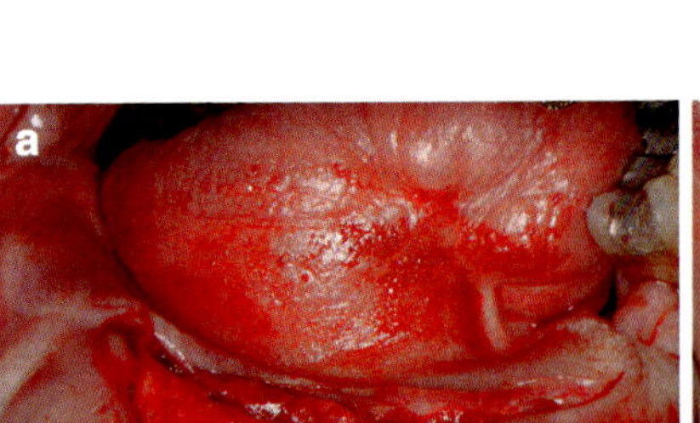
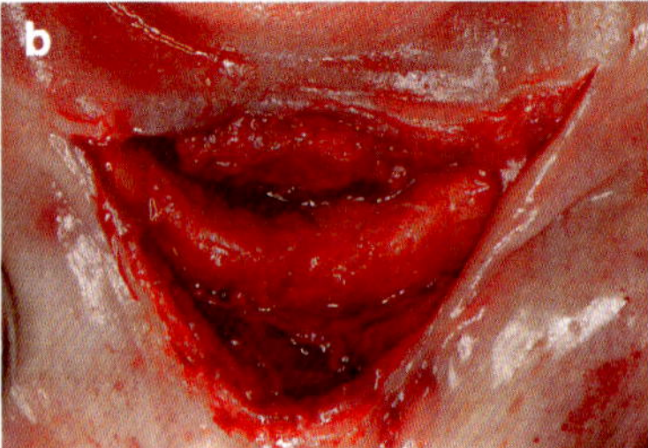
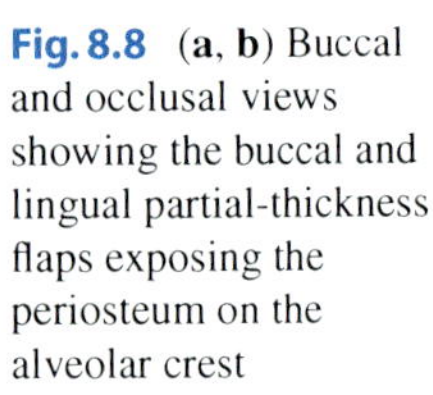

on the periosteum with interrupted 5-0 silk sutures (Fig. 8.10a, b). The buccal flap was sutured apically to the periosteum, and the lingual flap was left unsutured as it will reattach itself spontaneously during the healing phase. The patient is seen 2 weeks postoperatively to remove the sutures and assess initial healing. Three months later, the band of KG has been significantly increased (Fig. 8.11). A full-thickness envelope flap is elevated, and two implants are placed in regions #32 and 42 with 5-mm-long healing abutments in a one-stage surgical procedure (Fig. 8.12). The buccal and lingual flaps were sutured with 4-0 silk sutures (Fig. 8.13).

Another option that might be less technique-sensitive is to proceed with a free gingival graft once the implants are osseointegrated. The second case is a 65-year-old male who presented with a progressing gingival recession and inadequate band of KG (1 mm) on the buccal aspect of his midline implant (Fig. 8.14). An incision was performed at the mucogingival junction,

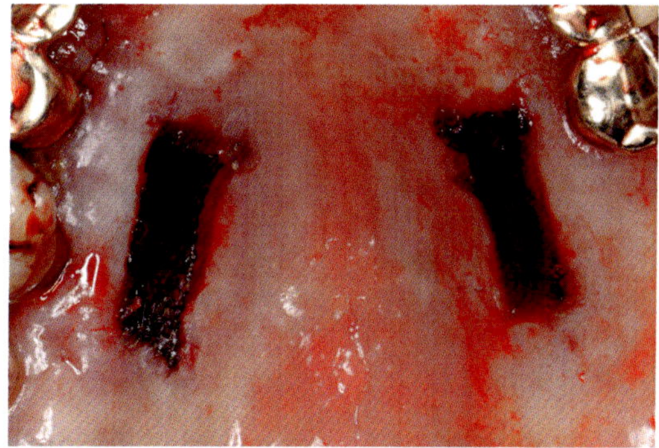

Fig. 8.9 Occlusal view showing the donor sites after harvesting

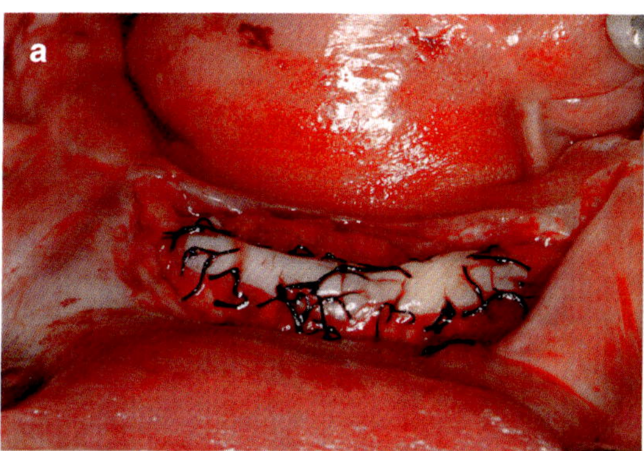

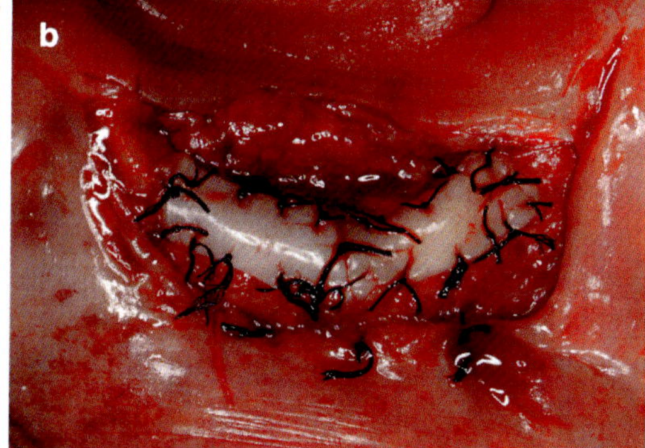

Fig. 8.10 (**a**, **b**) Buccal and occlusal views of the two free gingival grafts sutured to the periosteum

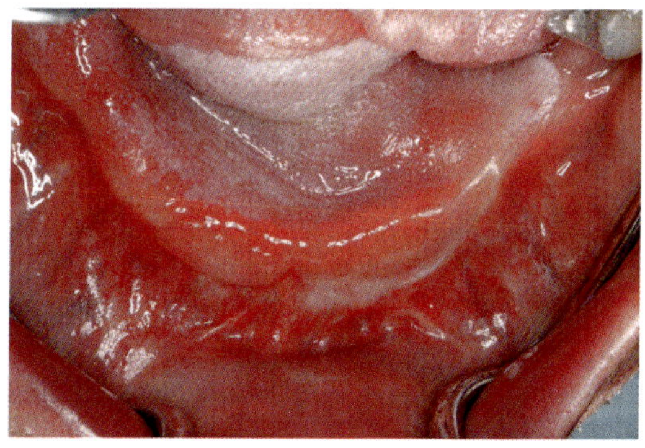

Fig. 8.11 Occlusal view showing the mandibular alveolar ridge three months after the free gingival grafts

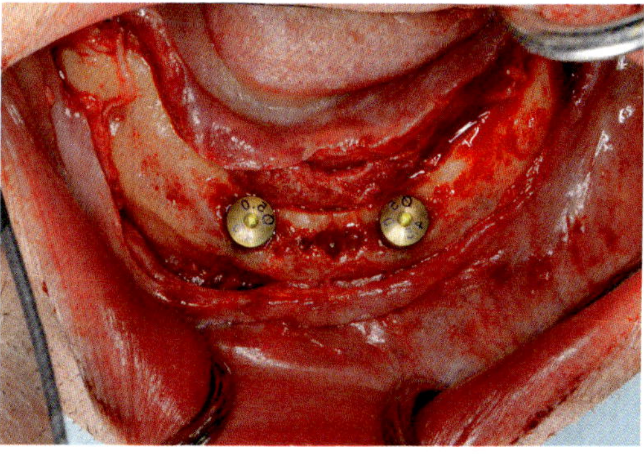

Fig. 8.12 Occlusal view showing the mandibular ridge after the placement of two endosseous implants in the #3.2 and 4.2 area

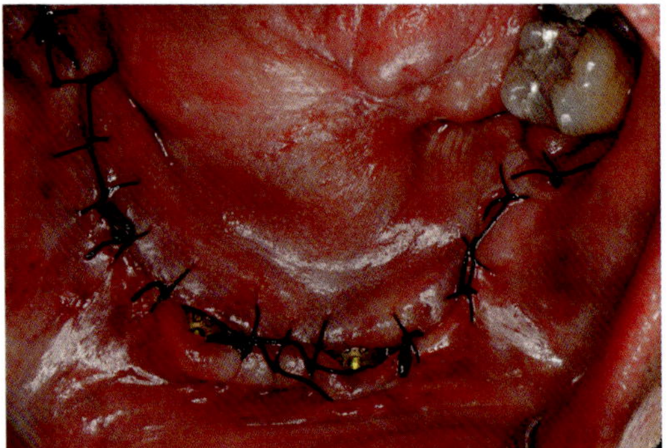

Fig. 8.13 The flaps were sutured with 4-0 silk sutures

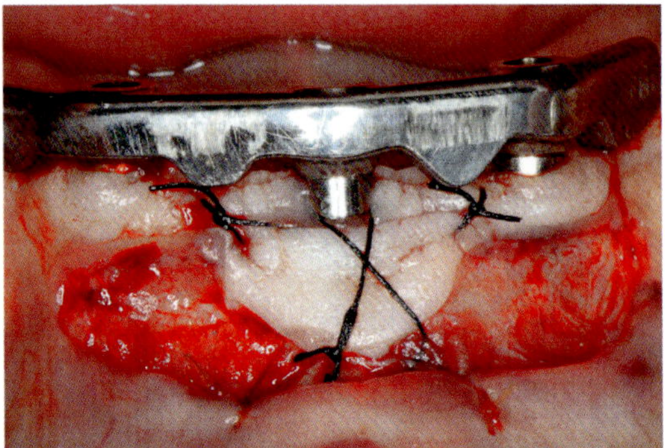

Fig. 8.15 Buccal view showing the free gingival graft sutured to the periosteum on the buccal aspect of the midline implant

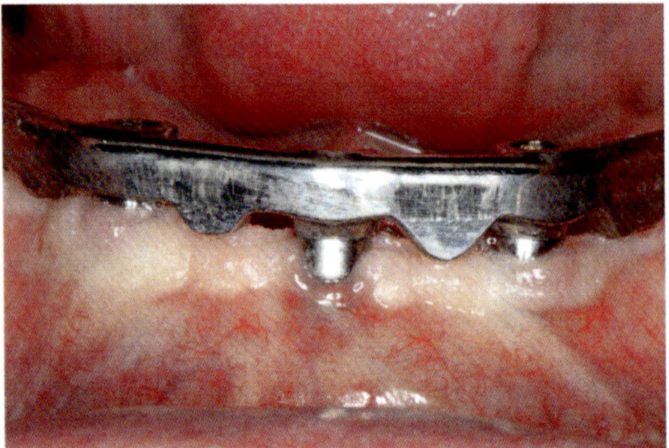

Fig. 8.14 Buccal view showing a retaining bar supported by three dental implants. A mucogingival defect is present on the buccal aspect of the midline implant

and a partial-thickness flap was elevated on the buccal aspect of the implant. A free gingival graft was harvested from the palate, close to the posterior gingival crest, and sutured on the buccal aspect of the implant (Fig. 8.15). A cellulose dressing with cyanoacrylate tissue adhesive was placed over the donor site after hemostasis was achieved (Fig. 8.16). A periodontal dressing (Coe-Pak®, GC America Inc., Alsip, IL, USA) was placed over the recipient site to protect the graft, and the patient was advised not to wear the denture for 1 week postoperatively, until the dressing is removed (Fig. 8.17a, b). After 1 week, surface necrosis of the graft is visible but it is attached to the periosteum (Fig. 8.18). The sutures were removed and the patient was told to brush gently with a soft bristle toothbrush. Two weeks later, the gingival graft is keratinized and the

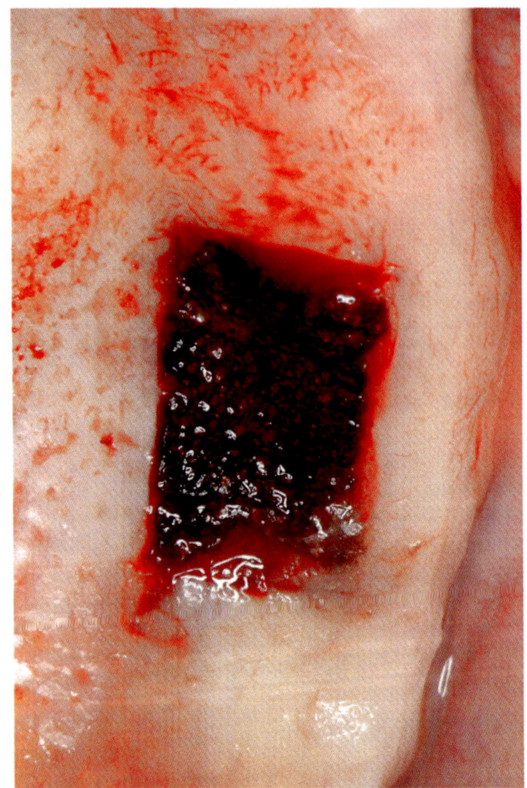

Fig. 8.16 Occlusal view showing the donor site after harvesting

band of KG has significantly increased (Fig. 8.19). Regular oral hygiene measures may be resumed around the implants and the bar. The donor site in the palate is almost completely healed as well (Fig. 8.20).

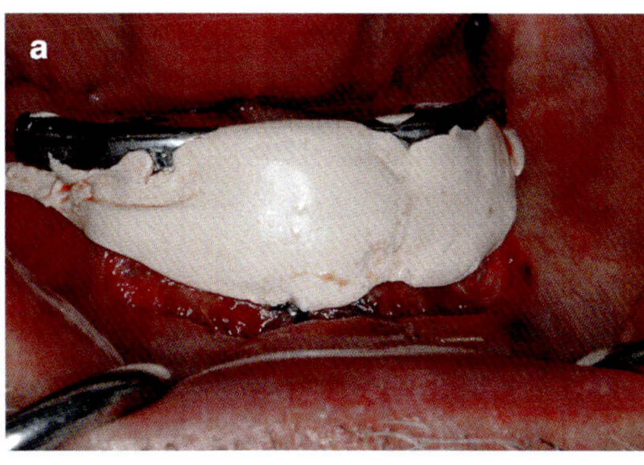
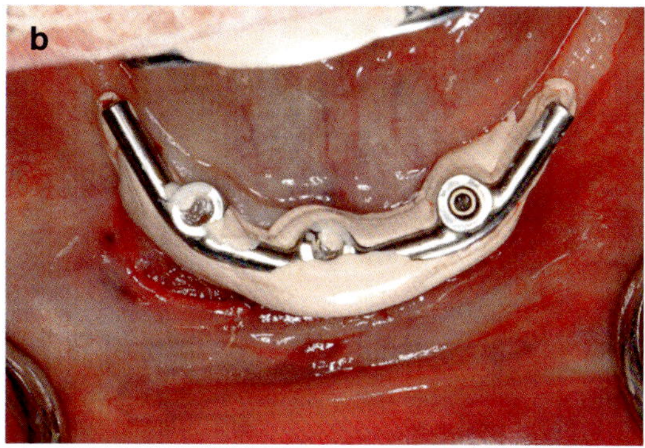

Fig. 8.17 (**a**, **b**) Buccal and occlusal views showing the periodontal dressing used to cover the free gingival graft

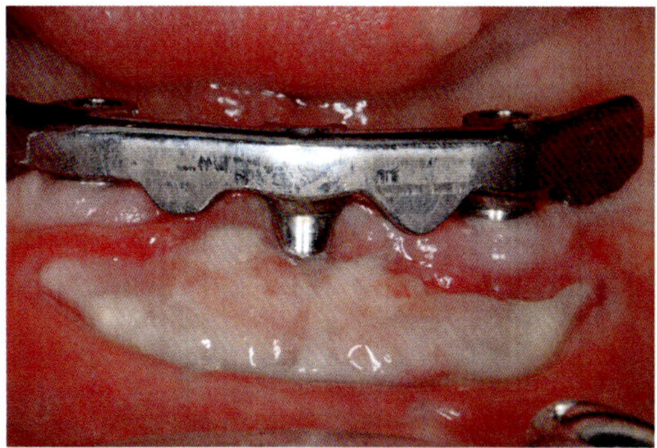

Fig. 8.18 Buccal view showing the free gingival graft after one week of healing

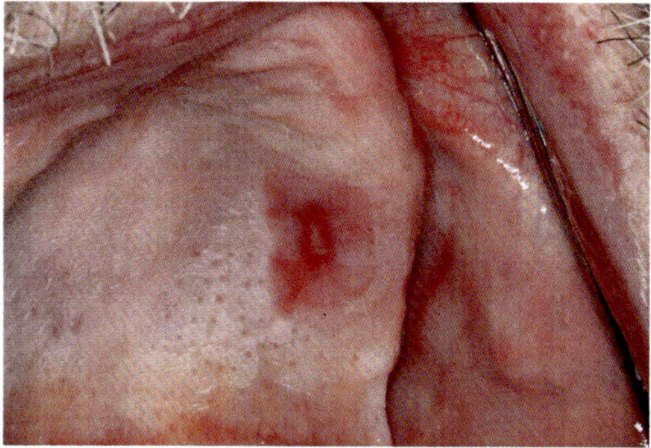

Fig. 8.20 Occlusal view showing the donor site after three weeks of healing

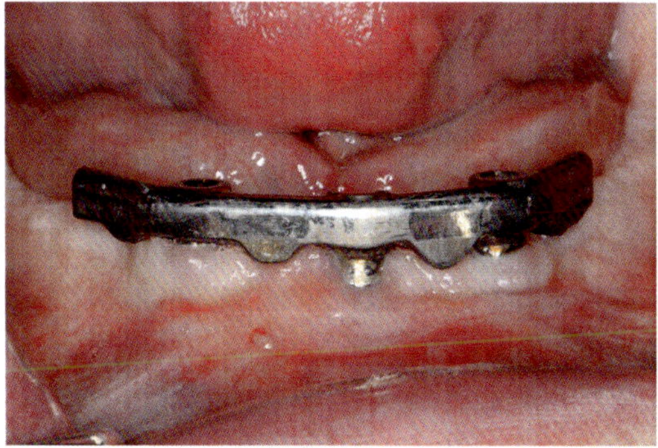

Fig. 8.19 Buccal view showing the free gingival graft after three weeks of healing

The apically positioned flap is a more conservative approach compared to the free gingival graft as there is no need for a donor site. However, a minimal buccolingual width of 1 mm of KG is required on the mandibular ridge to allow apically positioned suturing [99]. An incision is initially performed in the middle of the remaining band of KG. A partial-thickness flap is then raised on the buccal aspect of the ridge to expose the periosteum. The buccal flap is sutured to the underlying periosteum at the desired depth. The mandibular complete denture or overdenture should not be worn for at least two weeks. At the postoperative appointment, an increase in width of KG is usually noted. The granulation cells migrating into the wound area dictate the nature of the new tissues that will cover the exposed periosteum [101–103]. Since this exposed periosteum is entirely surrounded by KG, the epithelial cells from the oral mucosa cannot reach the area. Consequently, the connective tissue and epithelial cells come from the wound margins that are keratinized, allowing the formation of new KG to take place. This approach was described and illustrated in detail elsewhere [99].

8.6 Room Preparation and Surgical Instrumentation

As mentioned before, the better prepared the surgeon and his assistants are, the more efficient the dental team will be during the surgery. All team members play a crucial role in planning the surgery and preparing the surgical room. Highest level of asepsis must be respected before and during surgery. The surgical guide is often a duplicate of the patient's current denture and must clearly indicate where the ideal implant locations should be using lines with a permanent marker (Fig. 8.21a, b). Disinfection may be achieved by soaking it in a 0.12% chlorhexidine gluconate solution to achieve proper disinfection prior to surgery (Fig. 8.22). It must be available at the time of surgery since it will simplify significantly the implant placement procedure for the surgeon. Also, all the required radiographs should be displayed in the surgical room, and the medical history of the patient should be reviewed one last time immediately before the surgery with the patient as it may have changed. Sterile drapes on a table with implant surgery kit and surgical instruments in a cassette, implant motor with handpiece and irrigation system, electric motor with universal cutting burs for ridge recontour-

ing, surgical gloves and implants, and healing abutments should be in place (Fig. 8.23a–f).

The surgical cassette should include sharp and well-maintained instruments to facilitate handling of soft and hard tissues. The number of instruments should be kept to a minimum to facilitate not only sterilization but to render handling more efficient intraoperatively. Indeed, implant placement in the edentulous patient will often last longer than the single-tooth implant surgery due to its complexity, and care must be taken to reduce operatory time as much as possible. The surgical procedure can easily be performed using local anesthesia containing a vasoconstrictor such as epinephrine in a concentration of 1:100 K or 1:50 K. If a longer surgery (more than two hours) is planned, bupivacaine 0.5% may be used. An adequate quantity of carpules must be available for the duration of the surgical procedure (Fig. 8.24).

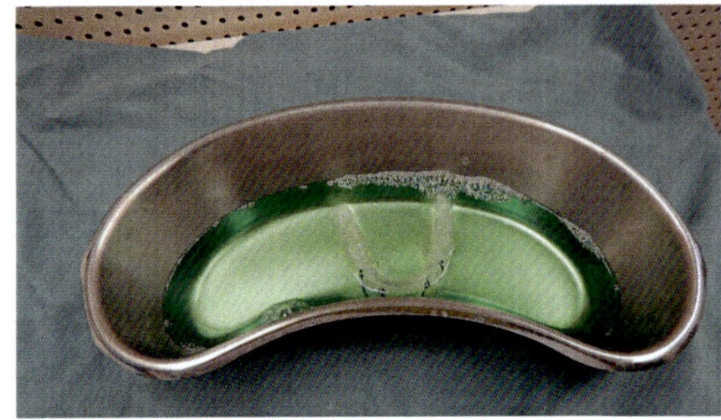

Fig. 8.22 Surgical guide soaking in a 0.12% chlorhexidine gluconate solution

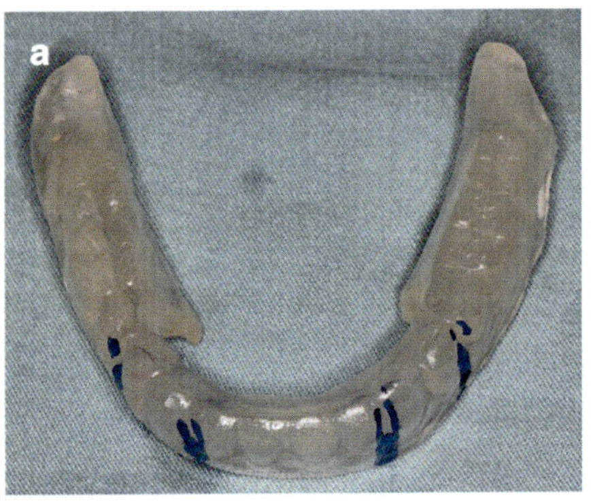
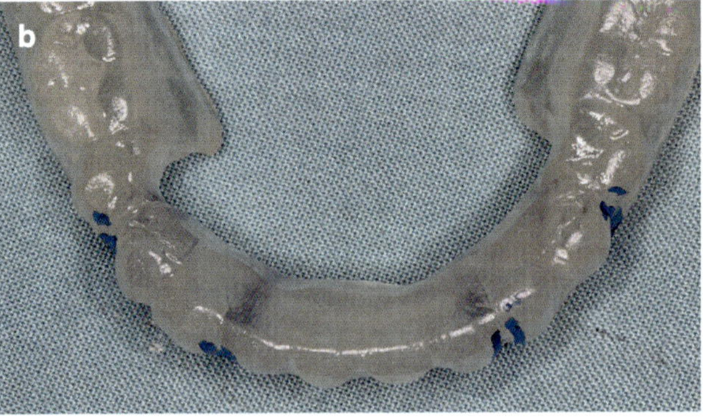

Fig. 8.21 (**a**, **b**) The surgical guide used for the placement of dental implants on the edentulous mandibular ridge

The surgical instruments listed here are commonly used during implant surgery on edentulous patients at the Université de Montréal dental clinics. Figure 8.25 shows the instruments from left to right in a surgical cassette (with their respective purpose(s).

Lower compartment (Fig. 8.25a):

- Mirror (tissue retraction, indirect view on the lingual aspect)
- UNC-15 periodontal probe
- Two blade handles
- Hirschfeld periosteal elevator (for muscle fibers and flap elevation)
- Goldman-Fox periosteal elevator (for flap elevation)
- Pritchard periosteal elevator (for lingual flap elevation and retraction)
- Orban knife (to facilitate flap elevation, especially flap corners)

- Wedelstaedt straight bone chisel (for osteoplasty around implant platform after insertion)
- Rhodes back-action bone chisel (for ridge osteoplasty and ridge debridement)
- Miller surgical curette (for curettage of residual tooth sockets and ridge debridement)
- Ochsenbein 1 (for ridge osteoplasty and ridge debridement)
- Ochsenbein 2 (for ridge osteoplasty and ridge debridement)
- Nabers probe (for mental foramen detection)
- Castroviejo needle holder (for suturing)
- Gerald tissue forceps (for delicate soft tissue handling)
- Corn suture pliers (for suturing membranes around implants if guided bone regeneration is indicated)
- Dressing pliers
- Anesthetic syringe

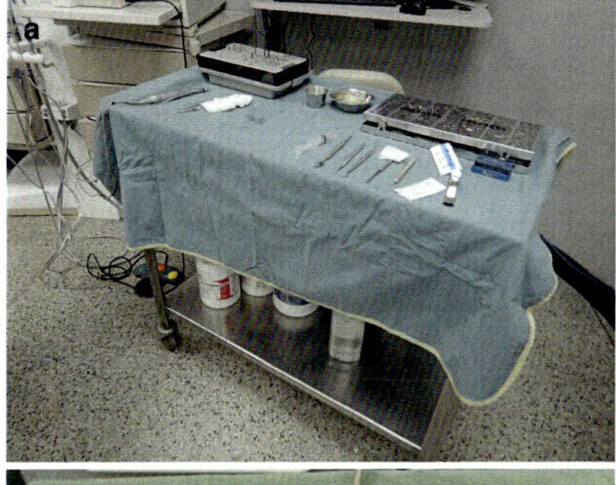

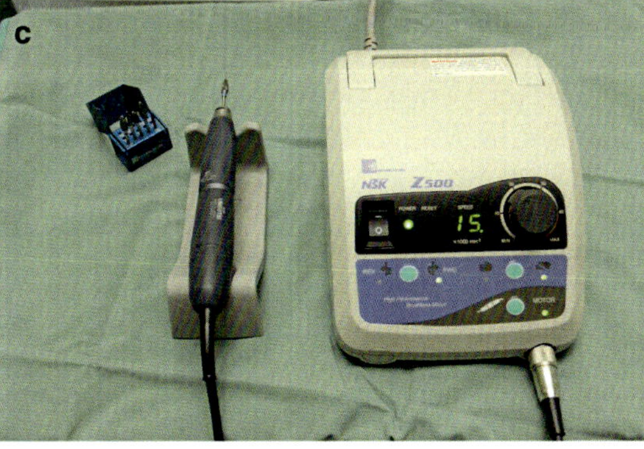

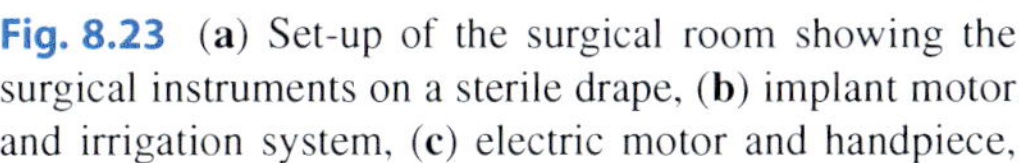

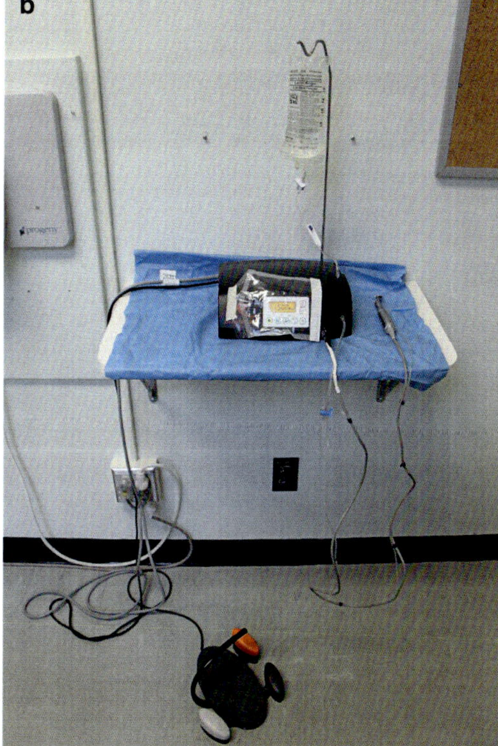

Fig. 8.23 (**a**) Set-up of the surgical room showing the surgical instruments on a sterile drape, (**b**) implant motor and irrigation system, (**c**) electric motor and handpiece, (**d**) set of universal cutting burs, (**e**) surgical gloves, and (**f**) implants and healing abutments

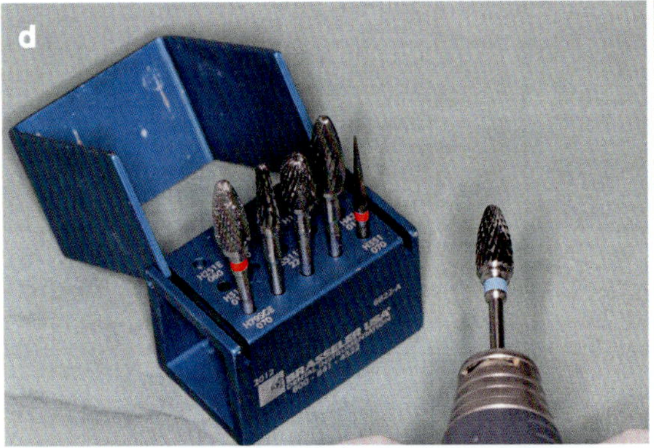
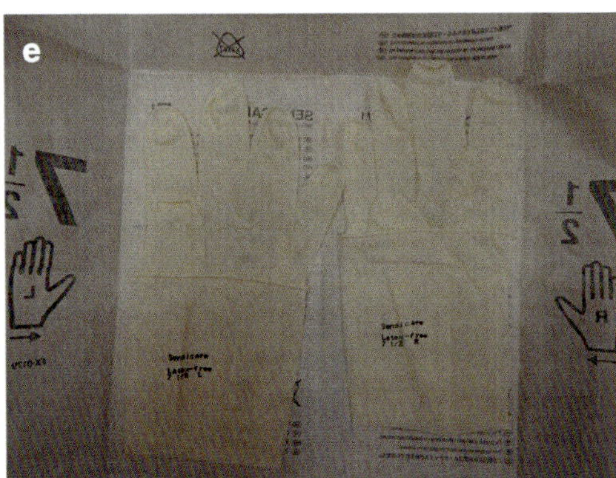
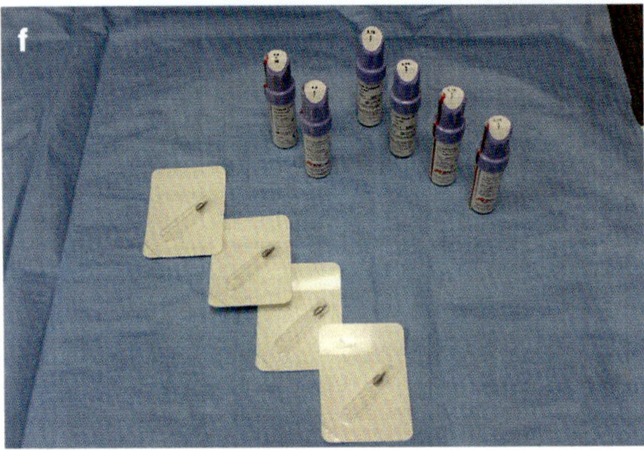

Fig. 8.23 (continued)

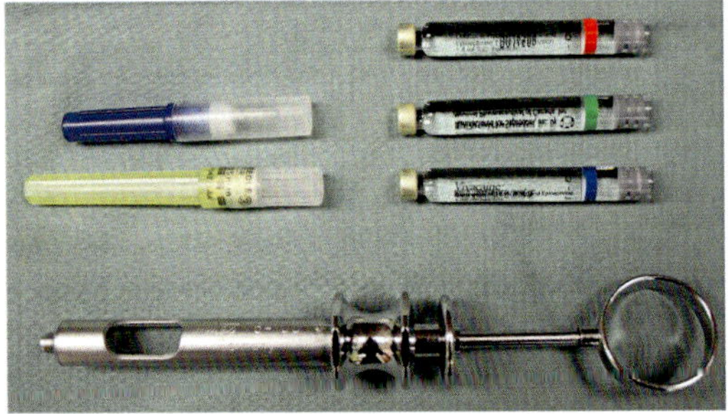

Fig. 8.24 From bottom to top: self-aspirating anesthetic syringe, long 27- and short 30-gauge needle, bupivacaine 0.5% 1:200 K epinephrine, lidocaine 2% 1:50 K epinephrine, and lidocaine 2% 1:100 K epinephrine

– Surgical suction tips with adapters
– Minnesota retractor (for buccal flap retraction)

Upper compartment (Fig. 8.25b):

– Crile-Wood needle holder (for suturing)
– Goldman-Fox scissors (for suture or tissue cutting)

– Curved Halsted-Mosquito hemostat (for hemorrhage control, root tip extraction, or small object grasp)

The implant system is usually selected according to the surgeon's preference. All components related to the implant surgical phase should be functional prior to surgery including implant motor and foot pedal, handpiece, tubing, sterile irrigation solution, and surgical implant kit. The latter should include all the necessary implant drills placed in the sequence of use to optimize surgical time and minimize surgical errors. Connection of the irrigation tubes should be verified in order to provide adequate irrigation during surgery.

It has been demonstrated that the extent of necrotic bone around the osteotomy site is proportional with the heat generated during implant bed preparation [104], and thermonecrosis has been reported in the literature [105, 106]. The heat generated may be reduced using different

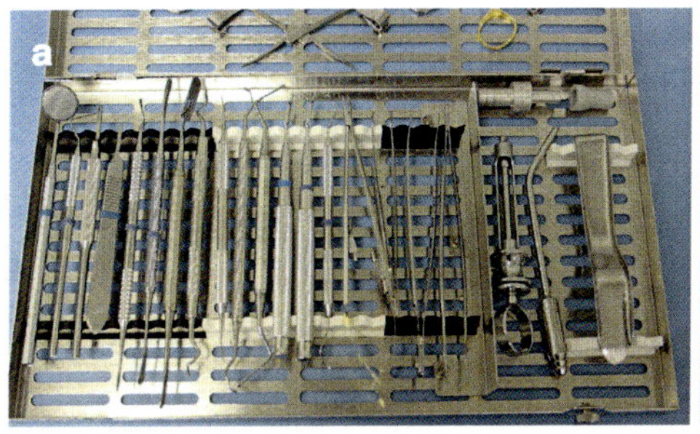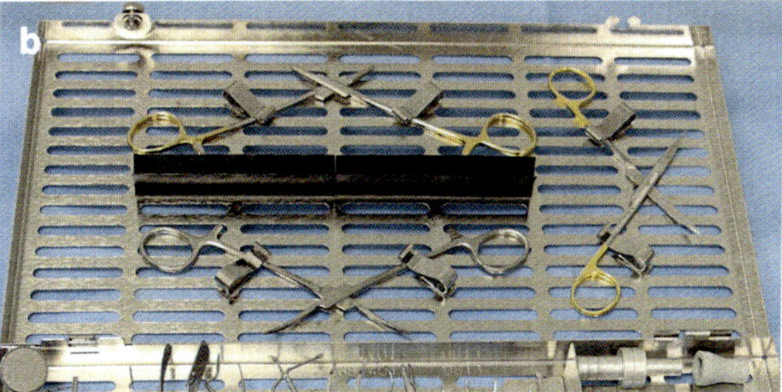

Fig. 8.25 Cassette containing the surgical instruments needed to perform the implant placement procedure. (**a**) Lower compartment of the cassette containing the surgical instruments. (**b**) Upper compartment of the cassette containing the remaining surgical instruments

measures. Sterile saline or physiologic water must be used with a patent irrigation system to allow cooling of the implant drill while performing the osteotomy to avoid overheating of the bone. External and internal irrigation systems are both efficient at reducing heat produced during the osteotomy preparation [107]. Although drill design and wear may affect cutting efficiency, durability, and heat generation [108, 109], no optimal geometrical design has been found so far to reduce heat intraoperatively [110]. The surgical drills used for site preparation should be sharp and provide efficient bone cutting properties without creating excessive heat and trauma to the bone. To minimize risks of overheating the bone associated with drill wear, one must respect the manufacturer's recommendations concerning the usage threshold, which may vary for each drill design. Consequently, keeping a logbook will allow the surgical team to determine the number of time each implant drill has been used and when it must be discarded and replaced.

More than 1300 types of dental implants varying in form, material, dimensions, surface properties, and geometry are available on the market [111]. No specific type of implant has shown superiority over another according to the most recent Cochrane systematic review [112]. However, there was a trend toward earlier failures for implants with turned surfaces. On the other hand, a 20% reduction in risk of developing peri-implantitis was found for implants with turned surfaces compared to implants with rough surfaces after 3 years in function (RR 0.80; 95% CI 0.67–0.96). Regarding the design of the abutment-implant junction, a significant smaller amount of crestal bone loss has been found for platform-switch implants compared to platform-matched implants in a recent systematic review, although most of the included studies had a small sample size with short follow-up periods (mean difference, −0.29 mm; 95% CI −0.38 to −0.19; $P < 0.00001$) [113]. In the authors' opinion, only implant systems that have sufficient well-designed clinical studies prior to marketing should be selected.

A reverse cutting needle is recommended for most surgical procedures in dentistry due to its capacity to cut through tissues with minimal risk of tears, especially when suturing the thin oral mucosa. Keeping the flap margins approximated may be a challenge in the edentulous mandible since the tissues are often mobile due to the presence of muscle insertion close to the top of the alveolar ridge and the frequent lack of KG. Suture strings with a 4-0 or 5-0 diameter provide sufficient resistance and adequate handling in the edentulous mandible. When long-term stability of the flaps is desired, such as in the case of the edentulous mandible after implant placement, a non- or slow-absorbable material is selected to prevent premature flap opening. Silk sutures are nonabsorbable braided materials fabricated with an organic protein called fibroin that is commonly used in dentistry. Other nonabsorbable sutures include monofilament synthetic sutures such as ePTFE, polypropylene, and nylon. Materials such as polyglactin 910, poliglecap-

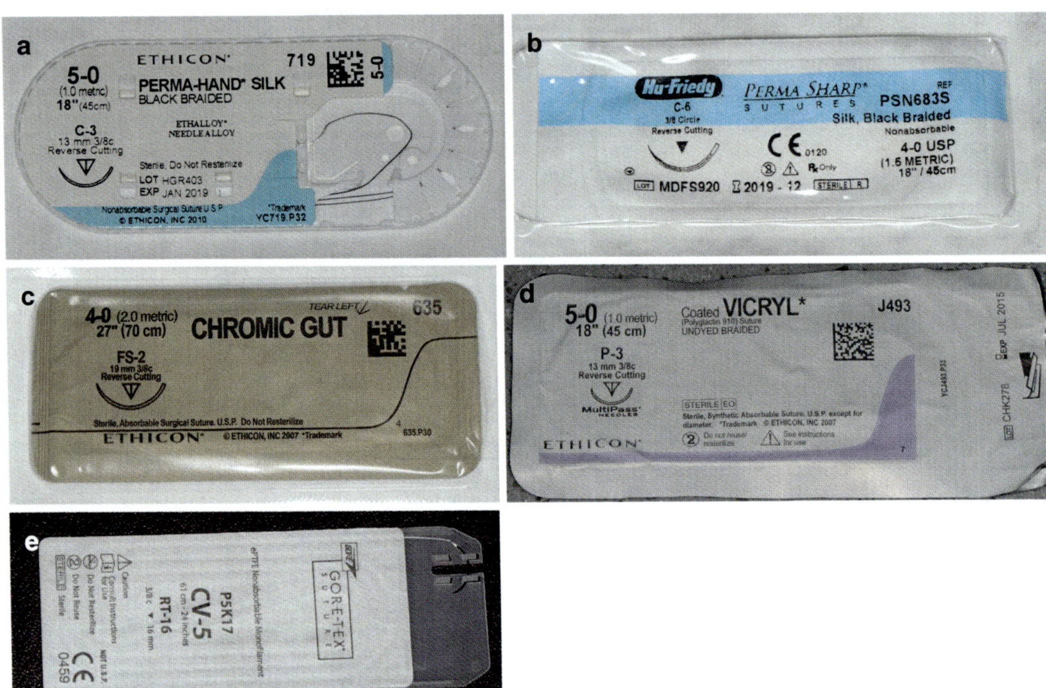

Fig. 8.26 Different suture materials used to suture the flaps during the implant placement procedure. (**a**) Nonabsorbable 5-0 silk with c-3 reverse cutting needle suture material. (**b**) Nonabsorbable 4-0 silk with c-6 reverse cutting needle suture material. (**c**) Absorbable 4-0 chromic gut with FS-2 reverse cutting needle suture material. (**d**) Absorbable 5-0 polyglactic 910 with P3 reverse cutting needle suture material. (**e**) Nonabsorbable CV-5 ePTFE with RT-16 reverse cutting needle suture material

rone 25, and chromic gut are absorbable sutures also commonly used in dentistry. Compared to silk, ePTFE has shown better patient comfort, superior intraoperative ease of handling, less pain after removal, and less plaque accumulation [114]. It has shown significantly less inflammatory infiltrate and smaller degree of slack of the suture loops compared to silk sutures [115]. Poliglecaprone 25 has shown a better biological response when compared to polyglactin 910 sutures in the rat model [116]. Also, its handling is similar to ePTFE, allowing easy intraoperative knot tightening due to its monofilament texture. Chromic gut sutures sustained their tensile strength better than polyglactin 910 sutures in an in vitro study [117]. In that same study, 4-0 sutures showed higher strength than 5-0 sutures. To date, no clinical studies have shown whether specific types of sutures or diameters have a beneficial effect on implant success rate. Hence, it is up to the surgeon's preferences to select a specific suture material. Figure 8.26a–e shows commonly used sutures at the Université de Montréal dental clinics.

8.7 Patient Preparation

Most implant placement surgical procedures should be done using a strict asepsis protocol. The surgeon needs to select an implant system that has demonstrated a high level of predictability in controlled clinical studies. Each implant system has its own specific armamentarium and protocol for use. It is therefore essential to follow the manufacturer's protocol in terms of drill sequence and rotating speed. The implants should ideally be inserted at the recommended torque from the manufacturer.

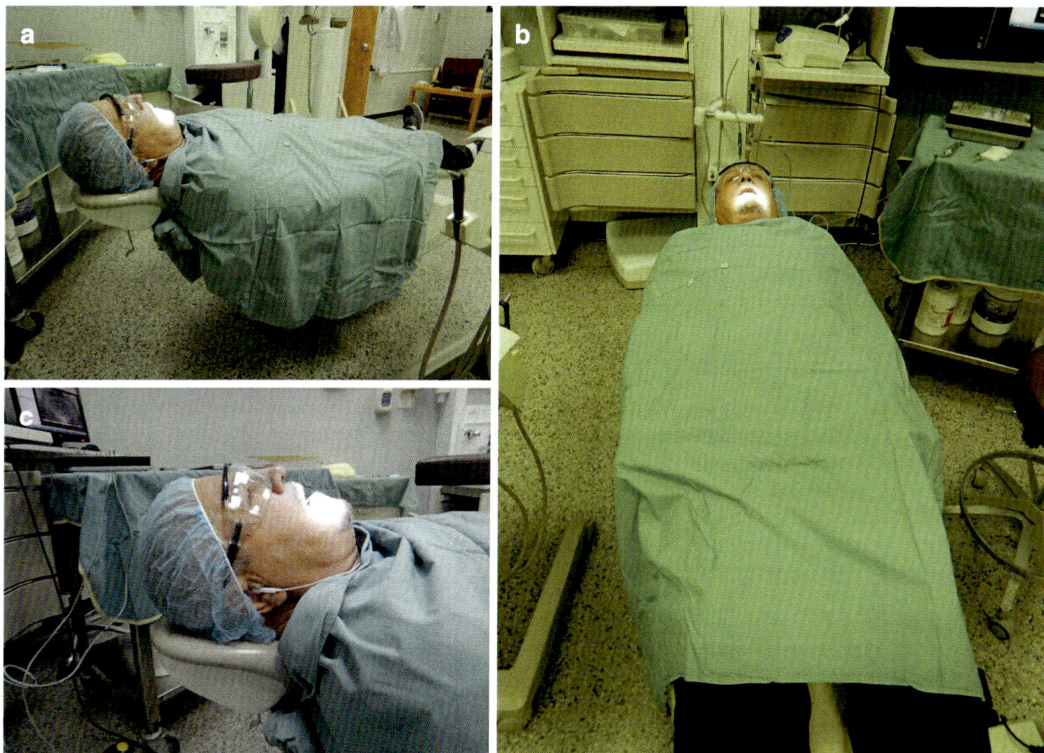

Fig. 8.27 (**a–c**) The patient is draped, the head is covered, and he wears protective eyewear

The procedure needs to be performed in an aseptic environment using sterile equipment. The patient is draped and wears protective eyewear (Fig. 8.27a–c). The surgeon and his assistant also wear a sterile uniform and protective eyewear (Fig. 8.28), although the use of non-sterile scrubs for the surgeon and his staff and smaller sterile drapes have shown no significant differences in implant survival rate compared to the standard sterile protocol [118, 119].

For all implant surgeries, it is recommended to give a preoperative analgesic to the patient such as acetaminophen (paracetamol in Europe) or, preferably, a nonsteroidal anti-inflammatory analgesic (NSAID). Indeed, preemptive intake of nonsteroidal anti-inflammatory analgesics (NSAIDS) has shown reduction of postoperative edema and reduction of additional postoperative analgesic intake as well as an increased delay before the first postoperative analgesic intake [120]. A preoperative antibiotic is given once preoperatively (e.g., 2 g amoxicillin) for all patients undergoing implant surgery as it was found to reduce the implant failure rate in the latest Cochrane review [121]. In addition, a 0.12% chlorhexidine rinse for 30 s prior to surgery is used to reduce the oral bacterial count [122].

Local anesthesia with a vasoconstrictor is recommended to achieve a long and deep anesthesia. The concentration of the vasoconstrictor 1:50 K epinephrine is the preferred choice to reduce bleeding during a surgical procedure [123]. Lidocaine 2% is generally used, but for longer surgeries, bupivacaine 0.5% with epinephrine may also be used to increase the duration of local anesthesia. Bilateral inferior alveolar nerve blocks with local buccal and lingual infiltrations will generally provide adequate anesthesia for mandibular implant placement. However, the amount of local anesthetic that can be safely administered to geriatric patients should be approximately 70% of the maximum dose recommended by the manufacturer due to their reduced metabolism [76].

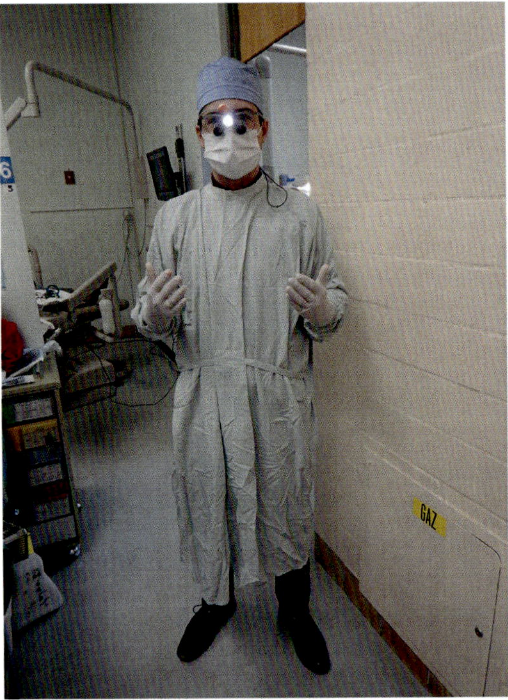

Fig. 8.28 Surgeon wearing a sterile gown and protective eyewear

8.8 Surgical Procedure for Implant Placement

8.8.1 Incisions and Flap Elevation

Once the local anesthesia has been established, the surgical procedure begins with the full-thickness incisions and the elevation of buccal and lingual mucoperiosteal flaps. Some factors must be considered when planning the flap design and the configuration of the incisions:

- The number of implants: If three to five implants have to be placed, an increased surgical access will be needed to localize the mental foramina. This approach allows the surgeon to place the most distal implant at a safe distance mesial to the mental foramina.

- Ridge recontouring: If the edentulous ridge requires osteoplasty to eliminate a knife-edge ridge and irregularities or to increase the inter-occlusal space, more access will be needed. In both situations, the incisions will be extended

further posteriorly to the first or second molar areas.

The surgical procedure demonstrated in this section is from a 65-year-old female seeking to improve the function and stability of her man-dibular complete denture with a bar with clip prosthetic system supported by four dental implants (Fig. 8.29a–c). A free gingival graft had been previously performed in the #4.3 and 4.4 area. The panoramic film shows that recent extractions were done and an adequate bone height to allow implant placement was present (Fig. 8.29d). The lateral cephalograph shows a knife-edge anterior alveolar ridge that will neces-sitate at least 7 mm of osseous reduction with osteoplasty before implant site preparation may be initiated to allow a flat and regular ridge sur-face (Fig. 8.29e). After bilateral inferior alveolar blocks, mental blocks, and buccal and lingual infiltrations are completed, the surgery may be initiated. The main incision is located in the cen-ter of the edentulous ridge and is contained within the keratinized gingiva (KG) (Fig. 8.30). This will distribute an equal amount of KG on the buc-cal and lingual aspects of every implant and therefore, optimizing the amount of postopera-tive KG around the implants. Another advantage of performing the incision within the KG is that it is easier to manage the flaps during suturing and in the authors' experience, it results in less edema and less discomfort for the patient.

Vertical releasing incisions on the buccal aspect of the ridge will improve access to the sur-gical area. The ideal location to perform the releasing incisions is generally in the first molar area. A periosteal elevator is then used to raise full-thickness buccal and lingual flaps. The eleva-tor must be seated against the bone to prevent trauma and tear to the soft tissues. The extension of the reflection must enable the surgeon to locate the position of the mental foramen and to per-form bone recontouring when indicated. The alveolar ridge must be thoroughly debrided of all soft and granulation tissues with curettes, perios-teal elevators, or bone chisels. This is especially true if the teeth were recently extracted and when the sockets are still recognizable such as in this

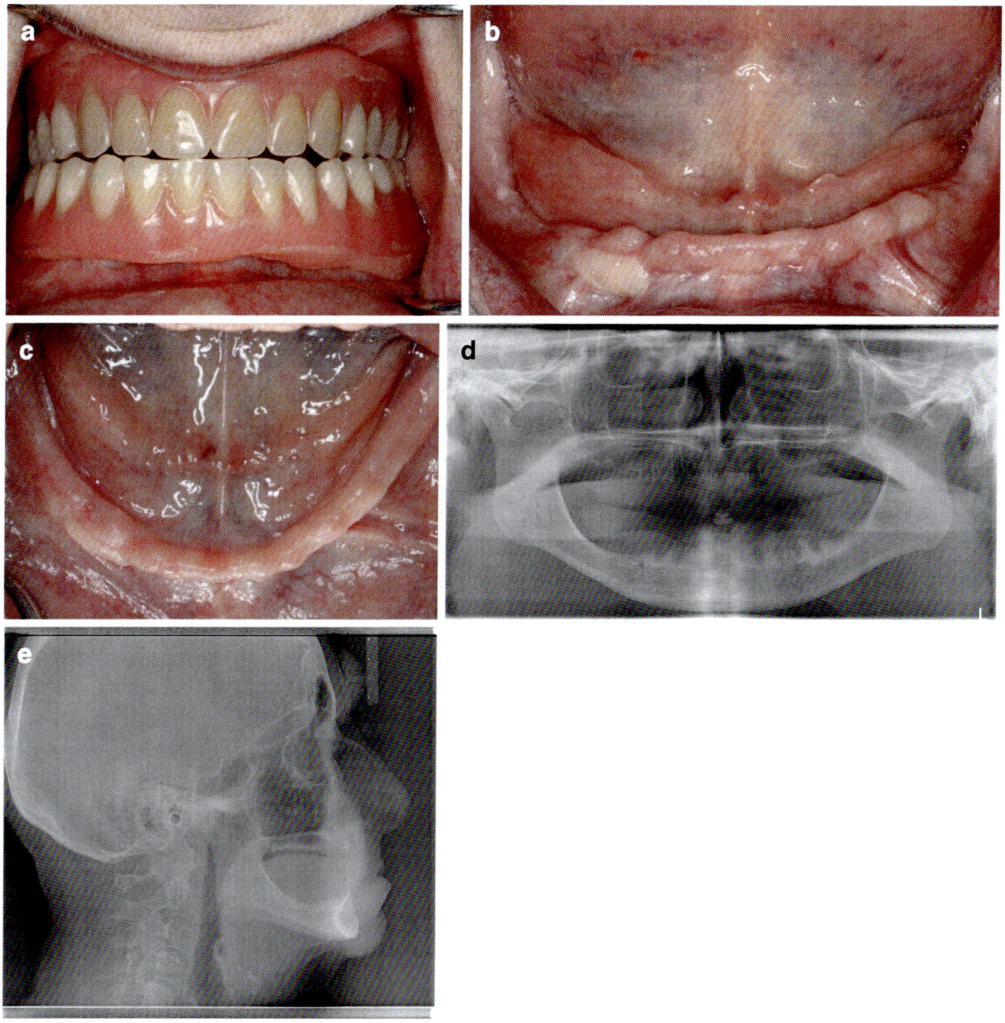

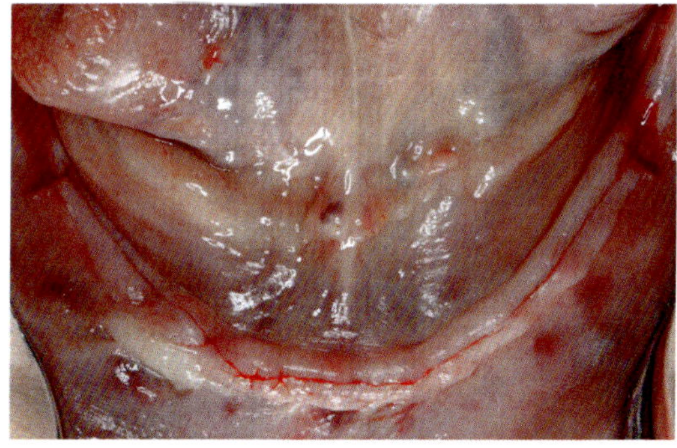

Fig. 8.29 (**a**) View of the dentures in occlusion, (**b**) buccal view of the edentulous mandible, (**c**) occlusal view of the edentulous mandible, (**d**) panoramic radiograph, and (**e**) lateral cephalograph

Fig. 8.30 Incision performed in the center of the KG and extending to the first molar areas. Two releasing incisions on the buccal aspect are performed bilaterally at the distal aspect of the main incision

case. The ridge shows severe buccolingual resorption and needs to be fully exposed before ridge recontouring can be done to remove all irregularities (Fig. 8.31a, b). This is a common finding in elderly edentulous patients.

If implants are to be placed near the mental foramen, its location and the possibility that an anterior loop may be present mesial to the mental foramen need to be considered before implant placement to avoid inferior alveolar nerve injury. Adequate radiographic interpretation regarding the location of the mental foramen and the presence and length of the anterior loop of the mental foramen is mandatory. The radio-

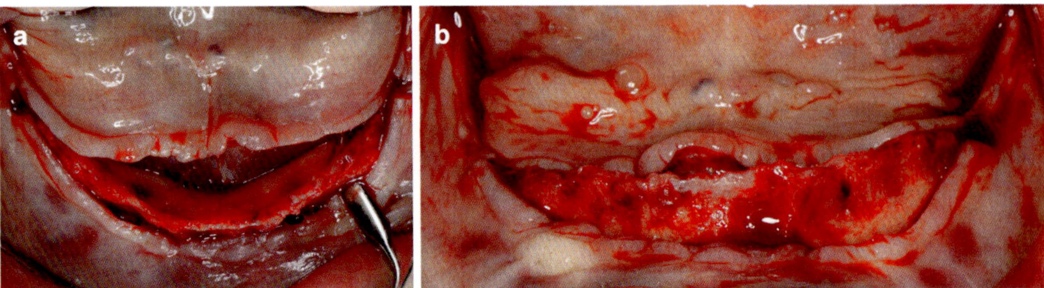

Fig. 8.31 (**a**) Occlusal view of the mandible with a full-thickness buccal and lingual flap exposing the alveolar bone. (**b**) Full-thickness flap showing the buccal aspect of the alveolar bone

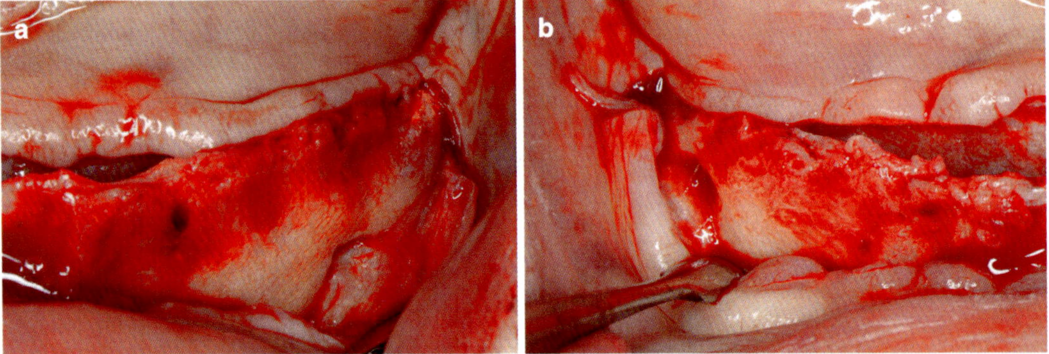

Fig. 8.32 Full-thickness flap exposing the coronal aspect of the (**a**) left mental nerve and (**b**) right mental nerve

graphs should be displayed so the surgeon can easily corroborate radiographic and clinical observations during the surgery. A periosteal elevator is used to raise a full-thickness flap up to the coronal margin of the foramen. Figure 8.32a, b shows the left and right mental nerves exposed. A blunt furcation probe (Nabers probe) may be gently inserted into the foramen to determine whether the distal aspect is patent [124]. If it is not patent, then the nerve entered on the mesial side, confirming the presence of an anterior loop.

If the absence of an anterior loop has been confirmed, an implant may be placed so that its distal aspect is 2 mm mesial to the mental foramen. If there is an anterior loop, it is recommended to preserve a distance of 2 mm mesial to the loop before placing the most distal implant. This distance may be measured from the mesial wall of the loop [12]. If there are doubts concerning the presence and/or extent of an anterior loop, it is recommended to obtain a CBCT.

8.8.2 Ridge Recontouring (Optional)

If ridge recontouring is required, it must be performed prior to any preparation of the osteotomy sites for the implants. Careful manipulation of the lingual flap is very important in order to prevent any trauma to the periosteum and the adjacent important blood supply located in the floor of the mouth. A high-speed surgical handpiece or a straight electric handpiece is used to recontour the ridge and remove irregularities with copious irrigation (Fig. 8.33a, b). Osteoplasty is needed until the thickness of the edentulous ridge allows the placement of the implants with 1 mm of bone on both buccal and lingual aspects of each

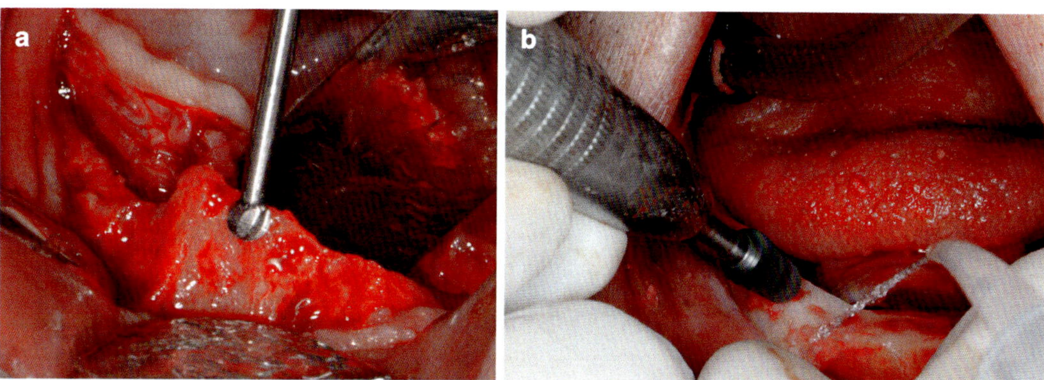

Fig. 8.33 Osteoplasty of the edentulous ridge being performed using (**a**) a #8 round carbide bur on a high-speed surgical handpiece or (**b**) a large carbide universal bur mounted on a straight surgical electric handpiece

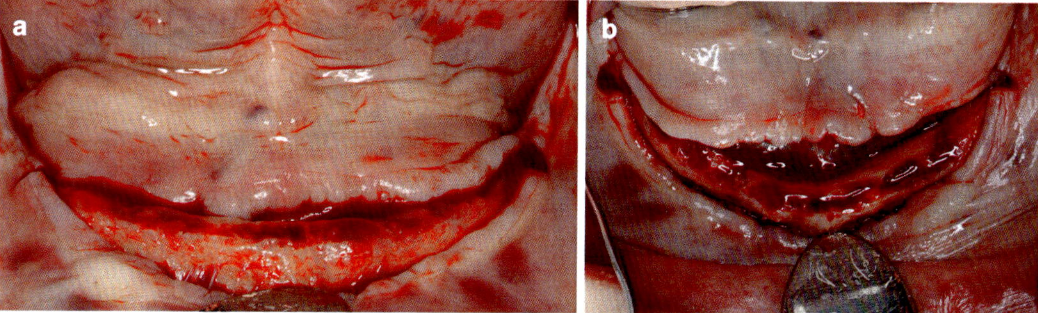

Fig. 8.34 (**a**) Buccal view and (**b**) occlusal view of the alveolar ridge after recontouring

implant. Figure 8.34a, b shows the edentulous ridge after bone recontouring.

Indications for ridge recontouring are:

- Thin and knife-edge alveolar ridge
- Alveolar sockets present
- Lack of interocclusal space for prosthetic components (this situation may be found when the ridge shows very little resorption or when the teeth were recently extracted)
- Uneven alveolar ridge
- Presence of a prominent genial tubercle

8.8.3 Osteotomy Site Preparation

Once the alveolar ridge has been debrided and leveled, the implant osteotomy site may be initiated. The surgeon follows the sequence and protocol of the implant system selected. A series of drills, specific for each implant system, are used in sequence and according to the type of bone encountered.

Illustrated in this chapter are the sequences used for the placement of screw-type, threaded, self-tapping, external hex endosseous implants (Nobel Biocare Branemark MK III® implants, Nobel Biocare Inc., Kloten, Switzerland).

With a surgical guide in place, the surgeon marks all the implant sites using a round or spear-point bur. This marking bur will facilitate the next step, which is the first osteotomy preparation with a 2 mm twist drill (Fig. 8.35). This drill establishes the desired depth and the alignment of the implants. While drilling in the interforaminal area, caution must be exercised to avoid perforating the lingual cortex, which could result in hemorrhaging from the blood supply of the floor of the mouth. Direct visualization of the ridge morphology will allow the surgeon to properly angulate the 2 mm twist drill. This will ensure that the implant osteotomy site is contained within the mandibular bone. Emphasis should be placed on the parallelism between all implants. This may be facilitated by asking the surgical assistant to verify the axis in the buccolingual direction, while the surgeon empha-

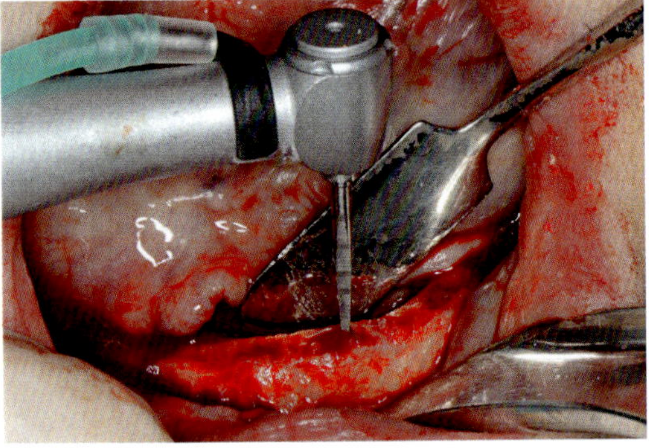

Fig. 8.35 The spear-point bur marking the sites of the implants on the edentulous ridge

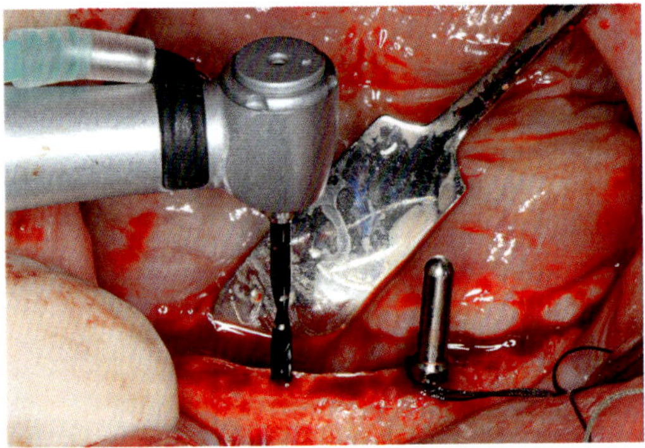

Fig. 8.36 The 2 mm twist drill preparing the osteotomy sites on the edentulous ridge

sizes on the mesiodistal angulation of the osteotomy drill or vice versa. Also, the surgeon may use two hands to maintain a constant axis of the bur and pressure on the handpiece. The implants should be inserted as perpendicular as possible to the occlusal plane and at a similar occlusal height on the alveolar crest in order to balance the load on the implants. Figure 8.36 shows the 2 mm twist drill preparing the osteotomy sites with a guide pin in place to facilitate parallelism between the osteotomy sites. An up-and-down movement of the drill at high speed (1000–1500 RPM) with a firm but not excessive pressure will allow the irrigation to reach the bone and, hence, adequate cooling of the osteotomy site being prepared. In the authors' opinion, it is easier to start with the midline implant(s) osteotomy preparations and, then, proceed posteriorly to the distal sites.

After the first osteotomy drill has been used, the surgeon may estimate the bone density using the Lekholm and Zarb classification [125]. A higher bone density type 1 or 2 will require slightly higher apical pressure on the twist drill than a bone density type 3 or 4. While preparing the osteotomy sites, the surgeon may want to assess the quality and the depth of the local anesthesia by communicating with the patient. This shows empathy and helps building a bond of trust between the surgeon and the patient. This will likely reduce the patient's anxiety during surgery.

A guide pin is then inserted in each osteotomy site, and with the surgical guide in place, it is possible to confirm the proper position, angulation, and parallelism of the implants' axis (Fig. 8.37a,

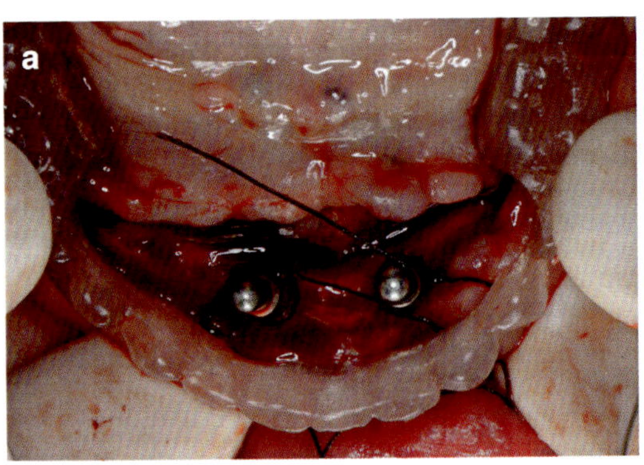
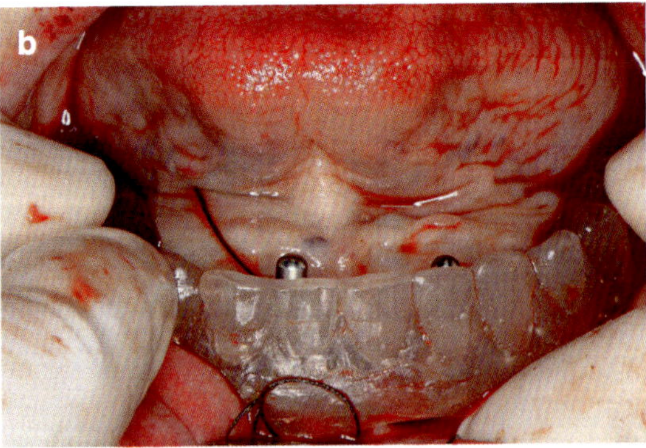

Fig. 8.37 (**a**) Occlusal view and (**b**) buccal view showing the first two osteotomy sites prepared

b). At this point, the two posterior sites may be prepared while keeping in place the midline guide pins as a guide. After completion of all osteotomy sites, guide pins are inserted in all osteotomy sites, and the positions are confirmed with the surgical guide (Fig. 8.38a–c).

A second twist drill (2.4/2.8 mm diameter) is then used to increase the diameter of the osteotomy site. At this point, it is still possible, if required, to adjust the angulation of the osteotomy site. In the presence of a low bone density that might not allow the implant to achieve an adequate primary stability, i.e., an insertion torque of 30 Ncm or higher, one option is to underprepare the site by skipping the final twist drill and attempt to insert the implant at this stage.

The final twist drill is 3 mm in diameter and completes the final preparation of the osteotomy sites. It is critical to maintain the same axis with the previous drill to ensure parallelism between the implants.

With the Branemark® implant system, the countersink drill is used to widen the crestal part of the osteotomy site and allow for the crestal placement of the implant platform (Fig. 8.39). The depth of the osteotomy sites is confirmed using the implant manufacturer's depth probe (Fig. 8.40). In addition, the osteotomy integrity may be confirmed with this probe to rule out any cortical perforation. At this point, the implants may be inserted. Figure 8.41 shows the four osteotomy sites prepared.

The implants used in this clinical case are 3.75 mm in diameter and are self-tapping. Therefore, it is not necessary to create screw threads (tap) in the osteotomy sites before the insertion of the implants. However, in the presence of dense cortical bone (type I), it is recommended to tap the sites, as it may be very difficult to insert the implants, which could generate excessive insertion torque leading to compression bone necrosis, although this phenomenon has been debated in the literature [126, 127]. Care must be taken to avoid contact of the implant surface with contaminated instruments to prevent postoperative infection and subsequent loss of osseointegration.

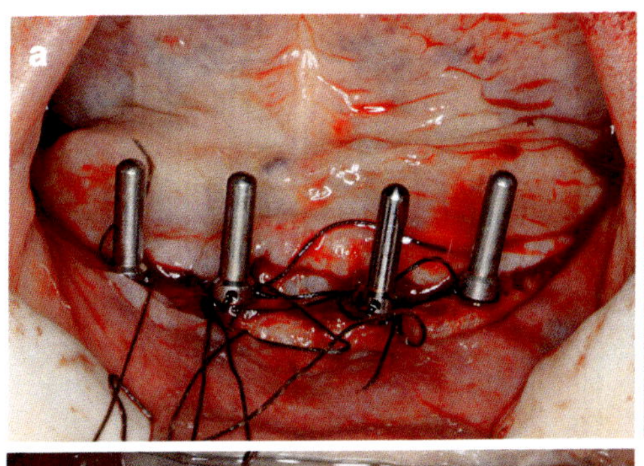
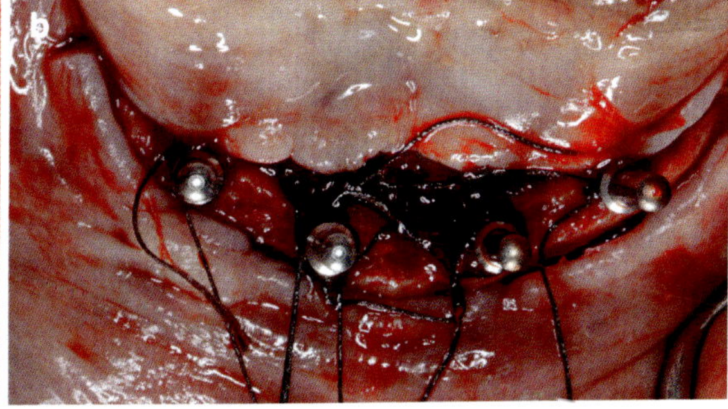
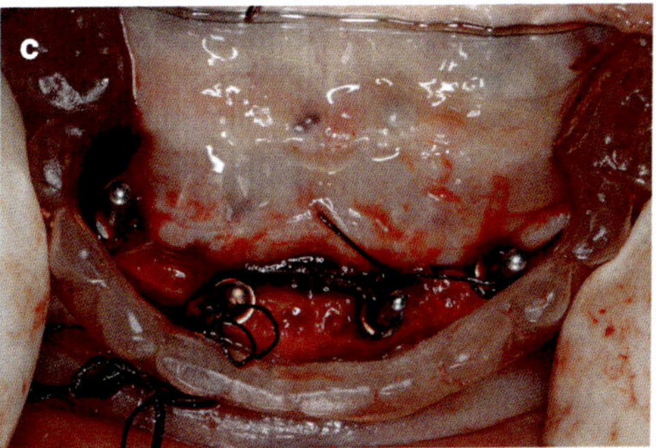

Fig. 8.38 (**a**) Buccal view and (**b**) occlusal view showing the four guide pins in place. (**c**) Occlusal view of the four guide pins inserted to confirm the proper position with the surgical guide in place

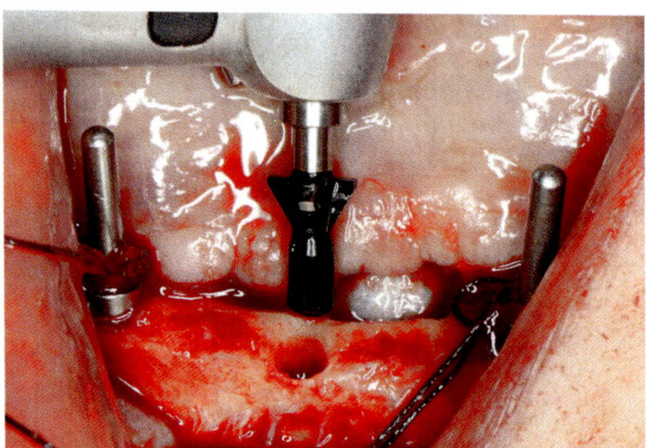

Fig. 8.39 The final bur, the countersink bur, is used to widen the crestal bone of all the osteotomy sites

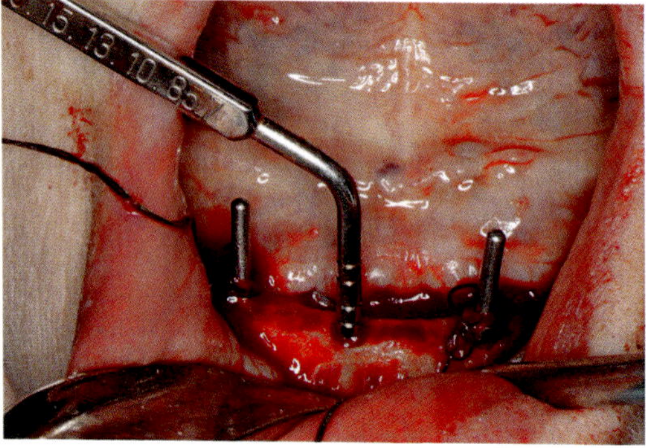

Fig. 8.40 Buccal view showing the depth probe confirming the adequate depth of each osteotomy site before inserting the implants

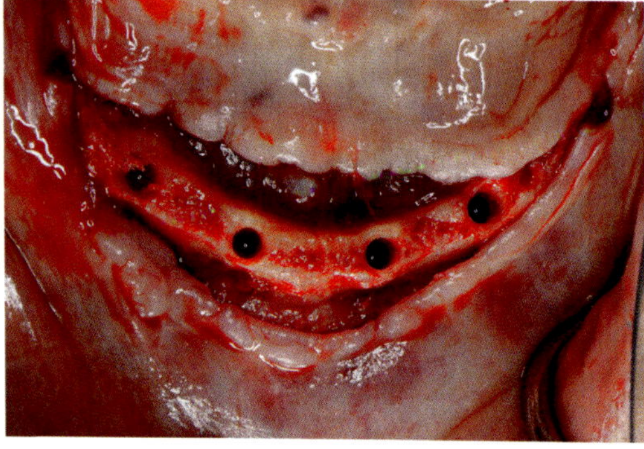

Fig. 8.41 Occlusal view showing the four osteotomy sites prepared

8.8.4 Implant Insertion

It is recommended to keep the guide pins in place to help with the insertion as the implant system illustrated here is self-tapping and the implants could be potentially misangulated if the established axis is not respected. The implant is inserted at low speed (25–30 RPM) and at a minimal torque of 30–35 Ncm in the osteotomy site until the top of the implant platform is located at the level of the crestal bone (Fig. 8.42a, b). The implant motor is set at a predetermined maximum torque and will stop automatically when it is reached. If the set torque is reached before the implant is fully seated, insertion can be completed with the use of a manual torque wrench. Otherwise, the surgeon may opt to tap the osteotomy site if excessive torque is required. The higher the bone density is, the more stable the implant will most likely be with a higher insertion torque needed to fully seat the implant into the osteotomy site.

If the implant reaches an adequate primary stability (insertion torque ≥ 30 Ncm), the healing abutments may be placed, and the surgeon will follow a one-stage protocol (Fig. 8.43). Before placing the healing abutment, it is important to verify if there are any bony steps around the implant platform, especially if the implant platform has been placed subcrestally as these steps will prevent the complete seating of the abutment on the platform. If these steps are present, a small round bur or bone chisel may be used to eliminate them and recontour the ridge around the implant. The healing abutment must then be fully seated on the implant platform. This procedure is repeated for each implant. When all the implants are in place, the flaps are adapted against the healing abutments and sutured with interrupted absorbable or nonabsorbable sutures. A radiograph may be taken to confirm the implant locations and verify if the healing abutments are well seated on the implant platform (Fig. 8.44).

Implants with an adequate primary stability will be able to withstand early loading forces, and the healing abutments will be kept in place during the osseointegration process until the restorative phase. This represents a major advantage for the patient, as it is not necessary to undergo a second surgical procedure. In this scenario, osseointegration occurs with the formation of a new peri-implant attachment and sulcus

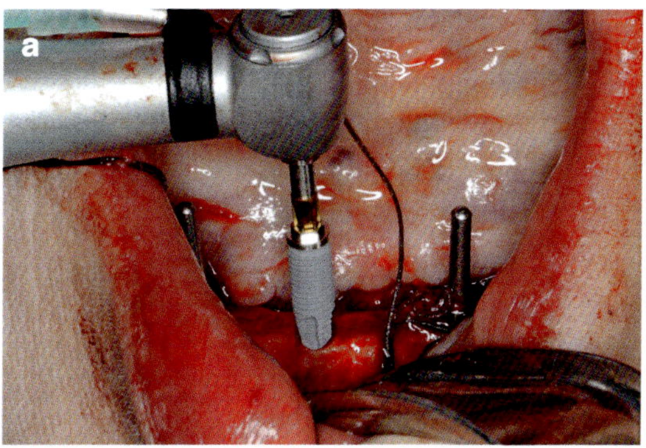
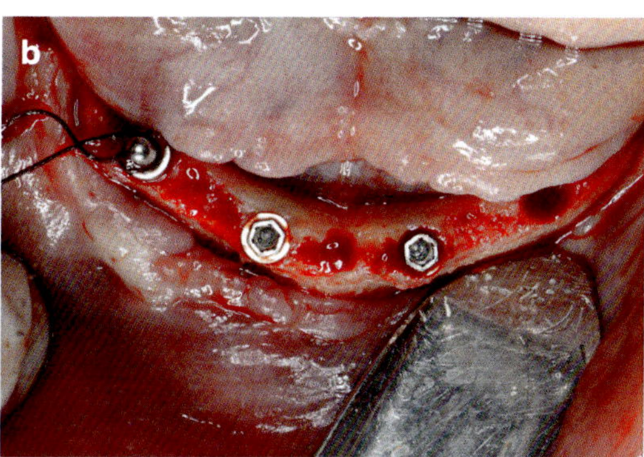

Fig. 8.42 (**a**) Buccal view showing the insertion of the first implant. The adjacent guide pins are kept in place to help the surgeon maintain the right position during this process. (**b**) Occlusal view showing two implants fully inserted and torqued in their osteotomy site

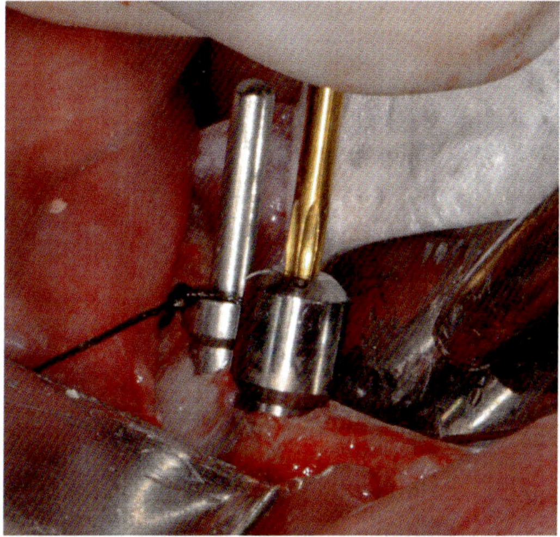

Fig. 8.43 Buccal view of a healing abutment placed on the implant

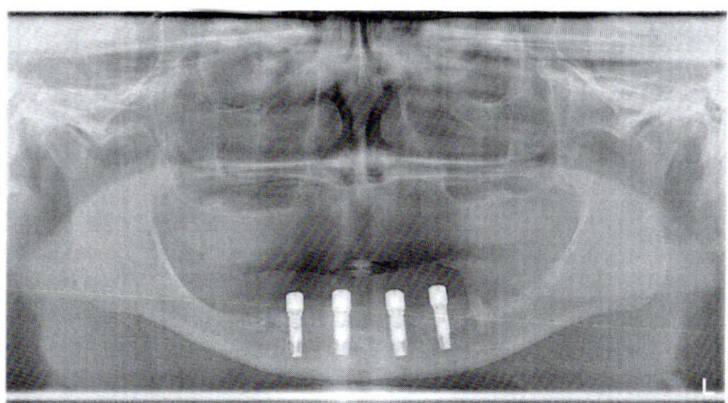

Fig. 8.44 Panoramic radiograph taken immediately after the placement of the implants

along the implant and the abutment. Another major advantage of the one-stage protocol is that the healing abutments will increase the stability of the lower removable prosthesis once it is relined with a soft lining material and well adapted to the mandibular ridge. Using long healing abutments will minimize the risks of soft tissue coronal migration during the first postoperative weeks, which could result in partial or complete coverage of the abutments. In most situations, healing abutments with a minimal height of 5 mm will be satisfactory to prevent this complication.

If it is not possible to achieve an adequate implant primary stability, it is preferable to install a cover screw on top of the implant instead of the healing abutment. The implant is then submerged until the osseointegration process is completed. In this two-stage protocol, a second surgical procedure is required to expose the implant and place the healing abutment two to six months after implant placement. In the event that the osteotomy site was fully prepared with the last drill and the implant is not stable, i.e., the implant is spinning while the healing abutment is screwed on, a larger-diameter implant may be placed. Nobel Biocare has a 4.0-mm-diameter Branemark MK III® (rescue) implant that is designed for those circumstances.

If a buccal dehiscence occurs after implant placement, a cover screw is placed on the implant, and a bone graft is packed on the buccal aspect of the implant and covered with a membrane to attempt bone regeneration (guided bone regeneration (GBR) procedure).

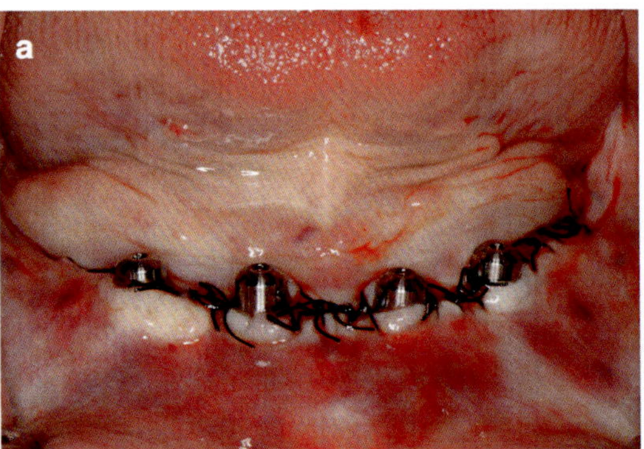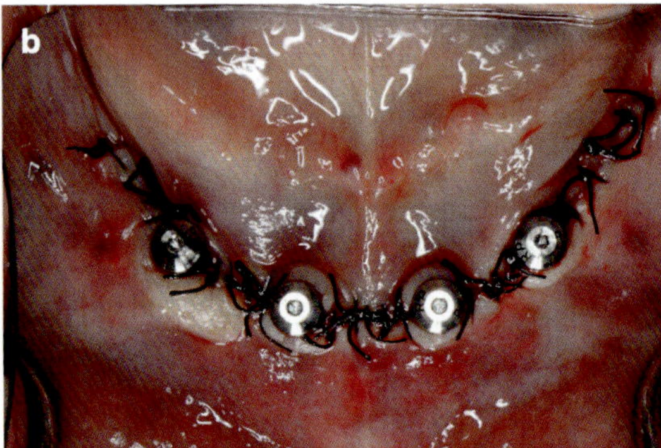

Fig. 8.45 (**a**) Buccal view and (**b**) occlusal view showing the flaps sutured against the four healing abutments

In this case, the implant is submerged with primary closure of the flaps, and a second-stage surgery will have to be done four to six months later to allow placement of a healing abutment. GBR procedures on implant buccal dehiscence defects have shown marginal bone level preservation after 18 months of healing compared to crestal bone loss when such defects were left untreated [128].

8.8.5 Suturing Techniques

For short surgical segments, as those observed between implants in the anterior area of the mandible, simple interrupted sutures are commonly used. In the posterior ridge area, continuous lock sutures are used to allow adequate flap adaptation while saving time. Interrupted sutures provide security in case one or more knots become slack due to postoperative swelling. Horizontal or vertical mattress sutures may also be used, especially if guided bone regeneration has been done around one or many implants, to provide primary closure and higher tensile strength and to prevent premature flap opening. The flaps need to be tightly closed with several sutures, as the tension on the buccal and lingual flaps is very strong in the anterior region of the mandible due to muscle insertions (Fig. 8.45a, b). An adequate band of KG is observed in this illustrated case on the buccal and lingual aspects of the implants.

8.9 Postoperative Care

At the end of the surgical appointment, the geriatric patient should remain seated for a few minutes before getting up from the dental chair in order to prevent an orthostatic hypotension episode, a condition during which the patient might become dizzy, light-headed, and nauseous and might develop a headache or blurred vision [129].

Written and verbal postoperative instructions are given to the patient and his/her designated escort after the surgical procedure. The patient and his/her escort must understand all instructions before leaving the surgical room. However, it is a good practice to discuss them with the patient in one of the appointments that precedes the surgical appointment. They should include the following topics:

- *Pain*: an analgesic agent is prescribed to the patient for the management of postoperative pain and discomfort. A nonsteroidal anti-inflammatory drug (NSAID) such as ibuprofen 400–600 mg or naproxen sodium 550 mg is routinely prescribed for at least the first two to three postoperative days if there are no medical contraindications. It should be prescribed along with acetaminophen (paracetamol) 500 mg if significant pain is expected since these two medications are more efficient for pain control when taken together than when either drug is taken alone [130]. Narcotics may be prescribed to elderly patients but with a lower dosage than the adult population since they are more at risk of developing respiratory depression. A relatively low number of medications ($\approx$12–20 tabs) should be given without any refill to encourage the patient to contact the surgeon if significant pain persists after three to four days. Increasing pain occurring three days after surgery may be a sign of postoperative infection, and an intraoral examination to verify the source of pain is recommended [131].

- *Infection control*: postoperative systemic antibiotics may be given although no scientific evidence has been supporting this practice for routine implant placement without additional bone grafting procedure. If there are no contraindications, amoxicillin 500 mg t.i.d. for one week may be prescribed if a GBR procedure was done simultaneously although this is a subject to debate [132]. If the patient presents a contraindication to penicillin, azithromycin 250 mg (two tabs stat and one tab per day for four days) may be prescribed.
- *Swelling*: the patient is encouraged to indirectly apply a cold pack on both sides of the lower jaw, on the skin adjacent to the surgical site, for alternating periods of 20 min for at least two hours as this may help reduce swelling and discomfort [133]. Swelling is expected and will peak 48 hours after the procedure. The surgeon may recommend to the patient to elevate his/her head above the heart level during the first two nights of sleep to reduce blood flow at the surgical site and swelling.
- *Bleeding*: minor bleeding is expected for the first 24 hours following the surgical procedure. Bruising of the chin is not unusual after this procedure.
- *Activities*: following a surgical procedure, the patient should refrain from doing intense activities. However, the patient may continue with his/her normal daily activities.
- *Eating*: the patient should be advised to refrain from drinking alcohol and eating spicy or hot food for the next 48 hours to prevent irritation

and swelling. For the first two postoperative weeks, a very soft diet is recommended to prevent flap reopening and food impaction. The patient is advised not to chew food with the healing abutments.

- *Prosthesis*: the patient is allowed to wear the upper prosthesis. For the first two postoperative weeks, the patient should refrain from wearing the lower denture and using any oral hygiene measure.
- *Oral hygiene*: a 0.12% gluconate chlorhexidine rinse is prescribed to the patient, and he/she is instructed to rinse for 30 s twice a day for at least two weeks. The patient should refrain from eating or drinking in one hour after using the rinse to maximize its bactericidal effect.
- *Smoking*: smokers should refrain from smoking one week before and eigth weeks after implant placement to decrease the risk of implant failure [134].

8.10 Postoperative Appointments

One week after the surgery, the patient may be seen to monitor soft tissue healing and oral hygiene (Fig. 8.46a, b). It is not uncommon to observe a slight opening between the buccal and lingual flaps with epithelial invagination, exposing the underlying granulation tissue. A significant postoperative swelling may cause this, especially when osteoplasty has been performed to flatten the mandibular ridge and for surgical procedures of longer duration. This may also be explained by a decrease in glycosaminoglycans, fibronectin synthesis, and type 1 binding of collagen, as well as the reduced efficiency of the immune system associated with older age [76]. Other age-related etiological factors related to delayed healing are poor nutrition, dehydration, reduced vascular perfusion, and polypharmacy [76]. If the flaps are not well approximated, as illustrated in this case, sutures should be left in place for another week to reduce the risk of creating a wider opening between the edges of the

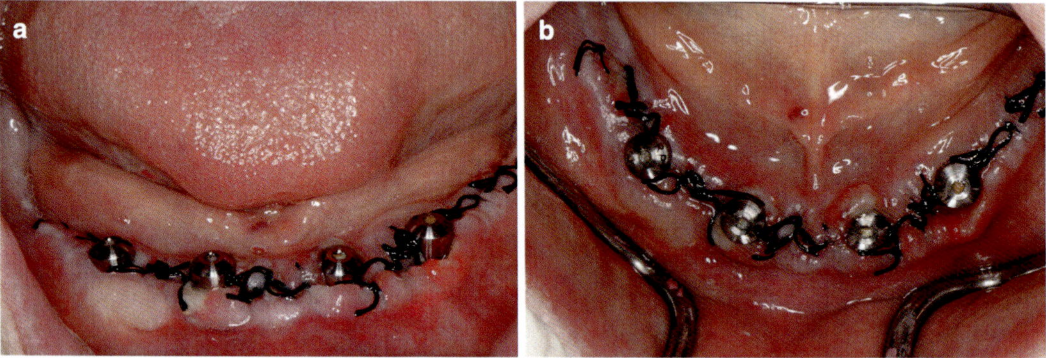

Fig. 8.46 (a) Buccal view and (b) occlusal view showing the mandible one week after the placement of the implants

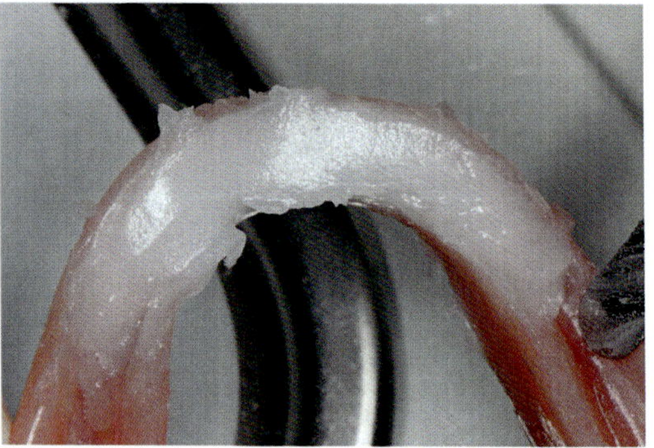

Fig. 8.47 The tissue conditioner material is applied under the lower denture

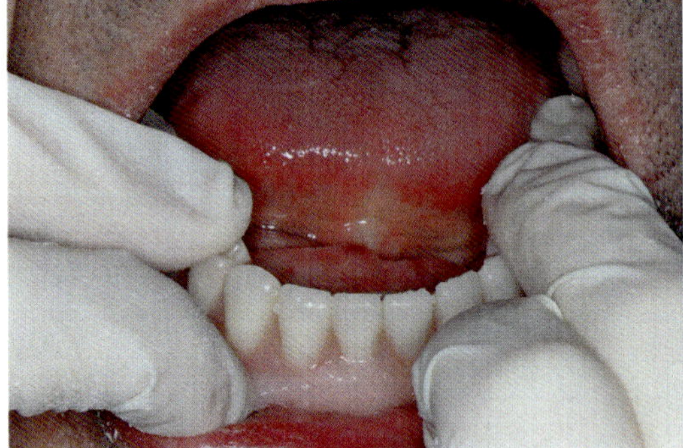

Fig. 8.48 The denture is seated on the ridge, and with finger pressure, the tissue conditioner is allowed to flow around the healing abutments

flaps. If a large opening (>2 mm) is present between the edges of the flaps, more sutures may be added to approximate them and cover the exposed alveolar bone. If only minor exposure occurs at the first visit or if the alveolar bone is covered with granulation tissue, the area may be left to heal by secondary intention.

Two weeks postoperatively, the sutures are removed, and any residual plaque or calculus should be removed from the healing abutments with plastic or titanium curettes. The mandibular complete denture may be relined with a methacrylate-based soft liner (e.g., Visco-gel Temporary Soft Denture Liner®, Dentsply Sirona Co., York, PA, USA) that will allow the patient to wear the denture, to resume chewing, and to regain partially his/her masticatory function. Briefly, a blue marking stick may be used to locate the healing abutments on the denture base, if a one-stage surgery was performed. Then, the denture material

is removed from underneath the denture to allow space for the healing abutment and soft lining material. Once the denture is well seated and adapted on the mandibular ridge and the healing abutments, the soft lining material or tissue conditioner is placed in the newly shaped housing under the denture (Fig. 8.47). The denture is then placed on the ridge with finger pressure to allow the material to flow around the healing abutments (Fig. 8.48). Once the material has settled, excesses are removed with a #15 surgical blade, and care must be taken to remove the material that could have settled between the edges of the buccal and lingual flaps (Fig. 8.49). If a one-stage surgery was elected, the healing abutments placed on the implants will provide extra stability for the lower prosthesis during the osseointegration phase. The patient is instructed to clean the denture after every meal and remove it at night.

A third follow-up visit is scheduled four weeks postoperatively to monitor the soft tissue healing, the osseointegration process of the implants, the tightness of the healing abutments, and the comfort of the patient (Fig. 8.50a, b). If required, the soft liner might be changed to obtain better adaptation to the underlying soft tissues undergoing maturation. It might be required in some cases to repeat this procedure at the same time interval until the final prosthesis is in place. When the osseointegration is completed, the restorative phase may be undertaken.

In a two-stage scenario, a second surgical procedure to expose the cover screws is performed two to six months after surgery. If a GBR procedure was performed, it is advisable to wait at least four to six months before re-exposing the implants to allow adequate time for bone regeneration. To establish the presence of KG on both aspects of the healing abutments, it is recommended to use an incision in its center and raise a small full-thickness flap to access the cover screws and replace them with healing abutments. Because the band of KG is normally narrow on an edentulous mandible, using a soft tissue punch could result in the complete elimination of KG and lead to a mucogingival defect around the implants. For this reason, the authors discourage its use in edentulous mandibles. The flaps are sutured, and it is possible to reline the lower denture with a soft liner, which will allow the patient to wear it immediately. Only soft tissue healing is required before undergoing with the restorative phase as the osseointegration in now completed. This process takes about four weeks.

8.11 Surgical and Postsurgical Complications

Complications related with implant surgery may arise during (intraoperative) and after (postoperative) the surgical procedure. Additionally, there are long-term complications related to the peri-implant tissues and surgery. As with any other surgical procedures, prevention of complications begins with a complete medical history including past and current medications, management and control of the risk factors, a thorough clinical and radiographic evaluation, adequate surgical techniques, and proper postoperative instructions. Despite taking all those measures, there are still risks of complications. The most common ones are presented below.

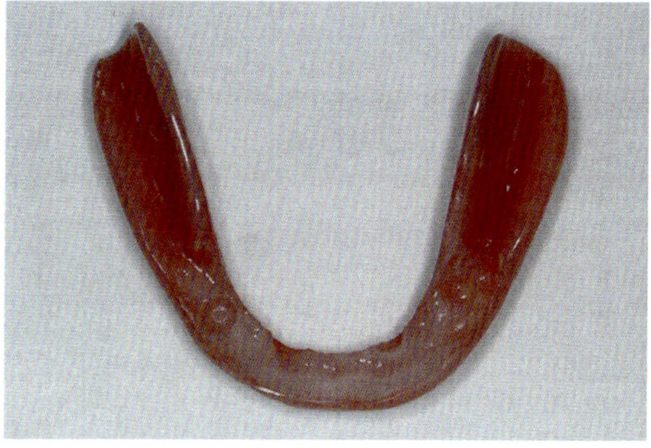

Fig. 8.49 Once the tissue conditioner has settled, the excesses are trimmed off

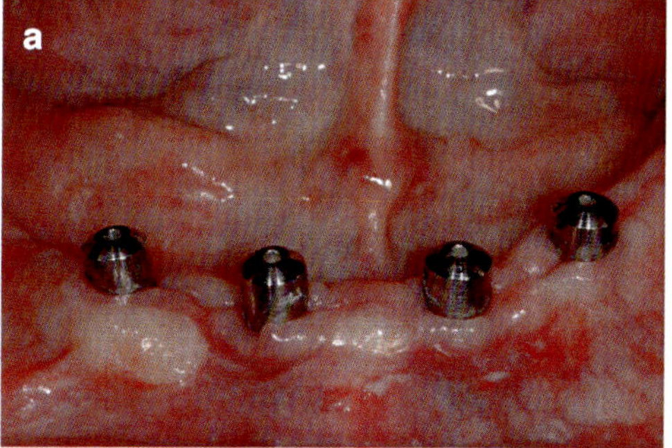

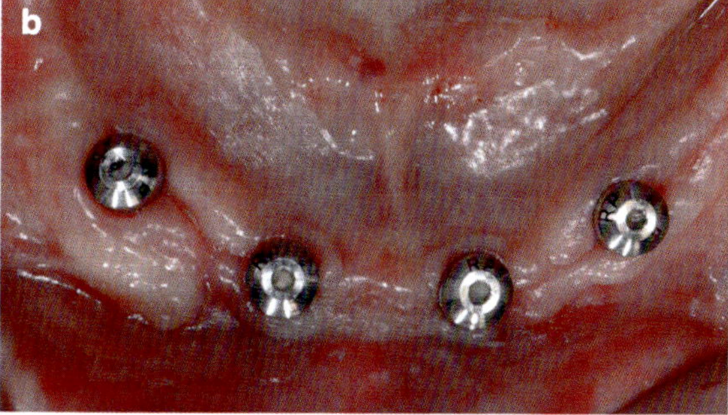

Fig. 8.50 (**a**) Buccal view and (**b**) occlusal view showing the mandible four weeks after the placement of the implants

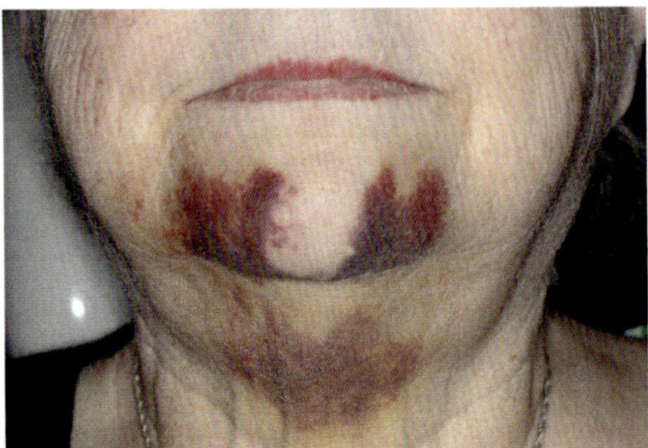

Fig. 8.51 Photograph taken one week after the surgical placement of the implants and showing a hematoma of the chin and neck

- *Hemorrhage, ecchymosis, and hematoma*: Minor bleeding is expected during and immediately after the surgical procedure. During the procedure, bleeding may be managed with the use of an anesthetic agent containing a vasoconstrictor such as epinephrine. Bleeding is related to the extent of flap reflection, the anatomy of the surgical area, and the systemic condition of the patient. The injury to small capillaries and blood vessels can cause bleeding in the tissues leading to an ecchymosis. This condition does not require therapy, and the patient needs only to be reassured that it will disappear by itself. Figure 8.51 shows an ecchymosis during the first week following the surgical placement of the implants. A hematoma is a collection of blood within a space or tissue that leads to the formation of an elevated and hard lump. Specific to this type of surgery is the vascularization in the anterior floor of the mouth. The implant surgeon must be careful not to perforate the lingual cortical plate or perforate the lingual flap, which could perforate the arteries in that area. There are two major blood vessels in the anterior region of the floor of the mouth, the sublingual and the submental arteries and their anastomosis through the mylohyoid muscle and multiple accessory foramina in the lingual cortical plate of the anterior mandible. The pattern of bone loss in the anterior mandible is mostly horizontal from the buccal side. This resorption generally results in a lingually angulated trajectory of the anterior region of the mandible. This angulation is prone to a lingual perforation during osteotomy site preparation leading to severed arteries and subsequent hemorrhage. This complication may be life threatening for the patient as it could cause an obstruction of the airway. If this situation arises during the surgery, the emergency medical services must be notified, as it is likely the patient will need intubation [135]. Patients taking anticoagulants or antiplatelet medications are more prone to this type of complication. Therefore, appropriate blood tests (INR, bleeding time, CBC) might be needed. For geriatric patients taking anticoagulants, no current guidelines have been published, but the authors recommend that the INR should be obtained within 72 h preoperatively and be lower than 3.0–3.5 before they undergo implant surgery. In patients taking anticoagulants, local hemostatic measures such as pressure for 30–60 min with a gauze soaked with 4.8% tranexamic acid immediately after surgery, gelatin sponges, or thrombin-containing biologic adhesive have been equally effective at preventing postoperative bleeding after implant surgeries [136]. A 4.8% tranexamic acid mouthwash may also be used during the two first postoperative days to prevent bleeding episodes. For geriatric patients taking these medications, it is recommended to communicate with the treating physician to assess their medical status.

- *Neurosensory disturbances*: Surgical trauma, disturbance to the nerve microcirculation, local inflammation, edema, and hematoma may lead to neural degenerative processes. If there has been no direct trauma to the mental nerve, the resulting neuropathies are usually temporary. Damage to a nerve may manifest as one of the following symptoms: paresthesia (numb feeling, burning, and prickling), hypoesthesia (reduced feeling), hyperesthesia (increased sensitivity), dysesthesia (painful sensation), or anesthesia (complete loss of feeling of the surrounding skin and mucosa) [137]. If such symptoms occur, the surgeon needs to determine if they are the results of the soft tissue manipulations and edema or the presence of the implant in close proximity to a nerve branch. If it is determined that the implant might have been placed too close or into a nerve canal, it must be removed [40]. If the cause is not related to the implant position, corticosteroids or anti-inflammatory medications might be prescribed empirically for one to two weeks postoperatively. Adequate mapping of the injured area using a blunt and sharp instrument must be noted in the patient's file in order to detect any subsequent reduction in signs and symptoms. If there is no improvement after two weeks, the patient must be referred to a specialist knowledgeable in neurosensory complications.

- *Damage to the soft tissues*: An implant placement surgery on an edentulous mandible requires an extensive access with a buccal and lingual flap, especially if an osteoplasty of the ridge is indicated. It is highly recommended to use large flap retractors during the surgical procedure to prevent the soft tissues from being in contact with the rotating instruments or other sharp instruments, which could result in soft tissue damage such as a tear or a flap perforation. Interrupted sutures may be used to consolidate any tissue tear or perforation before suturing the main flaps.

- *Flap opening and premature loss of sutures*: The buccal and lingual flaps in the anterior region of the mandible are subjected to tension from the muscles in the area. If the number of sutures is insufficient, if the suture entry points are too close to the incision, or if the tension is too strong, it is possible for the sutures to tear through the edges of the flaps resulting in a gap between them. This situation will expose the underlying bone and create discomfort for the patient and delay soft tissue healing. Depending on the severity of the gap created by this situation, the surgeon has two options. If the gap is narrow and the bone not exposed, the area may be left to heal by secondary intention. Figure 8.52 is showing a minor opening between the edges of the flaps one week after the surgical procedure. On the other hand, if the gap is wide (>2 mm) and the bone exposed, there is a need to place new sutures to bring the edges of the flaps to a

close. If the flap is slow to reattach to the bone and the bone is exposed, perforations in the cortical bone may be required to encourage bleeding to the area and enhance flap adhesion through fibrin clot formation. Figure 8.53 is showing perforations through the cortical bone. The flap is then sutured over the perforation (Fig. 8.54).

- *Loss of a healing abutment*: During the surgical procedure, the healing abutments are screwed hand-tight on the implants and will be kept in place during the osseointegration phase. Occasionally, a healing abutment may become loose and even lost. The patients need to be informed of that possibility, and they must notify the surgeon immediately when it occurs. The surgeon needs to ensure there is no soft tissue caught under the abutment before tightening it back to the seated position on the platform of the implant. If the healing abutment is loss, the soft tissues will cover the implant platform rapidly (Fig. 8.55). In this case, a midline incision is made, and a conservative flap is elevated to expose the implant platform and provide the access to place the healing abutment (Fig. 8.56). The flap is then sutured around the healing abutment (Fig. 8.57).

- *Soft tissue overgrowth*: In the weeks following the surgical placement of the implants, the edges of the flaps may creep and cover the healing abutments (Fig. 8.58). This complication may arise when extensive reduction of the alveolar ridge is performed. Using healing abutments that are at least 5 mm long may prevent this complication. At the end of the initial healing period (≈four weeks), if soft tissue irregularities and/or gingival overgrowth remain, a minor gingivoplasty/gingivectomy may be required around the healing abutments.

- *Loss of a dental implant*: Although the success rate of dental implants in the edentulous mandible is highly favorable (99.5%) [138], osseointegration occasionally fails to occur. This leads to an early implant loss. Depending on the situation, there are different options available:
  - A wider diameter implant may be placed in the osteotomy site after a thorough curet-

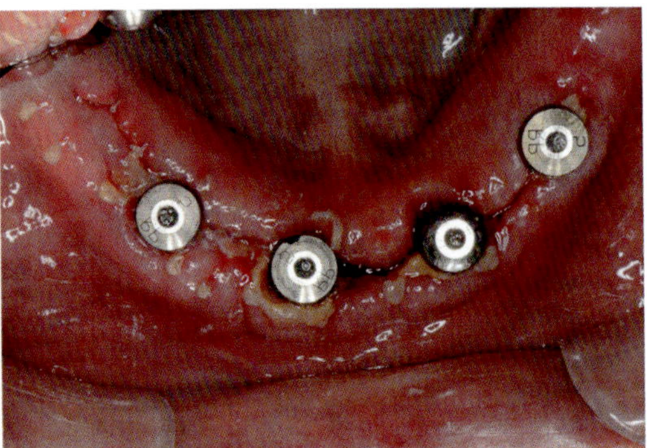

Fig. 8.52 Occlusal view showing the mandible one week after the placement of the implants

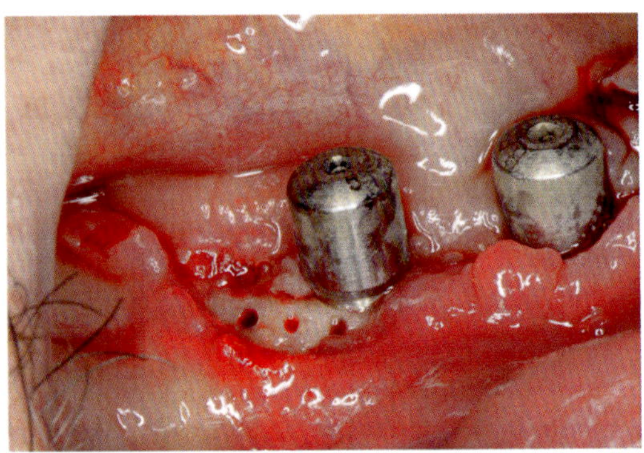

Fig. 8.53 Buccal view showing an area where the cortical bone became exposed two weeks after the surgical procedure. Perforations were performed through the cortical plate to promote bleeding to the area

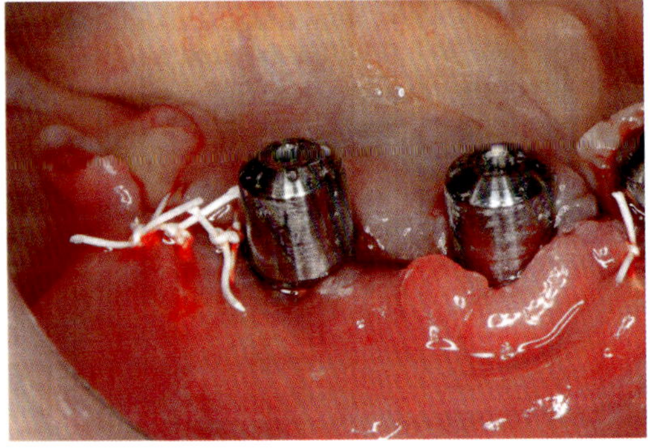

Fig. 8.54 Buccal view showing the area after the flaps were sutured over the perforations that were performed

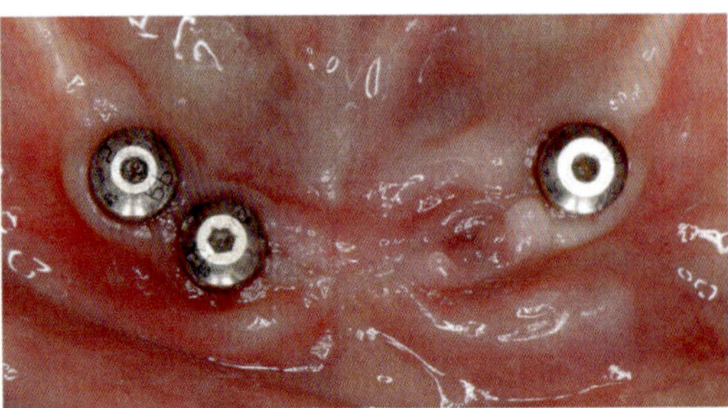

Fig. 8.55 Occlusal view showing the loss of a healing abutment

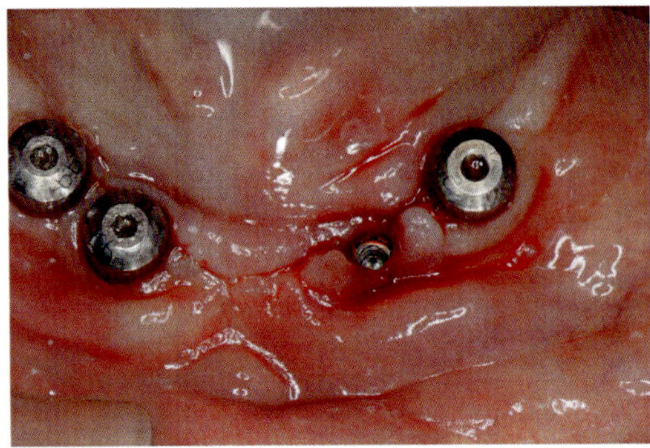

Fig. 8.56 Occlusal view showing the area after a small flap was performed to expose the platform of the implant

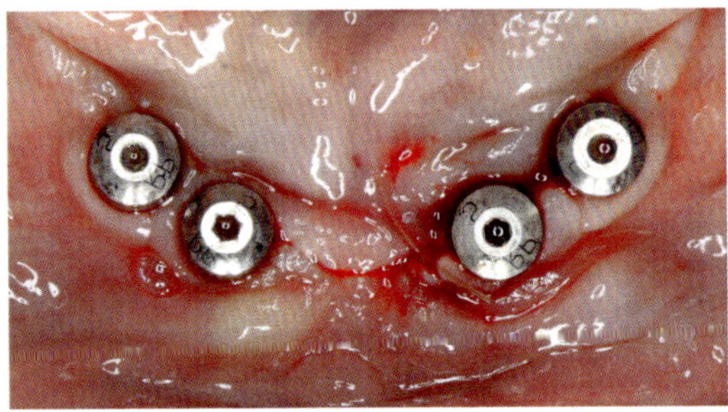

Fig. 8.57 Occlusal view showing the area after the placement of the healing abutment and the sutures

tage and irrigation if minimal bone resorption occurs.

- Another implant may be inserted adjacent to the failed implant if the restorative design of the prosthesis allows it.
- If the previous options are not possible, a bone graft must be placed and covered with a resorbable membrane into the implant socket. Another implant may be placed after four to six months of healing.

• *Mandibular fracture*: This is a serious and rare complication in the atrophic mandible. When a fracture of the mandible is detected shortly

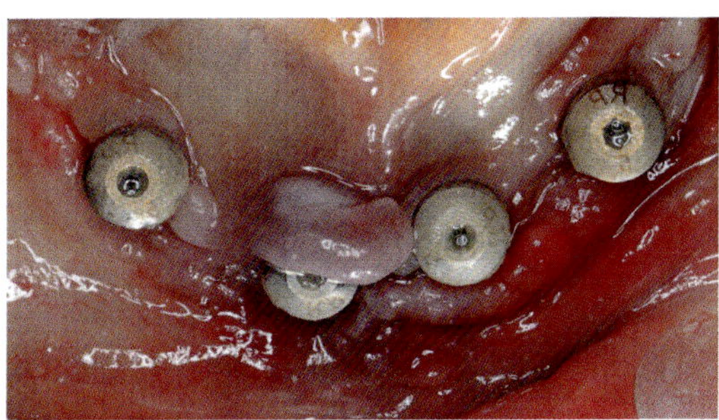

Fig. 8.58 Occlusal view showing a soft tissue overgrowth covering part of a healing abutment

after the implant placement surgery, it is likely the result of a weakened area where the implant was placed. The risk factors that predispose a mandible to a fracture associated with the placement of an implant are osteoporosis, trauma, and stress at the implant location [139]. To reduce the risk of mandibular fracture, it is recommended to avoid long and wide implants in the atrophic mandible [140]. Furthermore, atrophic mandibles that have less than 7 mm of bone height and 6 mm of width are at increased vulnerability to fracture [141]. When a fracture occurs, the surgeon needs to perform a fracture reduction and decide if the implant may be kept [140].

- *Peri-implant diseases*: Peri-implant mucositis is defined as the inflammation of peri-implant tissues without loss of attachment and the supporting bone, while peri-implantitis is also an inflammatory disease involving the peri-implant tissues but also exhibits supporting bone and peri-implant attachment loss. Their prevalence has been recently estimated to be 43% and 22%, respectively, at the implant level [142]. Although the etiology is primarily bacterial plaque accumulation, other contributing factors might be patient-, surgical-, and prosthetic-related. A periodic peri-implant examination and debridement will minimize the incidence of these complications. The patient must maintain optimal oral hygiene, and thorough hygiene instructions with adjuvants must be presented to all implant rehabilitated patients. Since geriatric patients might often have difficulty to adequately maintain plaque-free implant surfaces, end-tuft manual or electric brushes are often recommended. A minimal peri-implant maintenance frequency of five to six months is recommended to prevent peri-implant diseases [143].

- In peri-implant mucositis cases, a peri-implant pocket is often present with a probing depth ≥ 5 mm with signs of inflammation such as erythema or bleeding upon probing but without peri-implant crestal bone loss. This lesion is reversible with nonsurgical periodontal therapy. A thorough subgingival debridement and improvement of oral hygiene will generally reduce the inflammation around the affected implant(s) and resolve the disease. In peri-implantitis cases, deep peri-implant pockets (≥ 5 mm) with bleeding upon probing are observed with crestal bone loss that may be visible on the radiographs. Subgingival debridement with or without application of a local or systemic antibiotic might control or stabilize the disease. Usually, a postoperative chlorhexidine rinse is prescribed, and the patient is seen four to six weeks later for a reevaluation to assess the peri-implant tissue health. If the peri-implant pocket and inflammation persist, a surgical approach is recommended. Several treatment options have been described including bone and soft tissue augmentation, resective peri-implant surgery including implantoplasty, or a combination of these approaches depending on the intrabony defect morphology. These procedures have shown positive outcomes [144]. In the presence of horizontal bone loss around implants with a small or absent intrabony component, resective surgery with decontamination of the implant surface is indicated.

- To illustrate this clinical situation, a 71-year-old female came for a consultation regarding a fistula located on the buccal aspect of a midline mandibular implant supporting a fixed implant-assisted prosthesis (Fig. 8.59). There were 7 mm peri-implant pockets with bleeding upon probing on the mesiobuccal, buccal, and distobuccal aspect of the implant #3.2, and the periapical radiograph showed crestal bone loss around the implant (Figs. 8.60 and 8.61). The

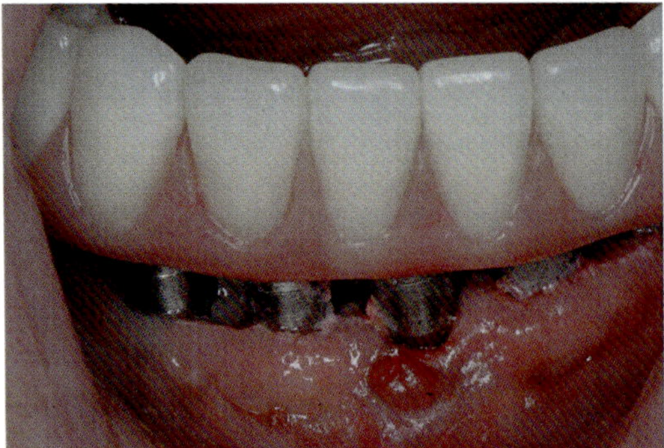

Fig. 8.59 A fistula is present on the buccal aspect of an implant in #3.2 position supporting a fixed implant-assisted prosthesis for a 71-year-old female patient

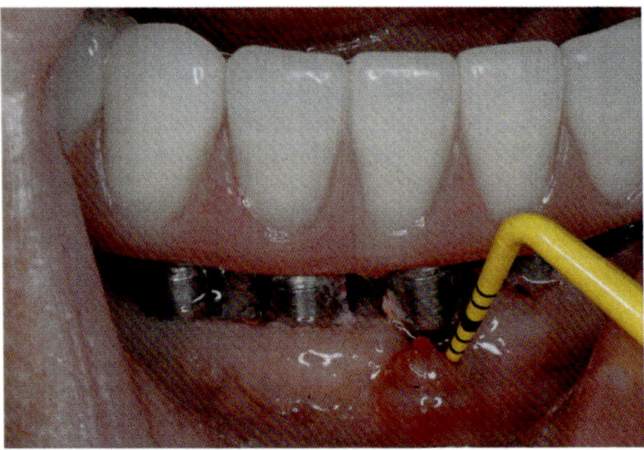

Fig. 8.60 A 7 mm probing depth is present on the mesio-, mid-, and distobuccal aspect of the implant with bleeding upon probing

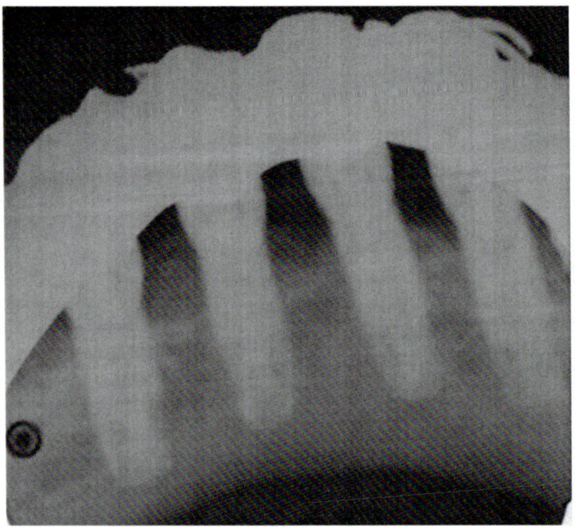

Fig. 8.61 A periapical radiograph reveals alveolar bone loss around the implant in the #3.2 position

implant threads were felt with the implant probe in the peri-implant pockets. Six weeks after initial periodontal debridement under local anesthesia with local antibiotic application, the patient comes back at the clinic for a reevaluation, but the deep peri-implant pockets are still present. Therefore, after removing the prosthesis to facilitate access, a full-thickness flap is elevated, and the implant and surrounding bone are debrided. An 8 mm horizontal bone loss is observed on the mesial, buccal, and distal aspect of implant #3.2 (Fig. 8.62). An implantoplasty is done to eliminate the exposed implant threads as they represent a contributing factor to plaque accumulation when they are exposed in the mouth. The implant surface is then empirically decontaminated with citric acid 30% and saline irrigation. A slight osteoplasty is done to facilitate apical repositioning of the gingival flaps (Fig. 8.63). Interrupted sutures are placed with minimal tension to allow passive flap adaption on the underlying bone (Fig. 8.64). The prosthesis is put back into place immediately after the surgery. The patient is seen one week postoperatively to remove the sutures and resume oral hygiene (Fig. 8.65). The patient was seen every four months for periodic recalls, and two years later, a 3 mm peri-implant probing depth with optimal oral hygiene and healthy peri-implant tissues are observed around the previously treated implant (Fig. 8.66).

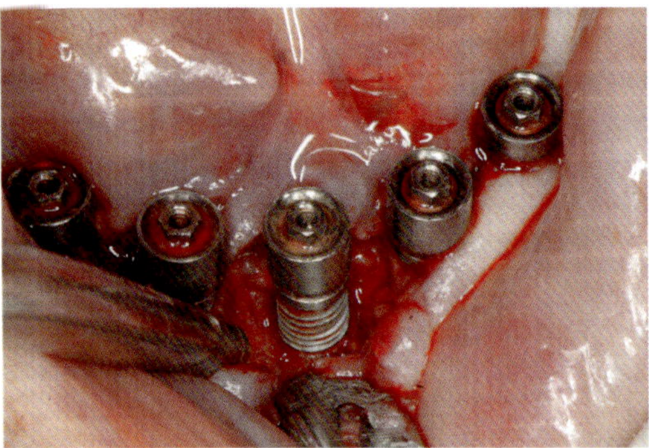

Fig. 8.62 The fixed prosthesis was removed, and upon elevation of a full-thickness flap, an 8 mm horizontal bone loss was found on the buccal aspect of the implant in #3.2 position

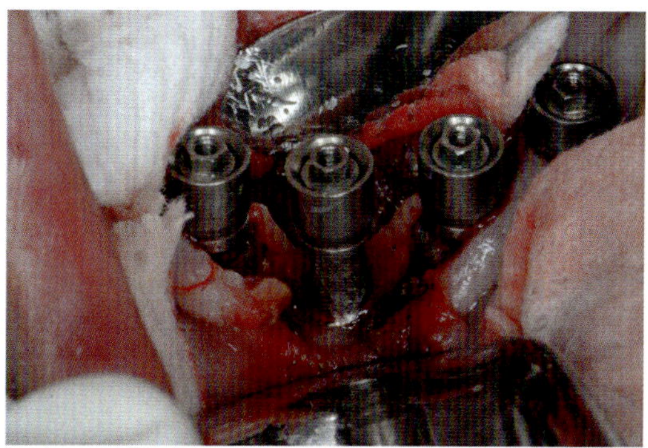

Fig. 8.63 A buccal view showing the implant surface after an implantoplasty and osteoplasty were performed

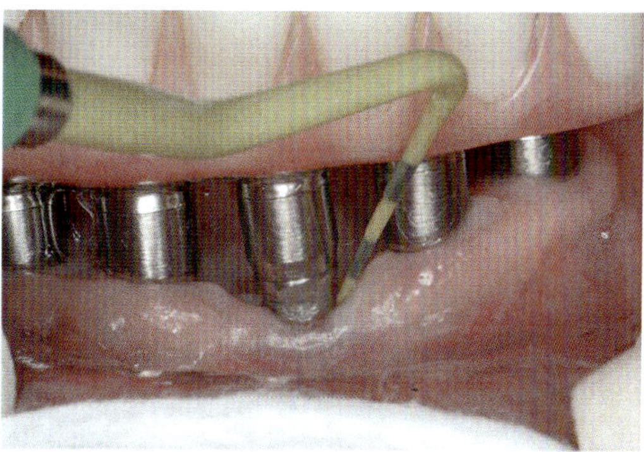

Fig. 8.66 A buccal view showing the buccal aspect of the implant in #3.2 position two years after the resective surgery

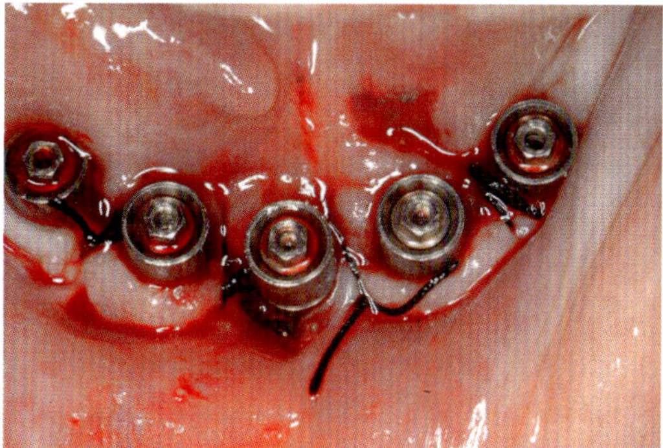

Fig. 8.64 A buccal view showing the flaps sutured around the abutments

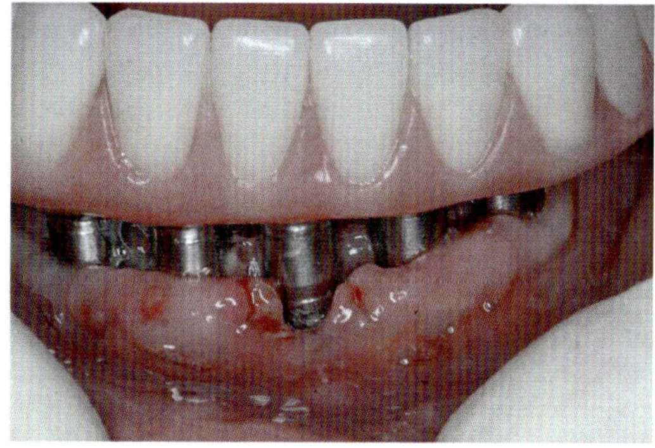

Fig. 8.65 A buccal view showing the surgical area one week after resective surgery

- If a three-wall intrabony defect is present with a minimal depth of 3 mm and the surgeon estimates that the access to the implant for surface decontamination is adequate, a guided bone regeneration procedure might be used to regenerate the supporting bone that has been lost. When indicated, this approach has resulted in greater pocket depth reduction and radiographic bone fill according to a recent systematic review [145]. However, peri-implantitis lesions with the presence of an intrabony defect with adequate morphology in the edentulous elderly patient are scarce due to the limited buccolingual width of the mandibular ridge often encountered.

Conclusion

In the presence of moderate to severe ridge resorption in the mandible, geriatric patients are often left with a mandibular removable denture that lacks stability, interferes with mastication, and causes soft tissue trauma and discomfort. Therefore, these symptoms can have significant psychological consequences on the elderly who is often in a fragile mental status. Implant dentistry has been a significant breakthrough in the treatment of edentulism for patients of all ages. Several options involving implants are available for geriatric patients with an edentulous mandible, offering them a great range of stability and comfort.

Despite severe mandibular ridge resorption, an adequate amount of bone is commonly found in the interforaminal region for the placement of dental implants. However, it is also an area where a significant blood and nerve supply can be found. Therefore, this anatomically challenging area must be operated with caution not to cause damage to those important structures. The dental team needs to follow a strict protocol involving comprehensive patient preparation, adequate radiographic and intraoral examinations, a meticulous implant placement surgery, a steady anxiety management and pain control protocol, as well as clear and concise pre- and postoperative instructions. The geriatric patient's and his/her escort's cooperation with the surgeon's instructions will affect the short- and long-term prognosis of the future implant-assisted prosthesis. As with any other treatments involving dental implants, there are short- and long-term complications, and most of them can be managed efficiently and predictably. The patient compliance to periodic hygiene recalls is of the utmost importance to maintain healthy peri-implant tissues and supporting bone around the implants. With regard to its good long-term prognosis, whether a fixed or removable mandibular rehabilitation is selected, this treatment modality should be offered to every geriatric patient suffering from edentulism in the mandible.

References

1. Niccoli T, Partridge L. Ageing as a risk factor for disease. Curr Biol. 2012;22(17):R741–52.
2. de Grandmont P, Feine JS, Tache R, Boudrias P, Donohue WB, Tanguay R, Lund JP. Within-subject comparisons of implant-supported mandibular prostheses: psychometric evaluation. J Dent Res. 1994;73(5):1096–104.
3. Tang L, Lund JP, Tache R, Clokie CM, Feine JS. A within-subject comparison of mandibular long-bar and hybrid implant-supported prostheses: psychometric evaluation and patient preference. J Dent Res. 1997;76(10):1675–83.
4. Sivaramakrishnan G, Sridharan K. Comparison of implant supported mandibular overdentures and conventional dentures on quality of life: a systematic review and meta-analysis of randomized controlled studies. Aust Dent J. 2016;61(4):482–8.
5. Hains F, Jones J. Treatment planning for the geriatric patient. In: Homl-Pedersen PWA, Ship JA, editors. Textbook of geriatric dentistry. 3rd ed. Chichester: Wiley; 2015. p. 165.
6. Alqutaibi AY. There is no evidence on the effect of the attachment system on implant survival rate, overdenture maintenance, or patient satisfaction. J Evid Based Dent Pract. 2015;15(4):193–4.
7. Hwang K, Lee WJ, Song YB, Chung IH. Vulnerability of the inferior alveolar nerve and mental nerve during genioplasty: an anatomic study. J Craniofac Surg. 2005;16(1):10–14; discussion 14.
8. Kim ST, Hu KS, Song WC, Kang MK, Park HD, Kim HJ. Location of the mandibular canal and the topography of its neurovascular structures. J Craniofac Surg. 2009;20(3):936–9.
9. Miller CS, Nummikoski PV, Barnett DA, Langlais RP. Cross-sectional tomography. A diagnostic technique for determining the buccolingual relationship of impacted mandibular third molars and the inferior alveolar neurovascular bundle. Oral Surg Oral Med Oral Pathol. 1990;70(6):791–7.
10. Yu SK, Lee MH, Jeon YH, Chung YY, Kim HJ. Anatomical configuration of the inferior alveolar neurovascular bundle: a histomorphometric analysis. Surg Radiol Anat. 2016;38(2):195–201.
11. Renton T, Dawood A, Shah A, Searson L, Yilmaz Z. Post-implant neuropathy of the trigeminal nerve. A case series. Br Dent J. 2012;212(11):E17.
12. Misch CE. Root form surgery in the edentulous mandible: stage I implant insertion. In: Misch CE, editor. Implant dentistry. 2nd ed. St. Louis: The CV Mosby Company; 1999. p. 347–70.
13. Kim YK, Park JY, Kim SG, Kim JS, Kim JD. Magnification rate of digital panoramic radiographs and its effectiveness for pre-operative assessment of dental implants. Dentomaxillofac Radiol. 2011;40(2):76–83.
14. Vazquez L, Nizam Al Din Y, Christoph Belser U, Combescure C, Bernard JP. Reliability of the vertical magnification factor on panoramic radiographs: clinical implications for posterior mandibular implants. Clin Oral Implants Res. 2011;22(12):1420–5.
15. Polland KE, Munro S, Reford G, Lockhart A, Logan G, Brocklebank L, McDonald SW. The mandibular canal of the edentulous jaw. Clin Anat. 2001;14(6):445–52.
16. Rosa MB, Sotto-Maior BS, Machado Vde C, Francischone CE. Retrospective study of the anterior loop of the inferior alveolar nerve and the incisive canal using cone beam computed tomography. Int J Oral Maxillofac Implants. 2013;28(2):388–92.
17. Uchida Y, Noguchi N, Goto M, Yamashita Y, Hanihara T, Takamori H, Sato I, Kawai T, Yosue T. Measurement of anterior loop length for the mandibular canal and diameter of the mandibular incisive canal to avoid nerve damage when installing endosseous implants in the interforaminal region: a second attempt introducing cone beam computed tomography. J Oral Maxillofac Surg. 2009;67(4):744–50.
18. Kqiku L, Sivic E, Weiglein A, Stadtler P. Position of the mental foramen: an anatomical study. Wien Med Wochenschr. 2011;161(9–10):272–3.
19. Ngeow WC, Yuzawati Y. The location of the mental foramen in a selected Malay population. J Oral Sci. 2003;45(3):171–5.
20. Wang TM, Shih C, Liu JC, Kuo KJ. A clinical and anatomical study of the location of the mental fora-

men in adult Chinese mandibles. Acta Anat (Basel). 1986;126(1):29–33.

21. Massey ND, Galil KA, Wilson TD. Determining position of the inferior alveolar nerve via anatomical dissection and micro-computed tomography in preparation for dental implants. J Can Dent Assoc. 2013;79:d39.

22. Rashid N, Yusuf H. Intermittent mental paraesthesia in an edentulous mandible. Br Dent J. 1997;182(5):189–90.

23. Kuzmanovic DV, Payne AG, Kieser JA, Dias GJ. Anterior loop of the mental nerve: a morphological and radiographic study. Clin Oral Implants Res. 2003;14(4):464–71.

24. Apostolakis D, Brown JE. The anterior loop of the inferior alveolar nerve: prevalence, measurement of its length and a recommendation for interforaminal implant installation based on cone beam CT imaging. Clin Oral Implants Res. 2012;23(9):1022–30.

25. Gomez-Roman G, Lautner NV, Goldammer C, McCoy M. Anterior loop of the mandibular canal-a source of possible complications. Implant Dent. 2015;24(5):578–85.

26. Juan del VL, Grageda E, Crespo SG. Anterior loop of the inferior alveolar nerve: averages and prevalence based on CT scans. J Prosthet Dent. 2016;115(2):156–60.

27. Lu CI, Won J, Al-Ardah A, Santana R, Rice D, Lozada J. Assessment of the anterior loop of the mental nerve using cone beam computerized tomography scan. J Oral Implantol. 2015;41(6):632–9.

28. Ritter L, Neugebauer J, Mischkowski RA, Dreiseidler T, Rothamel D, Richter U, Zinser MJ, Zoller JE. Evaluation of the course of the inferior alveolar nerve in the mental foramen by cone beam computed tomography. Int J Oral Maxillofac Implants. 2012;27(5):1014–21.

29. von Arx T, Friedli M, Sendi P, Lozanoff S, Bornstein MM. Location and dimensions of the mental foramen: a radiographic analysis by using cone-beam computed tomography. J Endod. 2013;39(12):1522–8.

30. Bavitz JB, Harn SD, Hansen CA, Lang M. An anatomical study of mental neurovascular bundle-implant relationships. Int J Oral Maxillofac Implants. 1993;8(5):563–7.

31. Benninger B, Miller D, Maharathi A, Carter W. Dental implant placement investigation: is the anterior loop of the mental nerve clinically relevant? J Oral Maxillofac Surg. 2011;69(1):182–5.

32. Uchida Y, Yamashita Y, Goto M, Hanihara T. Measurement of anterior loop length for the mandibular canal and diameter of the mandibular incisive canal to avoid nerve damage when installing endosseous implants in the interforaminal region. J Oral Maxillofac Surg. 2007;65(9):1772–9.

33. Mardinger O, Chaushu G, Arensburg B, Taicher S, Kaffe I. Anatomic and radiologic course of the mandibular incisive canal. Surg Radiol Anat. 2000;22(3–4):157–61.

34. Kalpidis CD, Setayesh RM. Hemorrhaging associated with endosseous implant placement in the anterior mandible: a review of the literature. J Periodontol. 2004;75(5):631–45.

35. McDonnell D, Reza Nouri M, Todd ME. The mandibular lingual foramen: a consistent arterial foramen in the middle of the mandible. J Anat. 1994;184(Pt 2):363–9.

36. Felisati G, Saibene AM, Di Pasquale D, Borloni R. How the simplest dental implant procedure can trigger an extremely serious complication. BMJ Case Rep. 2012;2012:bcr2012007373.

37. Jo JH, Kim SG, Oh JS. Hemorrhage related to implant placement in the anterior mandible. Implant Dent. 2011;20(3):e33–7.

38. Laboda G. Life-threatening hemorrhage after placement of an endosseous implant: report of case. J Am Dent Assoc. 1990;121(5):599–600.

39. Yildirim YD, Guncu GN, Galindo-Moreno P, Velasco-Torres M, Juodzbalys G, Kubilius M, Gervickas A, Al-Hezaimi K, Al-Sadhan R, Yilmaz HG, et al. Evaluation of mandibular lingual foramina related to dental implant treatment with computerized tomography: a multicenter clinical study. Implant Dent. 2014;23(1):57–63.

40. Greenstein G, Cavallaro J, Tarnow D. Practical application of anatomy for the dental implant surgeon. J Periodontol. 2008;79(10):1833–46.

41. Mraiwa N, Jacobs R, Moerman P, Lambrichts I, van Steenberghe D, Quirynen M. Presence and course of the incisive canal in the human mandibular interforaminal region: two-dimensional imaging versus anatomical observations. Surg Radiol Anat. 2003;25(5–6):416–23.

42. Romanos GE, Papadimitriou DE, Royer K, Stefanova-Stephens N, Salwan R, Malmstrom H, Caton JG. The presence of the mandibular incisive canal: a panoramic radiographic examination. Implant Dent. 2012;21(3):202–6.

43. Sahman H, Sekerci AE, Sisman Y, Payveren M. Assessment of the visibility and characteristics of the mandibular incisive canal: cone beam computed tomography versus panoramic radiography. Int J Oral Maxillofac Implants. 2014;29(1):71–8.

44. Raitz R, Shimura E, Chilvarquer I, Fenyo-Pereira M. Assessment of the mandibular incisive canal by panoramic radiograph and cone-beam computed tomography. Int J Dent. 2014;2014:187085.

45. Lee CY, Yanagihara LC, Suzuki JB. Brisk, pulsatile bleeding from the anterior mandibular incisive canal during implant surgery: a case report and use of an active hemostatic matrix to terminate acute bleeding. Implant Dent. 2012;21(5):368–73.

46. Romanos GE, Greenstein G. The incisive canal. Considerations during implant placement: case report and literature review. Int J Oral Maxillofac Implants. 2009;24(4):740–5.

47. Chan HL, Benavides E, Yeh CY, Fu JH, Rudek IE, Wang HL. Risk assessment of lingual plate perforation in posterior mandibular region: a virtual implant

placement study using cone-beam computed tomography. J Periodontol. 2011;82(1):129–35.

48. Chan HL, Brooks SL, Fu JH, Yeh CY, Rudek I, Wang HL. Cross-sectional analysis of the mandibular lingual concavity using cone beam computed tomography. Clin Oral Implants Res. 2011;22(2):201–6.

49. Bavitz JB, Harn SD, Homze EJ. Arterial supply to the floor of the mouth and lingual gingiva. Oral Surg Oral Med Oral Pathol. 1994;77(3):232–5.

50. Uchida Y, Goto M, Danjo A, Yamashita Y, Shibata K, Kuraoka A. Anatomical relationship between the sublingual fossa and the lateral lingual foramen. Int J Oral Maxillofac Surg. 2015;44(9):1146–51.

51. Nickenig HJ, Wichmann M, Eitner S, Zoller JE, Kreppel M. Lingual concavities in the mandible: a morphological study using cross-sectional analysis determined by CBCT. J Craniomaxillofac Surg. 2015;43(2):254–9.

52. Pietrokovski J, Chapman RJ. The form of the mandibular anterior lingual alveolar process in partially edentulous patients. J Prosthet Dent. 1981;45(4):371–5.

53. Kalpidis CD, Konstantinidis AB. Critical hemorrhage in the floor of the mouth during implant placement in the first mandibular premolar position: a case report. Implant Dent. 2005;14(2):117–24.

54. Mason ME, Triplett RG, Alfonso WF. Life-threatening hemorrhage from placement of a dental implant. J Oral Maxillofac Surg. 1990;48(2):201–4.

55. Mordenfeld A, Andersson L, Bergstrom B. Hemorrhage in the floor of the mouth during implant placement in the edentulous mandible: a case report. Int J Oral Maxillofac Implants. 1997;12(4):558–61.

56. Netter FH. Section 1: head and neck. Oral region: tongue. In: Hansen JT, editor. Atlas of human anatomy. Teterboro: ICON Learning Systems LLC; 2003. p. 55.

57. Netter FH. Section 1: head and neck. Oral region: muscles involved in mastication. In: Hansen JT, editor. Atlas of human anatomy. Teterboro: ICON Learning Systems LLC; 2003. p. 50.

58. Noia CF, Rodriguez-Chessa JG, Ortega-Lopes R, Cabral-Andrade V, Barbeiro RH, Mazzonetto R. Prospective study of soft tissue contour changes following chin bone graft harvesting. Int J Oral Maxillofac Surg. 2012;41(2):176–9.

59. Jung SY, Shin SY, Lee KH, Eun YG, Lee YC, Kim SW. Analysis of mandibular structure using 3d facial computed tomography. Otolaryngol Head Neck Surg. 2014;151(5):760–4.

60. Murlimanju BV, Prakash KG, Samiullah D, Prabhu LV, Pai MM, Vadgaonkar R, Rai R. Accessory neurovascular foramina on the lingual surface of mandible: incidence, topography, and clinical implications. Indian J Dent Res. 2012;23(3):433.

61. Kolsuz ME, Orhan K, Bilecenoglu B, Sakul BU, Ozturk A. Evaluation of genial tubercle anatomy using cone beam computed tomography. J Oral Sci. 2015;57(2):151–6.

62. Misch CE. The division c mandible: mandibular complete and unilateral subperiosteal implants. In: Misch CE, editor. Implant dentistry. 2nd ed. St. Louis: The CV Mosby Company; 1999. p. 434–5.

63. Tan WC, Krishnaswamy G, Ong MM, Lang NP. Patient-reported outcome measures after routine periodontal and implant surgical procedures. J Clin Periodontol. 2014;41(6):618–24.

64. Swenor BK, Ramulu PY, Willis JR, Friedman D, Lin FR. The prevalence of concurrent hearing and vision impairment in the United States. JAMA Intern Med. 2013;173(4):312–3.

65. Prince M, Bryce R, Albanese E, Wimo A, Ribeiro W, Ferri CP. The global prevalence of dementia: a systematic review and metaanalysis. Alzheimers Dement. 2013;9(1):63–75.e2.

66. Scheltens P, Blennow K, Breteler MM, de Strooper B, Frisoni GB, Salloway S, Van der Flier WM. Alzheimer's disease. Lancet. 2016;388(10043):505–17.

67. Small BJ, Hertzog C, Hultsch DF, Dixon RA, Victoria Longitudinal S. Stability and change in adult personality over 6 years: findings from the victoria longitudinal study. J Gerontol B Psychol Sci Soc Sci. 2003;58(3):P166–76.

68. Chalmers JM. Behavior management and communication strategies for dental professionals when caring for patients with dementia. Spec Care Dentist. 2000;20(4):147–54.

69. Bell RA, Arcury TA, Anderson AM, Chen H, Savoca MR, Gilbert GH, Quandt SA. Dental anxiety and oral health outcomes among rural older adults. J Public Health Dent. 2012;72(1):53–9.

70. Locker D, Liddell A, Burman D. Dental fear and anxiety in an older adult population. Community Dent Oral Epidemiol. 1991;19(2):120–4.

71. De Jongh A, Adair P, Meijerink-Anderson M. Clinical management of dental anxiety: what works for whom? Int Dent J. 2005;55(2):73–80.

72. Armfield JM, Heaton LJ. Management of fear and anxiety in the dental clinic: a review. Aust Dent J. 2013;58(4):390–407; quiz 531.

73. Alvis BD, Hughes CG. Physiology considerations in geriatric patients. Anesthesiol Clin. 2015;33(3):447–56.

74. American Society of Anesthesiologists. 2014. ASA physical status classification system. https://www.asahq.org/resources/clinical-information/asa-physical-status-classification-system. Accessed 1 July 2016.

75. Malamed S. The geriatric patient. In: Malamed S, editor. Sedation: a guide to patient management. 5th ed. St. Louis: Mosby; 2009. p. 517–8.

76. Turner M, Greenwood M. Oral and maxillofacial surgery for the geriatric patient. In: Homl-Pedersen P, Walls A, Ship JA, editors. Textbook of geriatric dentistry. 3rd ed. Chichester: Wiley; 2015. p. 256–64.

77. Rashid F, Awad MA, Thomason JM, Piovano A, Spielberg GP, Scilingo E, Mojon P, Muller F, Spielberg M, Heydecke G, et al. The effective-

ness of 2-implant overdentures—a pragmatic international multicentre study. J Oral Rehabil. 2011;38(3):176–84.

78. Thomason JM, Kelly SA, Bendkowski A, Ellis JS. Two implant retained overdentures—a review of the literature supporting the McGill and York consensus statements. J Dent. 2012;40(1):22–34.

79. Moraschini V, Velloso G, Luz D, Barboza EP. Implant survival rates, marginal bone level changes, and complications in full-mouth rehabilitation with flapless computer-guided surgery: a systematic review and meta-analysis. Int J Oral Maxillofac Surg. 2015;44(7):892–901.

80. D'Haese J, Van De Velde T, Elaut L, De Bruyn H. A prospective study on the accuracy of mucosally supported stereolithographic surgical guides in fully edentulous maxillae. Clin Implant Dent Relat Res. 2012;14(2):293–303.

81. Di Giacomo GA, da Silva JV, da Silva AM, Paschoal GH, Cury PR, Szarf G. Accuracy and complications of computer-designed selective laser sintering surgical guides for flapless dental implant placement and immediate definitive prosthesis installation. J Periodontol. 2012;83(4):410–9.

82. Arisan V, Karabuda CZ, Ozdemir T. Implant surgery using bone- and mucosa-supported stereolithographic guides in totally edentulous jaws: surgical and post-operative outcomes of computer-aided vs. standard techniques. Clin Oral Implants Res. 2010;21(9):980–8.

83. Engquist B, Astrand P, Anzen B, Dahlgren S, Engquist E, Feldmann H, Karlsson U, Nord PG, Sahlholm S, Svardstrom P. Simplified methods of implant treatment in the edentulous lower jaw. A controlled prospective study. Part i: one-stage versus two-stage surgery. Clin Implant Dent Relat Res. 2002;4(2):93–103.

84. Lang NP, Loe H. The relationship between the width of keratinized gingiva and gingival health. J Periodontol. 1972;43(10):623–7.

85. Dorfman HS, Kennedy JE, Bird WC. Longitudinal evaluation of free autogenous gingival grafts. J Clin Periodontol. 1980;7(4):316–24.

86. Kennedy JE, Bird WC, Palcanis KG, Dorfman HS. A longitudinal evaluation of varying widths of attached gingiva. J Clin Periodontol. 1985;12(8):667–75.

87. Wennstrom JL. Lack of association between width of attached gingiva and development of soft tissue recession. A 5-year longitudinal study. J Clin Periodontol. 1987;14(3):181–4.

88. Atsuta I, Yamaza T, Yoshinari M, Mino S, Goto T, Kido MA, Terada Y, Tanaka T. Changes in the distribution of laminin-5 during peri-implant epithelium formation after immediate titanium implantation in rats. Biomaterials. 2005;26(14):1751–60.

89. Buser D, Weber HP, Donath K, Fiorellini JP, Paquette DW, Williams RC. Soft tissue reactions to non-submerged unloaded titanium implants in beagle dogs. J Periodontol. 1992;63(3):225–35.

90. Gerber JA, Tan WC, Balmer TE, Salvi GE, Lang NP. Bleeding on probing and pocket probing depth in relation to probing pressure and mucosal health around oral implants. Clin Oral Implants Res. 2009;20(1):75–8.

91. Berglundh T, Lindhe J, Ericsson I, Marinello CP, Liljenberg B, Thomsen P. The soft tissue barrier at implants and teeth. Clin Oral Implants Res. 1991;2(2):81–90.

92. Atsuta I, Ayukawa Y, Kondo R, Oshiro W, Matsuura Y, Furuhashi A, Tsukiyama Y, Koyano K. Soft tissue sealing around dental implants based on histological interpretation. J Prosthodont Res. 2016;60(1):3–11.

93. Carcuac O, Abrahamsson I, Albouy JP, Linder E, Larsson L, Berglundh T. Experimental periodontitis and peri-implantitis in dogs. Clin Oral Implants Res. 2013;24(4):363–71.

94. Brito C, Tenenbaum HC, Wong BK, Schmitt C, Nogueira-Filho G. Is keratinized mucosa indispensable to maintain peri-implant health? A systematic review of the literature. J Biomed Mater Res B Appl Biomater. 2014;102(3):643–50.

95. Gobbato L, Avila-Ortiz G, Sohrabi K, Wang CW, Karimbux N. The effect of keratinized mucosa width on peri-implant health: a systematic review. Int J Oral Maxillofac Implants. 2013;28(6):1536–45.

96. Lin GH, Chan HL, Wang HL. The significance of keratinized mucosa on implant health: a systematic review. J Periodontol. 2013;84(12):1755–67.

97. Adibrad M, Shahabuei M, Sahabi M. Significance of the width of keratinized mucosa on the health status of the supporting tissue around implants supporting overdentures. J Oral Implantol. 2009;35(5):232–7.

98. Kaptein ML, De Lange GL, Blijdorp PA. Peri-implant tissue health in reconstructed atrophic maxillae—report of 88 patients and 470 implants. J Oral Rehabil. 1999;26(6):464–74.

99. Elkhaweldi A, Rincon Soler C, Cayarga R, Suzuki T, Kaufman Z. Various techniques to increase keratinized tissue for implant supported overdentures: retrospective case series. Int J Dent. 2015;2015:104903.

100. Bjorn H. Free transplantation of gingiva propria. Sven Tandlak Tidskr. 1963;22:684–9.

101. Karring T, Cumming BR, Oliver RC, Loe H. The origin of granulation tissue and its impact on postoperative results of mucogingival surgery. J Periodontol. 1975;46(10):577–85.

102. Karring T, Lang NP, Loe H. The role of gingival connective tissue in determining epithelial differentiation. J Periodontal Res. 1975;10(1):1–11.

103. Karring T, Ostergaard E, Loe H. Conservation of tissue specificity after heterotopic transplantation of gingiva and alveolar mucosa. J Periodontal Res. 1971;6(4):282–93.

104. Weinlaender M. Bone growth around dental implants. Dent Clin North Am. 1991;35(3):585–601.

105. Eriksson AR, Albrektsson T. Temperature threshold levels for heat-induced bone tissue injury: a vital-microscopic study in the rabbit. J Prosthet Dent. 1983;50(1):101–7.

106. Eriksson RA, Albrektsson T, Magnusson B. Assessment of bone viability after heat trauma. A histological, histochemical and vital microscopic study in the rabbit. Scand J Plast Reconstr Surg. 1984;18(3):261–8.

107. Benington IC, Biagioni PA, Briggs J, Sheridan S, Lamey PJ. Thermal changes observed at implant sites during internal and external irrigation. Clin Oral Implants Res. 2002;13(3):293–7.

108. Ercoli C, Funkenbusch PD, Lee HJ, Moss ME, Graser GN. The influence of drill wear on cutting efficiency and heat production during osteotomy preparation for dental implants: a study of drill durability. Int J Oral Maxillofac Implants. 2004;19(3):335–49.

109. Koo KT, Kim MH, Kim HY, Wikesjo UM, Yang JH, Yeo IS. Effects of implant drill wear, irrigation, and drill materials on heat generation in osteotomy sites. J Oral Implantol. 2015;41(2):e19–23.

110. Mohlhenrich SC, Modabber A, Steiner T, Mitchell DA, Holzle F. Heat generation and drill wear during dental implant site preparation: systematic review. Br J Oral Maxillofac Surg. 2015;53(8):679–89.

111. Binon PP. Implants and components: entering the new millennium. Int J Oral Maxillofac Implants. 2000;15(1):76–94.

112. Esposito M, Ardebili Y, Worthington HV. Interventions for replacing missing teeth: different types of dental implants. Cochrane Database Syst Rev. 2014;7:CD003815.

113. Chrcanovic BR, Albrektsson T, Wennerberg A. Platform switch and dental implants: a meta-analysis. J Dent. 2015;43(6):629–46.

114. Pons-Vicente O, Lopez-Jimenez L, Sanchez-Garces MA, Sala-Perez S, Gay-Escoda C. A comparative study between two different suture materials in oral implantology. Clin Oral Implants Res. 2011;22(3):282–8.

115. Leknes KN, Roynstrand IT, Selvig KA. Human gingival tissue reactions to silk and expanded polytetrafluoroethylene sutures. J Periodontol. 2005;76(1):34–42.

116. Gartti-Jardim EC, de Souza AP, Carvalho AC, Pereira CC, Okamoto R, Magro Filho O. Comparative study of the healing process when using Vicryl(r), Vicryl Rapid(r), Vicryl Plus(r), and Monocryl(r) sutures in the rat dermal tissue. Oral Maxillofac Surg. 2013;17(4):293–8.

117. Vasanthan A, Satheesh K, Hoopes W, Lucaci P, Williams K, Rapley J. Comparing suture strengths for clinical applications: a novel in vitro study. J Periodontol. 2009;80(4):618–24.

118. Cardemil C, Ristevski Z, Alsen B, Dahlin C. Influence of different operatory setups on implant survival rate: a retrospective clinical study. Clin Implant Dent Relat Res. 2009;11(4):288–91.

119. Scharf DR, Tarnow DP. Success rates of osseointegration for implants placed under sterile versus clean conditions. J Periodontol. 1993;64(10):954–6.

120. Ong CK, Lirk P, Seymour RA, Jenkins BJ. The efficacy of preemptive analgesia for acute postoperative pain management: a meta-analysis. Anesth Analg. 2005;100(3):757–73, table of contents.

121. Esposito M, Grusovin MG, Worthington HV. Interventions for replacing missing teeth: antibiotics at dental implant placement to prevent complications. Cochrane Database Syst Rev. 2013;(7):CD004152.

122. Veksler AE, Kayrouz GA, Newman MG. Reduction of salivary bacteria by pre-procedural rinses with chlorhexidine 0.12%. J Periodontol. 1991;62(11):649–51.

123. Buckley JA, Ciancio SG, McMullen JA. Efficacy of epinephrine concentration in local anesthesia during periodontal surgery. J Periodontol. 1984;55(11):653–7.

124. Greenstein G, Tarnow D. The mental foramen and nerve: clinical and anatomical factors related to dental implant placement: a literature review. J Periodontol. 2006;77(12):1933–43.

125. Lekholm U, Zarb GA. Patient selection and preparation. In: Branemark PI, Zarb GA, Albrektsson T, editors. Tissue integrated prostheses: osseointegration in clinical dentistry. Chicago: Quintessence Publishing Company; 1985. p. 199–209.

126. Bashutski JD, D'Silva NJ, Wang HL. Implant compression necrosis: current understanding and case report. J Periodontol. 2009;80(4):700–4.

127. Khayat PG, Arnal HM, Tourbah BI, Sennerby L. Clinical outcome of dental implants placed with high insertion torques (up to 176 Ncm). Clin Implant Dent Relat Res. 2013;15(2):227–33.

128. Jung RE, Herzog M, Wolleb K, Ramel CF, Thoma DS, Hammerle CH. A randomized controlled clinical trial comparing small buccal dehiscence defects around dental implants treated with guided bone regeneration or left for spontaneous healing. Clin Oral Implants Res. 2017;28(3):348–54.

129. Lanier JB, Mote MB, Clay EC. Evaluation and management of orthostatic hypotension. Am Fam Physician. 2011;84(5):527–36.

130. Ong CK, Seymour RA, Lirk P, Merry AF. Combining paracetamol (acetaminophen) with nonsteroidal antiinflammatory drugs: a qualitative systematic review of analgesic efficacy for acute postoperative pain. Anesth Analg. 2010;110(4):1170–9.

131. Durand R, Tran SD, Mui B, Voyer R. Managing postoperative pain following periodontal surgery. J Can Dent Assoc. 2013;79:d66.

132. Powell CA, Mealey BL, Deas DE, McDonnell HT, Moritz AJ. Post-surgical infections: prevalence associated with various periodontal surgical procedures. J Periodontol. 2005;76(3):329–33.

133. Greenstein G. Therapeutic efficacy of cold therapy after intraoral surgical procedures: a literature review. J Periodontol. 2007;78(5):790–800.

134. Bain CA. Smoking and implant failure—benefits of a smoking cessation protocol. Int J Oral Maxillofac Implants. 1996;11(6):756–9.

135. Isaacson TJ. Sublingual hematoma formation during immediate placement of mandibular endosseous implants. J Am Dent Assoc. 2004;135(2):168–72.

136. Madrid C, Sanz M. What influence do anticoagulants have on oral implant therapy? A systematic review. Clin Oral Implants Res. 2009;20(Suppl 4):96–106.

137. Kraut RA, Chahal O. Management of patients with trigeminal nerve injuries after mandibular implant placement. J Am Dent Assoc. 2002;133(10):1351–4.

138. Schwartz-Arad D, Kidron N, Dolev E. A long-term study of implants supporting overdentures as a model for implant success. J Periodontol. 2005;76(9):1431–5.

139. Tolman DE, Keller EE. Management of mandibular fractures in patients with endosseous implants. Int J Oral Maxillofac Implants. 1991;6(4):427–36.

140. Laskin DM. Nonsurgical management of bilateral mandibular fractures associated with dental implants: report of a case. Int J Oral Maxillofac Implants. 2003;18(5):739–44.

141. Park SH, Wang HL. Implant reversible complications: classification and treatments. Implant Dent. 2005;14(3):211–20.

142. Jepsen S, Berglundh T, Genco R, Aass AM, Demirel K, Derks J, Figuero E, Giovannoli JL, Goldstein M, Lambert F, et al. Primary prevention of peri-implantitis: managing peri-implant mucositis. J Clin Periodontol. 2015;42(Suppl 16):S152–7.

143. Monje A, Aranda L, Diaz KT, Alarcon MA, Bagramian RA, Wang HL, Catena A. Impact of maintenance therapy for the prevention of peri-implant diseases: a systematic review and meta-analysis. J Dent Res. 2016;95(4):372–9.

144. Mahato N, Wu X, Wang L. Management of peri-implantitis: a systematic review, 2010-2015. Springerplus. 2016;5:105.

145. Chan HL, Lin GH, Suarez F, MacEachern M, Wang HL. Surgical management of peri-implantitis: a systematic review and meta-analysis of treatment outcomes. J Periodontol. 2014;85(8):1027–41.

Bone Grafting

9

Zeeshan Sheikh, Siavash Hasanpour, and Michael Glogauer

Abstract

Successful dental implant placement for restoration of edentulous ridges depends on the quality and quantity of alveolar bone available in all spatial dimensions. There are several surgical grafting techniques used in combination with natural or synthetic materials to achieve alveolar ridge augmentation. The commonly available bone tissue replacement materials include autografts, allografts, xenografts, and alloplasts. Polymers (natural and synthetic) are widely used as barrier membrane materials in guided tissue regeneration (GTR) and guided bone regeneration (GBR) applications. However, there is no single ideal technique or graft material to choose in clinical practice currently. Treatment protocols and materials that involve less invasive and more reproducible vertical and horizontal bone augmentation procedures are actively sought. This chapter focuses on existing surgical techniques, natural tissues, and synthetic biomaterials commonly used for bone grafting in order to successfully restore edentulous ridges with implant-supported prostheses.

9.1 Preamble

Patients who become edentulous late in their lives provide unique challenges to clinicians who are to treat them and restore their dentition. These elderly patients have great difficulty in getting used to complete dentures, and when provided with the option, they seem to be more reluctant in accepting dental implants [1]. Even when such patients agree to getting dental implants placed, there are several anatomical and surgical limitations encountered. How successful dental implants ultimately are crucially depends upon the degree of osseointegration in sufficient and healthy bone [2, 3]. Dental implant osseointegration is dependent on a wound-healing response that could be less successful in older than in younger patients [4, 5]. Bone volume and quality are almost always reduced due to extended time after teeth are lost before implant placement [6, 7]. An average alveolar bone loss of 1.5–2 mm (vertical) and 40–50% (horizontal) occurs within 6 months after teeth are lost [8]. If the dentition is not restored and left

Z. Sheikh, Dip.Dh., B.D.S., M.Sc., Ph.D. (✉)
Faculty of Dentistry, Matrix Dynamics Group, University of Toronto, Toronto, ON, Canada

Lunenfeld-Tenebaum Research Institute, Mt. Sinai Hospital, Toronto, ON, Canada
e-mail: zeeshan.sheikh@utoronto.ca

S. Hasanpour • M. Glogauer
Faculty of Dentistry, Matrix Dynamics Group, University of Toronto, Toronto, ON, Canada

© Springer International Publishing AG, part of Springer Nature 2018
E. Emami, J. Feine (eds.), *Mandibular Implant Prostheses*,
https://doi.org/10.1007/978-3-319-71181-2_9

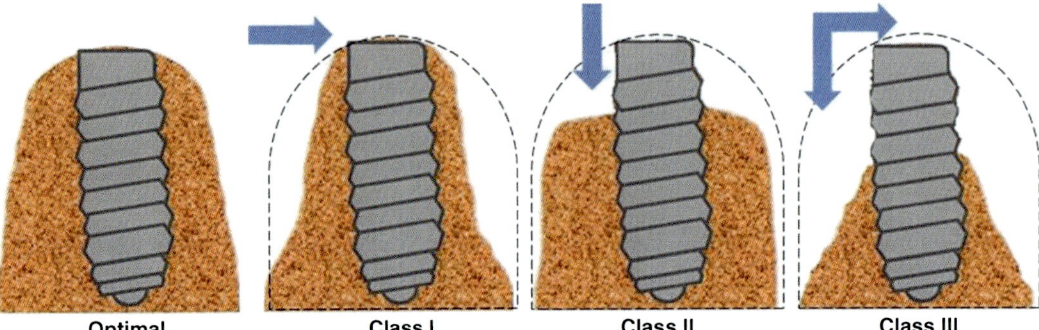

Fig. 9.1 Alveolar bone insufficiency for dental implant placement. When there is adequate alveolar ridge height and width, this allows for successful dental implant placement with optimal clinical results. In class I ridge defects, there is horizontal bone loss with adequate height leading to insufficient bone volume for successful regular diame-ter implant placement. In class II there is vertical bone loss with adequate width, leading to insufficient bone volume for proper placement of regular length implants. In class III there is bone loss in both vertical and horizontal dimensions not allowing placement implants in all spatial dimensions

untreated, then bone loss occurs continuously, and in the first 3 years, up to 60% of alveolar ridge volume is lost [9, 10]. This lack of sufficient bone volume, height, and quality poses extreme challenges to the final treatment outcome (Fig. 9.1) [11, 12]. A variety of bone grafting surgical techniques with and without the use of biomaterials have been explored to try successfully place dental implants in resorbed alveolar bone [13, 14]. Multiple bone grafting techniques and natural and synthetic graft materials have been tested for this purpose [14, 15], and this chapter discusses the various bone grafting techniques currently available to achieve alveolar ridge augmentation for allowing success-ful placement of dental implants.

9.2 Principles of Bone Regeneration and Various Grafting Techniques

Bone grafting procedures for alveolar ridge aug-mentation are based on biological principles of bone tissue regeneration. The osteoblasts (bone-forming cells) and osteoclasts (bone-resorbing cells) are the two basic cellular units that play a role in bone tissue formation and remodeling. The osteoblasts are derived from the mesenchy-mal stem cells (bone marrow stromal stem cells), while osteoclasts are derived from the hemato-poietic progenitors of monocytic lineage [16].

The key factors involved in differentiation of osteoblasts are estrogen, parathyroid hormone, vitamin D3, fibroblast growth factors (FGFs), and transforming growth factor-beta (TGF-β) [17–19]. Whereas, osteoclast differentiation depends on the activation of colony-stimulating factor-1 receptor/macrophage colony-stimulating factor/CD115 (MCSF, a colony-stimulating fac-tor receptor) and receptor activator of nuclear factor kappa-B (RANK) receptors [20], osteo-blasts regulate osteoclast differentiation and acti-vation of RANK ligand (RANKL) and its high-affinity decoy receptor, osteoprotegerin. Therefore, osteoblasts are essential to osteoclast differentiation by regulating the balance between RANKL and osteoprotegerin [21].

The presence and/or recruitment of osteoblast precursors and growth factors at sites of augmen-tation are essential for bone regeneration to occur. Some graft materials (cancellous autogenous grafts) and the recipient bed can provide the osteoblast precursors required [22], whereas the growth factors come from the vasculature and recipient bed. Active bone resorption and forma-tion throughout the graft dominate the early phase of bone regeneration at grafted sites [23]. The latter phase is mainly known to be character-ized by the osteoconductive processes [24]. Osteoconduction is a function of a bone graft substrate providing a three-dimensional (3D) scaffold area promoting ingrowth of host capillaries and osteoprogenitor cells [25]. Biomaterials that imitate natural bone chemistry and structure closely are considered ideal for cellular osteogenic differentiation. Graft macroporosity and pore interconnection have a major impact on osteoinduction potential as higher levels of porosity, appropriate pore shape, and sufficient interconnectivity are essential for ingrowth of blood vessels and bone matrix deposition [26].

During the initial first few weeks, new bone is synthesized by mature osteoblasts that are differentiated from osteoblast precursors under the influence of osteoinductors. The growth factors involved in formation of new bone act directly on osteoblast and fibroblast proliferation, mesenchymal cell differentiation, extracellular matrix deposition, and vascular proliferation [27].

Early stages of induction are influenced by the fibroblast growth factor (FGF) and platelet-derived growth factor (PDGF) by stimulating fibroblast and osteoblast proliferation. Bone morphogenetic proteins (BMPs) affect later stages of osteoinduction such as vascular proliferation and mesenchymal cell differentiation, whereas transforming growth factor-beta (TGF-β) does not affect mesenchymal cell differentiation but acts on cellular proliferation, matrix deposition, and vascularization [14]. The various bone grafting techniques employed for alveolar ridge augmentation are discussed in subsequent sections.

9.2.1 Distraction Osteogenesis

Distraction osteogenesis (DO) is used to achieve alveolar bone volume gain in all dimensions. In DO new bone is formed by mechanical elongation of bone callus through progressive separation of two bone fragments surrounding the callus under tension [28]. This is achieved in three phases: (1) the latency phase, in which soft tissues heal after the distractor is placed surgically (this phase usually lasts about 7 days); (2) the distraction phase, in which the bone fragments are separated at a rate of 0.5–1 mm/day incrementally; and (3) the consolidation phase, where the bone formed gets mineralized and matured [29, 30]. Devices used for DO can be intraosseous or extraosseous [31].

However, devices with extraosseous distraction configuration affixed to the cortical plate are more frequently used than intraosseous devices [32, 33]. There is sufficient literature reporting the potential of DO to achieve alveolar ridge augmentation as this technique can result in significantly greater and stable bone height gain compared to other vertical augmentation techniques [34, 35]. High rate of complications is associated with DO [36, 37] with vector control being the major problem which often leads to lingual inclination of the transport segment in the mandible [38]. Although DO allows for greater alveolar bone regeneration from native bone, the sensitivity of the technique and strict anatomical requirements have limited its use in clinical practice.

9.2.2 Osteoperiosteal Flap Techniques

Vascularized segmental osteotomy performed on alveolar bone is used to accomplish the osteoperiosteal flap (OPF) technique which is based on the biologic principles of vascularization studies and understanding of Le Fort I management techniques [39]. The major blood supply of the alveolar bone is from the bone marrow and periosteum. In geriatric patients with the atrophy of the ridge, there is decreased bone marrow blood flow. In OPF technique, vascularization in bone fragments via the periosteum. Osteoperiosteal flaps through segmental osteotomies are used in combination with interpositional grafts in the gap generated by transposition of the flap in the desired position to achieve vertical ridge gain [14]. OPF combined with interpositional grafts via the osteotomy-based techniques are being used commonly for treating alveolar ridges with height deficiencies and allow for preservation of the attached gingiva and the papillae [40, 41].

9.2.3 Block Grafting Techniques

Onlay bone grafting with bone blocks was first introduced in the early 1990s and was used to try augmenting maxillary and mandibular edentulous ridges [42]. In the classic block grafting technique, autologous bone blocks are immobilized to the recipient alveolar ridge by securing with osteosynthesis screws [43, 44]. Autologous bone grafting has been used for the treatment of severely resorbed edentulous mandible and maxilla [45, 46]. The mandibular ramus or mental region (intraoral) and the iliac crest (extraoral) are the most commonly used autologous donor sites for block grafting [47, 48]. Autogenous bone procured from the iliac crest has been used to gain ridge height, but high resorption rate before implant placement and after loading is observed [49]. This is possibly due to the low cortical-to-trabecular ratio in the graft material, endochondral versus intramembranous ossification memory, and differing osteoblast mechanosensing memory between the donor and recipient sites [14]. Other extraoral donor sites for obtaining block grafts include the tibia, ribs, and cranial vault but are not commonly used due to the high donor site morbidity associated with them [50, 51].

The mandibular ramus and the symphysis are the common sites for harvesting intraoral block grafts [52]. Although the symphysis gives greater bone volume, the morbidity is significantly higher when compared to the ramus grafts which include postoperative pain, neurosensory disturbances in the chin region, temporary mental nerve paresthesia, altered sensation in mandibular anterior teeth, and risk of mandibular fracture [53, 54]. Hence, the symphysis is used for cases that require thicker block grafts that otherwise are not possible to obtain from other intraoral donor sites. Close contact and stabilization of block grafts to the recipient bed are crucial and achieved by using osteosynthesis screws [55–57]. Revascularization and remodeling of bone can also be stimulated via inlay shaping and decortication of the recipient bed [58]. Ridge augmentation with allograft onlay blocks has demonstrated reasonable success [59], and the use of barrier membranes in combination with block grafts has been shown to improve clinical outcome [60–62].

9.2.4 Guided Bone Regeneration (GBR)

Guided bone regeneration (GBR) works on the principle of separation of particulate grafts from the surrounding tissues allowing for bone to regenerate, which naturally occurs at a rate slower than that of soft tissues [63, 64]. Since the major problem with particulate graft techniques is the high graft resorption rate and the anatomical limitations for graft containment [65], barrier membranes are commonly used in GBR technique to stabilize graft materials, to limit their resorption, and to serve as a separating barrier [64]. Local anatomy and type of bone graft tissues and materials used determine the choice of a specific membrane used for GBR. However, in some specific cases, barrier membranes are not used as the graft material can be used alone to fill the defect area [66].

Initially, the principles of GBR were applied to atrophic alveolar ridges for implant site development [67]. GBR has since been used to treat a variety of intraoral bone defect sites and is a routine technique employed in clinical practice [68]. GBR for alveolar ridge augmentation in the vertical direction is extremely technique sensitive, which limits the clinical success, and failure usually occurs due to wound dehiscence [69]. Another limitation of vertical GBR is the ability for bone generation along the long axis of applied force [14]. Barrier membranes combined with particulate and/or block grafts have resulted in more predictable clinical outcomes [70]. It has been demonstrated that there is less resorption of block grafts when used in combination with expanded polytetrafluoroethylene (ePTFE) barrier membranes [71].

Barrier membranes used alone for GBR are associated with membrane compression into the defect space by overlying soft tissues [72]. To overcome this problem, membranes made from still materials such as titanium or metal-reinforced expanded polytetrafluoroethylene (ePTFE) have been developed [73]. Treatment of complex vertical defects requires stable and stiff titanium or metal-reinforced PTFE membranes [65]. A problem associated with use of titanium

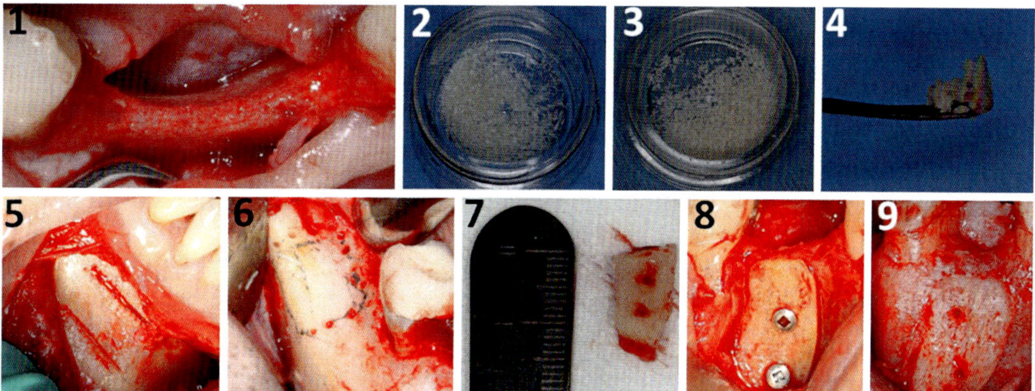

Fig. 9.2 Conventional methods of horizontal bone augmentation. Long-term edentulism can result in disuse bone atrophy resulting in residual ridge resorption of the alveolus. Areas with inadequate buccal-lingual represent a significant treatment challenge and often require horizontal bone augmentation either prior to or during implant surgery (1). Particulate demineralized freeze-dried bone allograft (DFDBA) (2) and particulate mineralized freeze-dried bone allograft (FDBA) (3) are commonly used in horizontal bone augmentation. Particulate graft materials are packed into the defect (4) and covered with biologically compatible membranes prior to achieving primary closure to allow for adequate buccal-lingual width needed for implant therapy. Alternatively, autologous block grafts harvested from the patient's chin or ramus (5, 6, 7) can be fixated to deficient areas using fixation screws (8) which allows for considerable gain in bone width following healing (9) (Periodontology Graduate Clinics, Faculty of Dentistry, University of Toronto)

membranes in GBR is the fibrous ingrowth and exposure of the membrane [74]. GBR therapy by using titanium-reinforced non-resorbable membranes in combination with dental implants has been carried out with varying levels of clinical success [74].

9.2.5 Minimally Invasive Approaches to GBR

Minimally invasive approach to perform GBR is preferred to prevent or reduce postoperative complications and graft exposure [75]. Kent et al. in the late 1970s developed a subperiosteal tunneling technique which involved a relatively small surgical incision in the alveolar ridge to elevate the periosteum and inject a low viscosity hydroxyapatite particle paste [76]. It has been observed that the hydroxyapatite particles are usually unstable and diffuse adjacently into tissues causing fibrous capsule formation which inhibits bone formation [77]. However, minimally invasive tunneling along with screw and/or barrier membrane-mediated graft stabilization can result in relatively predictable alveolar bone

augmentation in vertical direction [76, 78]. Calcium phosphates such as injectable brushite cement pastes with controlled viscosity have been investigated for minimally invasive augmentation procedures [79]. Novel graft biomaterials with improved viscosity offer potential for this technique, but results are controversial with insufficient data (Fig. 9.2).

9.3 Natural Tissues and Synthetic Biomaterials Used for Bone Grafting

There are various graft options available and used for alveolar bone grafting and divided into natural transplants (autografts, allografts, and xenografts) and synthetic materials (alloplasts) (Table 9.1) [14]. These graft materials are used because they are either osteogenic, osteoinductive, or osteoconductive [80]. Most grafts undergo macrophage- or osteoclast-mediated resorption before bone deposition by osteoblasts [23, 81]. As discussed before, bone deposition is expedited by osteoinductive ability and adequate blood flow throughout the graft, providing the

Table 9.1 Available tissue and biomaterial options for alveolar bone grafting

Bone replacement graft materials
1. Human bone graft tissues
(a) Autografts
• Extraoral
• Intraoral
(b) Allografts
• Fresh and/or frozen bone
• Freeze-dried bone allograft (FDBA)
• Demineralized freeze-dried bone allograft (FDBA)
2. Nonhuman natural tissues and materials
(a) Xenografts
• Bovine hydroxyapatite
• Coralline calcium carbonate
3. Synthetic materials (alloplasts)
(a) Bioactive glasses
(b) Bioceramics
• Hydroxyapatite
• Other calcium phosphates (tricalcium phosphate, brushite, monetite)

appropriate nutrients and growth factors essential for osteoblast differentiation and function. This section discusses the various graft tissues and biomaterials used commonly for bone grafting procedures.

9.3.1 Autogenous Grafts

Autogenous bone grafts (autografts) are harvested from a site in the same individual and transplanted to another site. Although these provide the most osteogenic organic materials, donor site morbidity, increase in postsurgical recovery time, and the limited amount of graft volume that can be obtained are the disadvantages [13]. Autografts used for bone alveolar bone grafting may be of intraoral or extraoral origin. The various harvesting sites for autografts are the mandibular ramus and corpus; the tuber, spina nasalis, and crista zygomatico-alveolaris from the maxilla; and the tibia and iliac crest [82]. Although autografts of iliac origin provide optimum osteoinductive, osteoconductive, and osteogenic potential [83], there is less morbidity associated with intraoral donor sites when compared to extraoral sites [48]. Mandibular autografts are used very commonly as bone blocks, chips, and/or milled particles [48, 84]. The most common extraoral harvest site that provides relatively large amounts of autologous cortical-cancellous bone is the pelvic rim [85]. Cortical autografts have high initial strength which after about 6 months of implantation is ~50% weaker than the normal bone tissue [86]. On the other hand, cancellous autografts are mechanically weaker because of their porous architecture initially but with time gain strength [80]. Also, the cancellous autografts have been shown to revascularize sooner than cortical grafts around the fifth day postimplantation due to their spongy architecture [80]. Alveolar bone and ridge augmentation in vertical and horizontal dimensions carried out using particulate autografts with GBR has been successful for placing dental implants [87, 88]. However, block grafts outperform particulate grafts with regard to revascularization, bone remodeling, bone-to-implant contact, and bone fill potential [87].

9.3.2 Allogeneic Grafts

Graft tissues obtained from genetically nonidentical members of the same species are known as allogeneic grafts (allografts). These grafts are available in larger quantities for use and do not have the usual drawbacks of autografts. Allografts (cortical and cancellous) of various particle size ranges are used routinely for bone augmentation procedures with minimal risk of disease transmission [89–91]. Allografts are available as cortical granules, cortical chips, cortical wedges, and cancellous powder prepared as frozen, freeze-dried, mineralized, and demineralized bone tissue [92].

9.3.2.1 Fresh or Frozen Iliac Cancellous Bone and Marrow Allogeneic Grafts

Atrophic maxillary ridges when grafted with human block grafts of tibia and fresh-frozen chips show features representative of mature and compact osseous tissue surrounded by marrow spaces [93, 94]. Fresh and/or frozen cancellous bone and marrow tissues demonstrate the highest osteoconductive and osteoinductive potential among all allografts [95, 96]. However, due to the risk of disease transmission, use of fresh or frozen iliac allografts is now obsolete.

9.3.2.2 Mineralized Freeze-Dried Bone Allogeneic Grafts (FDBA)

Freeze-dried bone allografts (FDBA) are mineralized and are used commonly for the treatment of periodontal defects with reasonable success [97–100]. The process of freeze-drying affects the immune recognition in the host by distorting the 3D presentation of the human leukocyte antigens on surface of graft particles [101, 102]. FDBA have inferior mechanical properties and osteoinductive potential when compared with fresh or frozen allografts [103]. FDBA are known to be osteoconductive and can be combined with autografts to enhance the osteogenic potential [104, 105]. Cortical FDBA have a higher volume of bone matrix, more osteoinductive potential via growth factors stored in the matrix [106]. The use of FDBA blocks for alveolar ridge grafting has demonstrated presence of vital bone with a lamellar organization [107, 108]. FDBA used in combination with resorbable barrier membranes can be used as a replacement to autogenous block grafts for ridge augmentation prior to implant placement [109].

9.3.2.3 Demineralized Freeze-Dried Bone Allogeneic Grafts (DFDBA)

Demineralized freeze-dried bone allografts (DFDBA) are used for grafting procedures alone or in combination with FDBA and/or autografts very frequently. DFDBA grafts undergo resorption quickly [110, 111] and have osteoinductive potential attributed to the morphogenetic proteins (BMPs) stored in the matrix [112]. Growth factors and differentiation factors have also been shown to be present in DFDBA preparations [113, 114]. DFDBA grafts obtained from the younger individuals have higher osteogenic potential in comparison with grafts from older individuals resulting in variation in BMP levels

in different DFDBA batches [115, 116]. DFDBA has been shown to have less new bone formation in comparison to autogenous grafts used in similar grafting procedures [117].

9.3.3 Xenogeneic Grafts

Xenogeneic grafts or xenografts are tissues used for bone grafting obtained from nonhuman species. Bone xenografts were first reported in aseptic bone cavities in 1889 [118]. Xenograft materials after implantation are usually osteoconductive and show variable ability to be resorbed and replaced by new bone over time [119, 120]. The commonly used xenograft in dentistry is Bio-Oss®, which is a commercially available bovine bone processed to yield natural bone mineral without any organic component [121]. The inorganic phase of bovine bone remaining after low-heat treatment and chemical extraction of organic component mainly consists of hydroxyapatite that retains the micro- and/or macroporous structural morphology [122]. Although this heat and chemical treatment removes most of the osteogenic components from the bovine bone, it is extremely important as this eliminates any potential risk of disease transmission (bovine spongiform encephalopathy) and graft rejection [123, 124]. Bovine-derived bone particles and block grafts have been used for the treatment of human ridge augmentation procedures and intrabony defect filling [125, 126]. The advantage of using bovine bone as graft materials is the higher osteoconductive potential compared with synthetically derived materials. The major disadvantage of these grafts is the inherent brittleness and lack of toughness as they routinely are prone to failure and breakage during the screw fixation or after implantation leading to less than optimal clinical results [126, 127].

Calcium carbonate grafts are of natural coralline origin and are composed mostly of aragonite which is more than 98% calcium carbonate. Having a pore size of 100–200 µm, very similar to that is observed in cancellous bone, and relatively high porosity of ~45% allows for greater resorption and new bone formation and infiltration within the graft area [91, 128]. Coralline calcium carbonate demonstrates high osteoconductivity since transformation to carbonate is not required like most other graft materials, allowing for new bone deposition to occur rapidly [129].

Coralline calcium carbonate has the potential for greater defect fill in periodontal regeneration applications and does not undergo fibrous encapsulation [130–132].

9.3.4 Alloplasts

Alloplastic bone grafting materials are sought after because they provide an abundant amount without the problems associated with autografts [133]. These are fabricated in various forms and with varying physicochemical properties and can be both resorbable and non-resorbable [14, 15, 134–136]. Alloplastic materials are usually osteoconductive without having any osteogenic and osteoinductive potential and have been used successfully in periodontal reconstructive applications [135]. The most routinely used alloplastic materials are hydroxyapatite (HA), tricalcium phosphates (TCP), bioactive glasses, and dicalcium phosphates [80].

Synthetic HA is available and used in various forms: porous non-resorbable, solid non-resorbable, and resorbable (non-ceramic, porous) [137]. HA is non-osteogenic and mainly functions as an osteoconductive graft material. The ability of HA to resorb is dependent upon the processing temperature. At higher temperatures the HA synthesized is very dense and non-resorbable [138]. The dense HA grafts are osteoconductive and mostly used as an inert biocompatible filler and have been shown to result in defect filling greater than flap debridement used alone [139, 140]. When processed at lower temperatures, the particulate HA produced is porous with a slow resorption rate [141]. Early implant loading studies in augmented alveolar ridges with nanostructured hydroxyapatite have shown promise [142, 143]. Also, alveolar ridge augmentation with HA granules alone [143] or in combination with autografts has shown high success rates [144].

TCP has two crystallographic forms, α-TCP and β-TCP [79], with the latter more commonly used partially resorbable filler allowing replacement with new bone formation [135]. β-TCP have been shown to be inferior when compared with allografts in terms of resorption and bone formation [145]. There is strong evidence of TCP grafts undergoing fibrous tissue encapsulation [146]. There are studies that report new bone deposition with β-TCP [146–149] and alveolar ridge augmentation in vertical and horizontal dimensions with variable results [147–149].

Bioactive glass is composed of silicon dioxide, calcium oxide, sodium oxide, and phosphorus pentoxide [150], and when implanted as bone grafting materials, the pH of the local environment increases (>10), and a silicon-rich gel is formed on the bioactive ceramic surface with the outer layer serving as a bonding surface for osteogenic cells and collagen fibers [151]. The article sizes of bioactive glasses range from 90–710 μm to 300–355 μm [150, 152], and clinical reports of alveolar ridge grafting and augmentation with bioglass show bone formation in close contact to the particles [150]. However, bioglass is non-resorption which limits the ability of bioglass to work as a bioresorptive scaffold for vertical alveolar bone augmentation.

Dicalcium phosphate (DCP) compounds have a high solubility at physiological pH, and dicalcium phosphate dihydrate (DCPD or brushite) has been tested for both vertical bone augmentation and bone defect repair as injectable cements or as preset cement granules [153–155]. Several clinical studies have demonstrated that injectable brushite cements are capable of regenerating bone in buccal dehiscence defects, atrophic ridges, and maxillary sinus floor elevation procedures [156]. The amount of vertical bone growth obtained with brushite cement granules is seen to be higher than that obtained with commercial bovine HA materials in vivo [157]. However, brushite cements undergo phase conversion to insoluble HA upon implantation and this limits their resorption [79, 158]. Dicalcium phosphate anhydrous (DCPA or monetite) resorbs at faster rates compared to brushite [159–161] and has been shown not to convert to HA [157, 158, 162].

The clinical performance of monetite granules has been compared with commercially available bovine HA and demonstrated greater resorption in vivo and bone formation in the alveolar ridge sockets [154]. Monetite bioceramic materials have been investigated for alveolar bone augmentation as 3D printed onlay blocks, and it has been shown that sufficient bone volume and height gain can be achieved for dental implant placement [155, 163].

9.4 Barrier Membranes Used in Bone Grafting Procedures

The turnover rate of soft tissues is faster than that of bone tissue formation, so using barrier membranes during bone grafting ensures that soft tissues are prevented from infiltrating and occupying the defect space where new bone is to be regenerated. If used in combination with bone grafts, then the membranes serve to stabilize the graft materials [73]. Also, the membranes also function as graft preservation devices by reducing the rate of graft resorption [64, 164]. The natural or synthetic tissues and materials the barrier membranes get fabricated from are required to be biocompatible and not evoke any immune reactions or cytotoxity once implanted [165]. If these membranes are resorbable, then ideally they should biodegrade without leaving any residues, and the degradation rate should match with the tissue regeneration rate. The mechanical properties of these membranes should be adequate to withstand the surgical placement and their function in vivo. The barrier membranes used for alveolar bone grafting can be non-resorbable or resorbable.

9.4.1 Non-resorbable Barrier Membranes

The first non-resorbable barrier membranes investigated experimentally were fabricated using cellulose acetate filters (Millipore®) [166]. Following this, commercial membranes were later produced from Teflon® which is polytetrafluoroethylene (PTFE) [167]. The function of these non-resorb-

able membranes is temporary as they maintain their structural integrity upon placement and are later retrieved via surgery. This second procedure for retrieval increases the risk of surgical site morbidity and renders the regenerated tissues susceptible to damage and postsurgery bacterial contamination [168]. Membrane exposure due to flap sloughing during healing is also a frequent postsurgical complication observed [169]. As evidence of resorbable membranes being effective increases, non-resorbable membranes are losing their popularity in clinical practice, and their use is being limited to specific applications [170]. Two non-resorbable barrier membranes that are commonly used are the expanded (ePTFE) and the titanium-reinforced polytetrafluoroethylene (Ti-PTFE). PTFE is a nonporous inert and biocompatible fluorocarbon polymer [171]. The ePTFE is chemically similar to PTFE and has been used in vascular surgeries for several decades [172]. ePTFE is made by subjecting PTFE to high tensile stresses which results in expansion and the formation of a porous microstructure [173]. Barrier membranes fabricated with ePTFE are highly stable in biological systems and resist breakdown by host responses. The clinical effectiveness of ePTFE barrier membranes has been studied in numerous studies [174]. There is evidence of periodontal regeneration when ePTFE membranes are used, and these membranes gained popularity and were used routinely in the past [170]. In clinical situations which require larger areas of space maintenance, Ti-PTFE can be used which are stiffer having a central portion reinforced with titanium to prevent collapse [175]. An alternative approach is using a double layer of PTFE membrane with a titanium framework interposed (Cytoplast® Ti-250) which has shown to be successful for ridge augmentation and treatment of large defects in the alveolar process [176].

9.4.2 Resorbable Barrier Membranes

Clinical studies in the early 1990s reported the successful use of resorbable membranes for GBR [177–179]. In the last few decades, research has been focused upon development of bioresorbable barrier membranes that overcome the inherent limitations of their non-resorbable counterparts. Both natural and synthetic polymers have been investigated for this purpose with collagen and aliphatic polyesters being the mostly researched [180]. Currently, most commonly used resorbable membranes are made of collagen or by polyglycolide and/or polylactide or copolymers of them [181]. The available resorbable barrier membranes are mostly incapable in maintaining defect space on their own due to their lack of rigidity. For this reason these membranes are routinely used in combination with autogenous or synthetic bone graft substitutes [182, 183] with or without the support screws, reinforcements, and pins [184].

9.4.2.1 Natural Resorbable Barrier Membranes

Natural resorbable barrier membranes are fabricated mostly using collagen from tissues from human or animal sources. Collagen is used extensively in biomedical applications and can be acquired from animal skin, tendons, or intestines [180]. Collagen has numerous desirable biological properties such as having low immunogenicity, attracting and activating gingival fibroblast cells, and being hemostatic [185]. It has been shown that collagen membranes stimulate the fibroblast DNA synthesis [178]. Also, osteoblasts show higher levels of adherence to collagen membrane surfaces in comparison to other barrier membrane surfaces [186]. The biodegradation of commercially available collagen membranes is accomplished by endogenous collagenases into carbon dioxide and water [185]. These enzymes are produced mainly by the macrophages and polymorphonuclear leukocytes (PMNs) [23]. The degree of cross-linking of collagen fibers directly affects the rate of degradation with the relationship being inversely proportional [187].

AlloDerm® Regenerative Tissue Matrix (RTM) is a collagen Type I derived from human skin (cadavers). AlloDerm® has been shown to support tissue regeneration by allowing rapid revascularization and white cell migration. The

membrane thickness ranges from 0.9 to 1.6 mm, and clinical applications include gingival augmentation, root coverage, soft tissue ridge augmentation, and soft tissue augmentation around dental implants [188]. AlloDerm GBR® RTM is manufactured utilizing the same process used for AlloDerm® RTM, and the membrane thickness ranges from 0.5 to 0.9 mm used for graft protection, containment, and flap extension to achieve adequate primary closure [189]. Paroguide® is a collagen Type I membrane enriched with chondroitin sulfate. There are reports of periodontal ligament regeneration and alveolar bone regeneration, with no signs of inflammation [182, 190]. Avitene® is a microfibrillar hemostatic collagen Type I membrane derived from bovine corium. Histological evaluation after a clinical study has shown that this membrane was not very effective and is difficult to handle during the surgery [191]. Bio-Gide® is a barrier membrane synthesized from collagen Types I and III derived from porcine skin source. Bio-Gide® has been seen to resorb in about 8 weeks with studies demonstrating their regenerative potential [192]. BioMend Extend® is fabricated from Type I collagen derived from bovine Achilles tendon. The membrane is semi-occlusive, having a pore size 0.004 μm, and resorbs in 4–8 weeks after implantation. Clinical results have revealed limited clinical effectiveness, dependent upon form and size of the defect [193]. Cytoplast RTM® is synthesized with collagen Type I derived from bovine tendon and is a multilayered membrane which takes 26–38 weeks for complete resorption. It has an organized fiber orientation providing good handling and high tensile strength [194, 195]. Collagen membrane cross-linked by diphenylphosphoryl azide is a Type I collagen membrane, derived from calf pericardium and cross-linked by diphenylphosphoryl azide. Although histology reveals significant inflammatory reaction [196], clinical studies have shown effective tissue regeneration outcomes [190]. Collistat® is another collagen Type I material which has demonstrated guided regeneration potential with the membrane completely resorbing 7 days after implantation [197].

9.4.3 Synthetic Resorbable Barrier Membranes

The most commonly used biomaterials used to fabricate barrier membranes are the poly-α-hydroxy acids, which include polylactic polyglycolic acid and their copolymers [198]. The advantage of using polyhydroxy acids are that they undergo complete hydrolysis to water and carbon dioxide, which allows for complete removal from the implantation site [195]. However, the degradation rate varies depending on the presence glycols and lactides in the constitutional makeup [199]. Resolut LT® is a barrier membrane made of glycolide and lactic copolymer and a porous network of polyglycolide fiber that completely resorbs in about 5–6 months [171, 200]. Atrisorb® is a barrier membrane that is prepared chairside during the surgical procedure because it is made up of a polylactic polymer in a flowable form, dissolved in poly-DL-lactide and a solvent. This is flowed into a cassette containing 0.9% saline for ~5 min, after which the membrane having a thickness of 600–750 μm is obtained and cut to desired shape. Studies have reported its efficacy in the treatment of periodontal defects [201], and it resorbs completely in 6–12 months [202]. Epi-Guide® is a porous three-layered and three-dimensional barrier membrane fabricated using polylactic acid polymers (D,D-L,L-polylactic acid) and is completely resorbed in 6–12 months. The three-layered construction of the membrane attracts, traps, and retains fibroblasts and epithelial cells while maintaining space around the defect. Epi-Guide® is a self-supporting barrier membrane and can be used in situations without support from bone grafting materials [182, 203]. Guidor® is a double-layered resorbable barrier membrane composed of both polylactic acid and a citric acid ester known as acetyl tributylcitrate. The external layer of the barrier membrane is designed with rectangular perforations allowing the integration of the overlying gingival flap. This surface design successfully promotes tissue integration, and only limited gingival recession after usage has been reported [181, 204]. Between the internal and external layers, internal spacers are present that create space for tissue ingrowth. The internal layer has smaller circular perforations and outer spacers for maintaining the space between the membrane and the root surface. Studies have shown this membrane to be successful in the treatment of various periodontal defects [204]. Vicryl periodontal mesh® is made up of polyglactin 910 fibers which are copolymers of glycolide and L-lactide which form a tight woven mesh [205]. This barrier membrane has been shown to start resorbing after 2 weeks of implantation and completely resorbs in about 4 weeks [206]. Mempol® is a membrane manufactured from polydioxanon (PDS) with a bilayer structure. The first layer is covered with PDS loops 200 μm long to be used on the gingival side and is completely non-permeable [207, 208].

9.5 Considerations for Bone Grafting in Older Patients

Although there are studies that demonstrate success of dental implantation in elderly patients, the major limitations of these studies are that a relatively small number of patients are involved and almost no or very few comparisons are made between groups with respect to gender, implantation site, implant type, implant length, numbers, systemic health, smoking, alveolar ridge volume and height (quality and quantity), and occlusal load considerations [5]. Although these limitations exist, still it can be concluded that the age of the patient does not seem to be the major factor in determining the prognosis of dental implants. Alveolar bone quantity and quality and the use of appropriate surgical and prosthetic techniques by a skillful team are definitely more critical to a favorable outcome. Older patients undergoing implant therapy including bone augmentation require a thorough evaluation for systemic conditions that may affect and potentially compromise bone healing and osseointegration [209]. Success of bone grafting procedures and ultimately dental implantation has been known to be affected by diabetes mellitus, postmenopausal estrogen replacement therapy, and long-term smoking habits [5]. Additionally, patients may be using medications such as steroids and bisphosphonates that affect bone metabolism and can alter the clinical outcomes [210, 211].

Osseointegration of dental implants is crucially dependent on the bone healing response. Osteoporotic bone is characterized by a general reduction in bone quality and quantity and therefore can be expected to affect the success of dental implants in older patients. However, studies have not shown any strong evidence directly implicating osteoporosis as being a risk factor for implant failure in elderly patients [5]. There are strong reservations regarding surgical interventions in patients who have osteoporosis and are receiving long-term oral bisphosphonate therapy [212–214]. Also, it has been noted that implants placed in atrophic maxilla which has trabecular bone are at a greater risk for undergoing complications [215]. Soft tissue response in older patients is another major concern especially if oral hygiene is not maintained and deteriorates over time. Inability to remove plaque has been shown to lead to peri-mucositis and peri-implantitis [5]. Although autogenous bone grafts remain the gold standard for augmenting atrophic jaws and repairing bone defects, it has to be taken into consideration that autografting in older individuals leads to more complications and should be chosen after careful consideration. There are doubts over the bone quality available, donor site morbidity, and impaired healing response to be taken into consideration [215, 216].

9.6 Future Directions for Achieving Successful and More Predictable Bone Grafting

Currently, research on newer methodologies for bone grafting is focused on molecular, cellular, and gene therapeutics [217]. There is great potential for platelet-derived growth factor (PDGF) for use in bone regeneration [218]. Recombinant human PDGF-BB (rhPDGF-BB) and inorganic bone blocks have been investigated for bone augmentation in vertical dimensions and have shown increased vertical gain compared to controls [219]. PDGF in combination with ePTFE barrier membranes used around implants in preclinical animal models has also resulted in rapid and increased bone formation [218]. Promising results have also been observed by using collagen membranes and chitosan sponges with PDGF for achieving vertical ridge augmentation [220, 221]. Ideal dosing of PDGF and their appropriate carriers are still under research and extensive long-term studies are essential.

Separating platelet-rich plasma (PRP) from patient blood and added to the bone grafting tissues and materials is a new approach [222–224]. Initial results using this technique have shown greater volume and denser bone compared to autografts used alone for bone augmentation [225]. However, using PRP with other graft materials and its usefulness is still inconclusive [226, 227]. Bone morphogenetic proteins (BMPs) have generated a lot of interest recently and have shown promising results for intraoral applications such as sinus augmentation and alveolar ridge preservation [228–232]. The most commonly used and researched BMPs for bone regeneration applications are BMP-2 and BMP-7. BMP-2 has been approved by the FDA for clinical use in spinal fusion therapy [232, 233]. However, the dosage and carrier methods are still undergoing the regulatory approval process. Gene therapy is based on the principle of delivering to cells modified genetic material to boost their regenerative potential by increased production and concentration of differentiation factors and growth factors [234, 235]. A cellular tissue engineering approach is being investigated through which in vitro amplification of osteoblasts or osteoprogenitor cells grown on 3D constructs is carried out to increase the regenerative potential of bone [236–238]. Cell seeding of constructs with mesenchymal stem cells also has great potential to be used in the future [239, 240]. All these approaches have the potential for providing improved tissue regenerative results in alveolar ridge grafting and augmentation [235].

There are a variety of surgical techniques with various combinations of graft materials that can be utilized for achieving alveolar ridge augmentation. Currently, there is no single ideal technique or graft material that exists to choose from in clinical practice, and individualized approach to ridge grafting is followed. The development of novel synthetic bone graft materials is a challenge from an engineering and biological perspective. The next generation of graft materials is expected to demonstrate improvements in implant and biological tissue interfacing based on the recent gain in knowledge. Treatment protocols that are less invasive and technique sensitive and more reproducible need to be developed and require constant revisions in light of new developments in bone regeneration therapeutics.

References

1. Basker RM, Davenport JC, Thomason JM. Prosthetic treatment of the edentulous patient. Oxford: Wiley; 2011.
2. Albrektsson T, et al. The long-term efficacy of currently used dental implants: a review and proposed criteria of success. Int J Oral Maxillofac Implants. 1986;1(1):11–25.
3. Smith DE, Zarb GA. Criteria for success of osseointegrated endosseous implants. J Prosthet Dent. 1989;62(5):567–72.
4. Bryant SR, Zarb GA. Outcomes of implant prosthodontic treatment in older adults. J Can Dent Assoc. 2002;68(2):97–102.
5. De Baat C. Success of dental implants in elderly people—a literature review. Gerodontology. 2000;17(1):45–8.
6. Esposito M, et al. Interventions for replacing missing teeth: horizontal and vertical bone augmentation techniques for dental implant treatment. The Cochrane Library; 2009.
7. Khoury F, Buchmann R. Surgical therapy of peri-implant disease: a 3-year follow-up study of cases treated with 3 different techniques of bone regeneration. J Periodontol. 2001;72(11):1498–508.
8. Van der Weijden F, Dell'Acqua F, Slot DE. Alveolar bone dimensional changes of post-extraction sockets in humans: a systematic review. J Clin Periodontol. 2009;36(12):1048–58.
9. Tallgren A. The continuing reduction of the residual alveolar ridges in complete denture wearers: a mixed-longitudinal study covering 25 years. J Prosthet Dent. 2003;89(5):427–35.
10. Bernstein S, et al. Vertical bone augmentation: where are we now? Implant Dent. 2006;15(3):219–28.
11. Sheikh Z, Glogauer M. Successful ridge augmentation: the challenge of periodontal tissue engineering. EC Dent Sci. 2015;2:216–8.
12. Tolman DE. Advanced residual ridge resorption: surgical management. Int J Prosthodont. 1993;6(2):118–25.
13. McAllister BS, Haghighat K. Bone augmentation techniques. J Periodontol. 2007;78(3):377–96.
14. Sheikh Z, Sima C, Glogauer M. Bone replacement materials and techniques used for achieving vertical alveolar bone augmentation. Materials. 2015;8(6):2953–93.
15. Sheikh Z, et al. Biodegradable materials for bone repair and tissue engineering applications. Materials. 2015;8(9):5744–94.
16. Bilezikian JP, Raisz LG, Martin TJ. Principles of bone biology: two-volume set. San Diego: Academic; 2008.
17. Krishnan V, et al. Parathyroid hormone bone anabolic action requires Cbfa1/Runx2-dependent signaling. Mol Endocrinol. 2003;17(3):423–35.
18. Ornitz DM, Marie PJ. FGF signaling pathways in endochondral and intramembranous bone development and human genetic disease. Genes Dev. 2002;16(12):1446–65.
19. Wu X, Shi W, Cao X. Multiplicity of BMP signaling in skeletal development. Ann N Y Acad Sci. 2007;1116:29–49.
20. Teitelbaum SL, Ross FP. Genetic regulation of osteoclast development and function. Nat Rev Genet. 2003;4(8):638–49.
21. Lacey DL, et al. Osteoprotegerin ligand is a cytokine that regulates osteoclast differentiation and activation. Cell. 1998;93(2):165–76.
22. Finkemeier CG. Bone-grafting and bone-graft substitutes. J Bone Joint Surg Am. 2002;84(3):454–64.
23. Sheikh Z, et al. Macrophages, foreign body giant cells and their response to implantable biomaterials. Materials. 2015;8(9):5671–701.
24. Urist MR. Bone transplants and implants. In: Urist MR, editor. Fundamental and clinical bone physiology. Philadelphia: JB Lippincott; 1980. p. 331–68.
25. Cornell CN, Lane JM. Current understanding of osteoconduction in bone regeneration. Clin Orthop Relat Res. 1998;355:S267–73.
26. Mastrogiacomo M, et al. Role of scaffold internal structure on in vivo bone formation in macroporous calcium phosphate bioceramics. Biomaterials. 2006;27(17):3230–7.
27. Boyne PJ. Bone induction and the use of HTR polymer as a vehicle for osseous inductor materials. Compend Suppl. 1988;10:S337–41.
28. McCarthy JG, et al. Distraction osteogenesis of the craniofacial skeleton. Plast Reconstr Surg. 2001;107(7):1812–27.
29. Davies J, Turner S, Sandy JR. Distraction osteogenesis—a review. Br Dent J. 1998;185(9):462–7.
30. Ilizarov GA. Basic principles of transosseous compression and distraction osteosynthesis. Ortop Travmatol Protez. 1971;32(11):7–15.
31. Uckan S, Oguz Y, Bayram B. Comparison of intraosseous and extraosseous alveolar distraction osteogenesis. J Oral Maxillofac Surg. 2007;65(4):671–4.

32. Polo WC, et al. Posterior mandibular alveolar distraction osteogenesis utilizing an extraosseous distractor: a prospective study. J Periodontol. 2005;76(9):1463–8.

33. Chiapasco M, et al. Alveolar distraction osteogenesis for the correction of vertically deficient edentulous ridges: a multicenter prospective study on humans. Int J Oral Maxillofac Implants. 2004;19(3):399–407.

34. Hidding J, Lazar F, Zoller JE. Initial outcome of vertical distraction osteogenesis of the atrophic alveolar ridge. Mund Kiefer Gesichtschir. 1999;3(Suppl 1):S79–83.

35. Urbani G, et al. Distraction osteogenesis to achieve mandibular vertical bone regeneration: a case report. Int J Periodontics Restorative Dent. 1999;19(4):321–31.

36. Van Strijen P, et al. Complications in bilateral mandibular distraction osteogenesis using internal devices. Oral Surg Oral Med Oral Pathol Oral Radiol Endod. 2003;96(4):392–7.

37. Garcia AG, et al. Minor complications arising in alveolar distraction osteogenesis. J Oral Maxillofac Surg. 2002;60(5):496–501.

38. Batal HS, Cottrell DA. Alveolar distraction osteogenesis for implant site development. Oral Maxillofac Surg Clin North Am. 2004;16(1):91–109, vii.

39. Lynch SE. Tissue engineering: applications in oral and maxillofacial surgery and periodontics. Chicago: Quintessence Publishing Company; 2008.

40. Jensen OT, Kuhlke KL. Maxillary full-arch alveolar split osteotomy with island osteoperiosteal flaps and sinus grafting using bone morphogenetic protein-2 and retrofitting for immediate loading with a provisional: surgical and prosthetic procedures and case report. Int J Oral Maxillofac Implants. 2013;28(5):e260–71.

41. Kilic E, et al. Vertical ridge augmentation using sandwich osteotomy: 2 case reports. Gen Dent. 2013;61(6):e22–5.

42. Isaksson S, Alberius P. Maxillary alveolar ridge augmentation with onlay bone-grafts and immediate endosseous implants. J Craniomaxillofac Surg. 1992;20(1):2–7.

43. Barone A, Covani U. Maxillary alveolar ridge reconstruction with nonvascularized autogenous block bone: clinical results. J Oral Maxillofac Surg. 2007;65(10):2039–46.

44. Cordaro L, Amade DS, Cordaro M. Clinical results of alveolar ridge augmentation with mandibular block bone grafts in partially edentulous patients prior to implant placement. Clin Oral Implants Res. 2002;13(1):103–11.

45. Sailer HF. A new method of inserting endosseous implants in totally atrophic maxillae. J Craniomaxillofac Surg. 1989;17(7):299–305.

46. Breine U, Branemark PI. Reconstruction of alveolar jaw bone. An experimental and clinical study of immediate and preformed autologous bone grafts in combination with osseointegrated implants. Scand J Plast Reconstr Surg. 1980;14(1):23–48.

47. Proussaefs P, Lozada J. The use of intraorally harvested autogenous block grafts for vertical alveolar ridge augmentation: a human study. Int J Periodontics Restorative Dent. 2005;25(4):351–63.

48. Misch CM. Comparison of intraoral donor sites for onlay grafting prior to implant placement. Int J Oral Maxillofac Implants. 1997;12(6):767–76.

49. Tolman DE. Reconstructive procedures with endosseous implants in grafted bone: a review of the literature. Int J Oral Maxillofac Implants. 1995;10(3):275–94.

50. Pikos MA. Block autografts for localized ridge augmentation: part I. The posterior maxilla. Implant Dent. 1999;8(3):279–85.

51. Pikos MA. Block autografts for localized ridge augmentation: part II. The posterior mandible. Implant Dent. 2000;9(1):67–75.

52. Levin L, Nitzan D, Schwartz-Arad D. Success of dental implants placed in intraoral block bone grafts. J Periodontol. 2007;78(1):18–21.

53. Stubinger S, et al. Harvesting of intraoral autogenous block grafts from the chin and ramus region: preliminary results with a variable square pulse Er:YAG laser. Lasers Surg Med. 2008;40(5):312–8.

54. Pourabbas R, Nezafati S. Clinical results of localized alveolar ridge augmentation with bone grafts harvested from symphysis in comparison with ramus. J Dent Res Dent Clin Dent Prospects. 2007;1(1):7–12.

55. Lin KY, et al. The effect of rigid fixation on the survival of onlay bone grafts: an experimental study. Plast Reconstr Surg. 1990;86(3):449–56.

56. de Carvalho PS, Vasconcellos LW, Pi J. Influence of bed preparation on the incorporation of autogenous bone grafts: a study in dogs. Int J Oral Maxillofac Implants. 2000;15(4):565–70.

57. Urbani G, et al. Localized ridge augmentation with chin grafts and resorbable pins: case reports. Int J Periodontics Restorative Dent. 1998;18(4):363–75.

58. Albrektsson T. Repair of bone grafts. A vital microscopic and histological investigation in the rabbit. Scand J Plast Reconstr Surg. 1980;14(1):1–12.

59. Keith JD Jr. Localized ridge augmentation with a block allograft followed by secondary implant placement: a case report. Int J Periodontics Restorative Dent. 2004;24(1):11–7.

60. Jardini MA, De Marco AC, Lima LA. Early healing pattern of autogenous bone grafts with and without e-PTFE membranes: a histomorphometric study in rats. Oral Surg Oral Med Oral Pathol Oral Radiol Endod. 2005;100(6):666–73.

61. Ronda M, et al. Expanded vs. dense polytetrafluoroethylene membranes in vertical ridge augmentation around dental implants: a prospective randomized controlled clinical trial. Clin Oral Implants Res. 2014;25(7):859–66.

62. Urban IA, et al. Vertical ridge augmentation with titanium-reinforced, dense-PTFE membranes and a combination of particulated autogenous bone and anorganic bovine bone-derived mineral: a prospec-

tive case series in 19 patients. Int J Oral Maxillofac Implants. 2014;29(1):185–93.

63. Dahlin C, et al. Healing of bone defects by guided tissue regeneration. Plast Reconstr Surg. 1988;81(5):672–6.

64. Buser D, et al. Localized ridge augmentation with autografts and barrier membranes. Periodontol 2000. 1999;19:151–63.

65. Deshpande S, et al. Vertical and horizontal ridge augmentation in anterior maxilla using autograft, xenograft and titanium mesh with simultaneous placement of endosseous implants. J Indian Soc Periodontol. 2014;18(5):661–5.

66. Clarizio LF. Successful implant restoration without the use of membrane barriers. J Oral Maxillofac Surg. 1999;57(9):1117–21.

67. Simion M, et al. Vertical ridge augmentation around dental implants using a membrane technique and autogenous bone or allografts in humans. Int J Periodontics Restorative Dent. 1998;18(1):8–23.

68. Bhola M, Kinaia BM, Chahine K. Guided bone regeneration using an allograft material: review and case presentations. Pract Proced Aesthet Dent. 2008;20(9):551–7; quiz 558.

69. Zitzmann N, Schärer P, Marinello C. Factors influencing the success of GBR. J Clin Periodontol. 1999;26(10):673–82.

70. Malmquist JP. Successful implant restoration with the use of barrier membranes. J Oral Maxillofac Surg. 1999;57(9):1114–6.

71. Jensen OT, et al. Vertical guided bone-graft augmentation in a new canine mandibular model. Int J Oral Maxillofac Implants. 1995;10(3):335–44.

72. Schenk RK, et al. Healing pattern of bone regeneration in membrane-protected defects: a histologic study in the canine mandible. Int J Oral Maxillofac Implants. 1994;9(1):13–29.

73. Sheikh Z, Abdallah MN, Hamdan N, Javaid MA, Khurshid Z. Barrier membranes for tissue regeneration and bone augmentation techniques in dentistry. In: Matilinna KP, editor. Handbook of oral biomaterials. Singapore: Pan Stanford Publishing; 2014.

74. Rakhmatia YD, et al. Current barrier membranes: titanium mesh and other membranes for guided bone regeneration in dental applications. J Prosthodont Rcs. 2013;57(1):3–14.

75. Hasson O. Augmentation of deficient lateral alveolar ridge using the subperiosteal tunneling dissection approach. Oral Surg Oral Med Oral Pathol Oral Radiol Endod. 2007;103(3):e14–9.

76. Kent JN, et al. Correction of alveolar ridge deficiencies with nonresorbable hydroxylapatite. J Am Dent Assoc. 1982;105(6):993–1001.

77. Williams CW, Meyers JF, Robinson RR. Hydroxyapatite augmentation of the anterior portion of the maxilla with a modified transpositional flap technique. Oral Surg Oral Med Oral Pathol. 1991;72(4):395–9.

78. Kent JN. Reconstruction of the alveolar ridge with hydroxyapatite. Dent Clin North Am. 1986;30(2):231–57.

79. Tamimi F, Sheikh Z, Barralet J. Dicalcium phosphate cements: brushite and monetite. Acta Biomater. 2012;8(2):474–87.

80. Sheikh ZA, Javaid MA, Abdallah MN. Bone replacement graft materials in dentistry. In: Zafar S, Khurshid Z, editors. Dental biomaterials (principle and its application). Karachi: Paramount Publishing Enterprise; 2013.

81. Sheikh Z, et al. Mechanisms of in vivo degradation and resorption of calcium phosphate based biomaterials. Materials. 2015;8(11):7913–25.

82. Draenert FG, et al. Vertical bone augmentation procedures: basics and techniques in dental implantology. J Biomed Mater Res A. 2014;102(5):1605–13.

83. Cypher TJ, Grossman JP. Biological principles of bone graft healing. J Foot Ankle Surg. 1996;35(5):413–7.

84. Simion M, et al. Long-term evaluation of osseointegrated implants inserted at the time or after vertical ridge augmentation. A retrospective study on 123 implants with 1-5 year follow-up. Clin Oral Implants Res. 2001;12(1):35–45.

85. Nkenke E, et al. Morbidity of harvesting of bone grafts from the iliac crest for preprosthetic augmentation procedures: a prospective study. Int J Oral Maxillofac Surg. 2004;33(2):157–63.

86. Wilk R. Bony reconstruction of the jaws. In: Miloro M, editor. Peterson's principles of oral and maxillofacial surgery. Hamilton (London): BC Decker; 2004. p. 785–7.

87. Rocchietta I, et al. Vertical bone augmentation with an autogenous block or particles in combination with guided bone regeneration: a clinical and histological preliminary study in humans. Clin Implant Dent Relat Res. 2016;18(1):19–29.

88. Merli M, Lombardini F, Esposito M. Vertical ridge augmentation with autogenous bone grafts 3 years after loading: resorbable barriers versus titanium-reinforced barriers. A randomized controlled clinical trial. Int J Oral Maxillofac Implants. 2010;25(4):801–7.

89. Block MS, Degen M. Horizontal ridge augmentation using human mineralized particulate bone: preliminary results. J Oral Maxillofac Surg. 2004;62(9 Suppl 2):67–72.

90. Araujo PP, et al. Block allograft for reconstruction of alveolar bone ridge in implantology: a systematic review. Implant Dent. 2013;22(3):304–8.

91. Sterio TW, et al. A prospective, multicenter study of bovine pericardium membrane with cancellous particulate allograft for localized alveolar ridge augmentation. Int J Periodontics Restorative Dent. 2013;33(4):499–507.

92. Al Ruhaimi KA. Bone graft substitutes: a comparative qualitative histologic review of current osteoconductive grafting materials. Int J Oral Maxillofac Implants. 2001;16(1):105–14.

93. Contar CM, et al. Fresh-frozen bone allografts in maxillary ridge augmentation: histologic analysis. J Oral Implantol. 2011;37(2):223–31.

94. Contar CM, et al. Maxillary ridge augmentation with fresh-frozen bone allografts. J Oral Maxillofac Surg. 2009;67(6):1280–5.

95. Dias RR, et al. Corticocancellous fresh-frozen allograft bone blocks for augmenting atrophied posterior mandibles in humans. Clin Oral Implants Res. 2016;27(1):39–46.

96. Macedo LG, et al. Fresh-frozen human bone allograft in vertical ridge augmentation: clinical and tomographic evaluation of bone formation and resorption. Cell Tissue Bank. 2012;13(4):577–86.

97. Mellonig JT. Freeze-dried bone allografts in periodontal reconstructive surgery. Dent Clin North Am. 1991;35(3):505–20.

98. Kukreja BJ, et al. A comparative evaluation of platelet-rich plasma in combination with demineralized freeze-dried bone allograft and DFDBA alone in the treatment of periodontal intrabony defects: a clinicoradiographic study. J Indian Soc Periodontol. 2014;18(5):618–23.

99. Blaggana V, Gill AS, Blaggana A. A clinical and radiological evaluation of the relative efficacy of demineralized freeze-dried bone allograft versus anorganic bovine bone xenograft in the treatment of human infrabony periodontal defects: a 6 months follow-up study. J Indian Soc Periodontol. 2014;18(5):601–7.

100. Markou N, et al. Treatment of periodontal endosseous defects with platelet-rich plasma alone or in combination with demineralized freeze-dried bone allograft: a comparative clinical trial. J Periodontol. 2009;80(12):1911–9.

101. Quattlebaum JB, Mellonig JT, Hensel NF. Antigenicity of freeze-dried cortical bone allograft in human periodontal osseous defects. J Periodontol. 1988;59(6):394–7.

102. Friedlaender GE, Strong DM, Sell KW. Studies on the antigenicity of bone. I. Freeze-dried and deep-frozen bone allografts in rabbits. J Bone Joint Surg Am. 1976;58(6):854–8.

103. Kao ST, Scott DD. A review of bone substitutes. Oral Maxillofac Surg Clin North Am. 2007;19(4):513–21.

104. Committee on Research, Science and Therapy of the American Academy of Periodontology. Tissue banking of bone allografts used in periodontal regeneration. J Periodontol. 2001;72(6):834.

105. Mellonig JT. Human histologic evaluation of a bovine-derived bone xenograft in the treatment of periodontal osseous defects. Int J Periodontics Restorative Dent. 2000;20(1):19–29.

106. Sunitha Raja V, Naidu M. Platelet-rich fibrin: evolution of a second-generation platelet concentrate. Indian J Dent Res. 2008;19(1):42.

107. Jacotti M, et al. Ridge augmentation with mineralized block allografts: clinical and histological evaluation of 8 cases treated with the 3-dimensional block technique. Implant Dent. 2012;21(6):444–8.

108. Wallace S, Gellin R. Clinical evaluation of freeze-dried cancellous block allografts for ridge augmentation and implant placement in the maxilla. Implant Dent. 2010;19(4):272–9.

109. Lyford RH, et al. Clinical evaluation of freeze-dried block allografts for alveolar ridge augmentation: a case series. Int J Periodontics Restorative Dent. 2003;23(5):417–25.

110. Russell J, Scarborough N, Chesmel K. Ability of commercial demineralized freeze-dried bone allograft to induce new bone formation. J Periodontol. 1997;68(8):804–6.

111. Hopp SG, Dahners LE, Gilbert JA. A study of the mechanical strength of long bone defects treated with various bone autograft substitutes: an experimental investigation in the rabbit. J Orthop Res. 1989;7(4):579–84.

112. Mellonig JT, Bowers GM, Bailey RC. Comparison of bone graft materials. Part I. New bone formation with autografts and allografts determined by Strontium-85. J Periodontol. 1981;52(6):291–6.

113. Shigeyama Y, et al. Commercially-prepared allograft material has biological activity in vitro. J Periodontol. 1995;66(6):478–87.

114. Hauschka PV, Chen TL, Mavrakos AE. Polypeptide growth factors in bone matrix. Ciba Found Symp. 1988;136:207–25.

115. Dodson SA, et al. In vitro comparison of aged and young osteogenic and hemopoietic bone marrow stem cells and their derivative colonies. J Periodontol. 1996;67(3):184–96.

116. Jergesen HE, et al. Age effects on bone induction by demineralized bone powder. Clin Orthop Relat Res. 1991;268:253–9.

117. Scarano A, et al. Maxillary sinus augmentation with different biomaterials: a comparative histologic and histomorphometric study in man. Implant Dent. 2006;15(2):197–207.

118. Senn. Senn on the healing of aseptic bone cavities by implantation of antiseptic decalcified bone. Ann Surg. 1889;10(5):352–68.

119. Thaller SR, et al. Reconstruction of calvarial defects with anorganic bovine bone mineral (Bio-Oss) in a rabbit model. J Craniofac Surg. 1993;4(2):79–84.

120. McAllister BS, et al. Eighteen-month radiographic and histologic evaluation of sinus grafting with anorganic bovine bone in the chimpanzee. Int J Oral Maxillofac Implants. 1999;14(3):361–8.

121. Liu X, et al. Maxillary sinus floor augmentation and dental implant placement using dentin matrix protein-1 gene-modified bone marrow stromal cells mixed with deproteinized boving bone: a comparative study in beagles. Arch Oral Biol. 2016;64:102–8.

122. Jarcho M. Calcium phosphate ceramics as hard tissue prosthetics. Clin Orthop Relat Res. 1981;(157):259–78.

123. Sogal A, Tofe AJ. Risk assessment of bovine spongiform encephalopathy transmission through bone graft material derived from bovine bone used for dental applications. J Periodontol. 1999;70(9):1053–63.

124. Wenz B, Oesch B, Horst M. Analysis of the risk of transmitting bovine spongiform encephalopa-

thy through bone grafts derived from bovine bone. Biomaterials. 2001;22(12):1599–606.

125. Zitzmann NU, Naef R, Scharer P. Resorbable versus nonresorbable membranes in combination with Bio-Oss for guided bone regeneration. Int J Oral Maxillofac Implants. 1997;12(6):844–52.

126. Yildirim M, et al. Maxillary sinus augmentation using xenogenic bone substitute material Bio-Oss in combination with venous blood. A histologic and histomorphometric study in humans. Clin Oral Implants Res. 2000;11(3):217–29.

127. Felice P, et al. Vertical ridge augmentation of the atrophic posterior mandible with interpositional bloc grafts: bone from the iliac crest vs. bovine anorganic bone. Clinical and histological results up to one year after loading from a randomized-controlled clinical trial. Clin Oral Implants Res. 2009;20(12):1386–93.

128. Yukna RA. Clinical evaluation of coralline calcium carbonate as a bone replacement graft material in human periodontal osseous defects. J Periodontol. 1994;65(2):177–85.

129. Guillemin G, et al. The use of coral as a bone graft substitute. J Biomed Mater Res. 1987;21(5):557–67.

130. Piattelli A, Podda G, Scarano A. Clinical and histological results in alveolar ridge enlargement using coralline calcium carbonate. Biomaterials. 1997;18(8):623–7.

131. Gao TJ, et al. Morphological and biomechanical difference in healing in segmental tibial defects implanted with Biocoral or tricalcium phosphate cylinders. Biomaterials. 1997;18(3):219–23.

132. Kim CK, et al. Periodontal repair in intrabony defects treated with a calcium carbonate implant and guided tissue regeneration. J Periodontol. 1996;67(12):1301–6.

133. Hench LL. Bioactive materials: the potential for tissue regeneration. J Biomed Mater Res. 1998;41(4):511–8.

134. AlGhamdi AS, Shibly O, Ciancio SG. Osseous grafting part II: xenografts and alloplasts for periodontal regeneration—a literature review. J Int Acad Periodontol. 2010;12(2):39–44.

135. Shetty V, Han TJ. Alloplastic materials in reconstructive periodontal surgery. Dent Clin North Am. 1991;35(3):521–30.

136. Sheikh Z, et al. Chelate setting of alkali ion substituted calcium phosphates. Ceram Int. 2015;41(8):10010–7.

137. Tevlin R, et al. Biomaterials for craniofacial bone engineering. J Dent Res. 2014;93(12):1187–95.

138. Klein CP, et al. Biodegradation behavior of various calcium phosphate materials in bone tissue. J Biomed Mater Res. 1983;17(5):769–84.

139. Rabalais ML Jr, Yukna RA, Mayer ET. Evaluation of durapatite ceramic as an alloplastic implant in periodontal osseous defects. I. Initial six-month results. J Periodontol. 1981;52(11):680–9.

140. Meffert RM, et al. Hydroxylapatite as an alloplastic graft in the treatment of human periodontal osseous defects. J Periodontol. 1985;56(2):63–73.

141. Ricci JL, et al. Evaluation of a low-temperature calcium phosphate particulate implant material: physical-chemical properties and in vivo bone response. J Oral Maxillofac Surg. 1992;50(9):969–78.

142. Canullo L, Trisi P, Simion M. Vertical ridge augmentation around implants using e-PTFE titanium-reinforced membrane and deproteinized bovine bone mineral (bio-oss): a case report. Int J Periodontics Restorative Dent. 2006;26(4):355–61.

143. Sugar AW, et al. Augmentation of the atrophic maxillary alveolar ridge with hydroxyapatite granules in a Vicryl (polyglactin 910) knitted tube and simultaneous open vestibuloplasty. Br J Oral Maxillofac Surg. 1995;33(2):93–7.

144. Small SA, et al. Augmenting the maxillary sinus for implants: report of 27 patients. Int J Oral Maxillofac Implants. 1993;8(5):523–8.

145. Strub JR, Gaberthuel TW, Firestone AR. Comparison of tricalcium phosphate and frozen allogenic bone implants in man. J Periodontol. 1979;50(12):624–9.

146. Buser D, et al. Lateral ridge augmentation using autografts and barrier membranes: a clinical study with 40 partially edentulous patients. J Oral Maxillofac Surg. 1996;54(4):420–32; discussion 432–3.

147. Shalash MA, et al. Evaluation of horizontal ridge augmentation using beta tricalcium phosphate and demineralized bone matrix: a comparative study. J Clin Exp Dent. 2013;5(5):e253–9.

148. Wang S, et al. Vertical alveolar ridge augmentation with beta-tricalcium phosphate and autologous osteoblasts in canine mandible. Biomaterials. 2009;30(13):2489–98.

149. Nyan M, et al. Feasibility of alpha tricalcium phosphate for vertical bone augmentation. J Investig Clin Dent. 2014;5(2):109–16.

150. Schepers E, et al. Bioactive glass particulate material as a filler for bone lesions. J Oral Rehabil. 1991;18(5):439–52.

151. Hall EE, et al. Comparison of bioactive glass to demineralized freeze-dried bone allograft in the treatment of intrabony defects around implants in the canine mandible. J Periodontol. 1999;70(5):526–35.

152. Schepers EJ, Ducheyne P. Bioactive glass particles of narrow size range for the treatment of oral bone defects: a 1-24 month experiment with several materials and particle sizes and size ranges. J Oral Rehabil. 1997;24(3):171–81.

153. Tamimi F, et al. Minimally invasive maxillofacial vertical bone augmentation using brushite based cements. Biomaterials. 2009;30(2):208–16.

154. Tamimi F, et al. Resorption of monetite granules in alveolar bone defects in human patients. Biomaterials. 2010;31(10):2762–9.

155. Sheikh Z, et al. Controlling bone graft substitute microstructure to improve bone augmentation. Adv Healthc Mater. 2016;5(13):1646–55.

156. Gehrke S, Famà G. Buccal dehiscence and sinus lift cases–predictable bone augmentation with synthetic bone material. Implants. 2010;11:4.

157. Tamimi FM, et al. Bone augmentation in rabbit calvariae: comparative study between Bio-Oss (R) and a novel beta-TCP/DCPD granulate. J Clin Periodontol. 2006;33(12):922–8.

158. Sheikh Z, et al. In vitro degradation and in vivo resorption of dicalcium phosphate cement based grafts. Acta Biomater. 2015;26:338–46.

159. Gbureck U, et al. Resorbable dicalcium phosphate bone substitutes prepared by 3D powder printing. Adv Funct Mater. 2007;17(18):3940–5.

160. Tamimi F, et al. The effect of autoclaving on the physical and biological properties of dicalcium phosphate dihydrate bioceramics: brushite vs. monetite. Acta Biomater. 2012;8(8):3161–9.

161. Idowu B, et al. In vitro osteoinductive potential of porous monetite for bone tissue engineering. J Tissue Eng. 2014;5:2041731414536572.

162. Tamimi F, et al. Bone regeneration in rabbit calvaria with novel monetite granules. J Biomed Mater Res A. 2008;87A(4):980–5.

163. Tamimi F, et al. Craniofacial vertical bone augmentation: a comparison between 3D printed monolithic monetite blocks and autologous onlay grafts in the rabbit. Biomaterials. 2009;30(31): 6318–26.

164. Sheikh Z, et al. Protein adsorption capability on polyurethane and modified-polyurethane membrane for periodontal guided tissue regeneration applications. Mater Sci Eng C. 2016;68:267–75.

165. Sanctis MD, Zucchelli G, Clauser C. Bacterial colonization of bioabsorbable barrier material and periodontal regeneration. J Periodontol. 1996;67(11):1193–200.

166. Schenk RK, Buser D, Hardwick WR, Dahlin C. Healing pattern of bone regeneration in membrane-protected defects: a histologic study in the canine mandible. Int J Oral Max Impl. 1994;9:13–29.

167. Blumenthal NM. A clinical comparison of collagen membranes with e-PTFE membranes in the treatment of human mandibular Buccal class II furcation defects*. J Periodontol. 1993;64(10): 925–33.

168. Tatakis DN, Promsudthi A, Wikesjö UM. Devices for periodontal regeneration. Periodontology 2000. 1999;19(1):59–73.

169. Murphy KG. Postoperative healing complications associated with Gore-Tex Periodontal Material. Part I. Incidence and characterization. Int J Periodontics Restorative Dent. 1995;15(4):363–75.

170. Hämmerle CH, Jung RE. Bone augmentation by means of barrier membranes. Periodontology 2000. 2003;33(1):36–53.

171. Sculean A, Nikolidakis D, Schwarz F. Regeneration of periodontal tissues: combinations of barrier membranes and grafting materials–biological foundation and preclinical evidence: a systematic review. J Clin Periodontol. 2008;35(s8):106–16.

172. Kempczinski RF, et al. Endothelial cell seeding of a new PTFE vascular prosthesis. J Vasc Surg. 1985;2(3):424–9.

173. Bauer JJ, et al. Repair of large abdominal wall defects with expanded polytetrafluoroethylene (PTFE). Ann Surg. 1987;206(6):765.

174. Piattelli A, et al. Evaluation of guided bone regeneration in rabbit tibia using bioresorbable and non-resorbable membranes. Biomaterials. 1996;17(8):791–6.

175. Scantlebury TV. 1982-1992: a decade of technology development for guided tissue regeneration*. J Periodontol. 1993;64(11s):1129–37.

176. Jovanovic SA, Nevins M. Bone formation utilizing titanium-reinforced barrier membranes. Int J Periodontics Restorative Dent. 1995;15(1):56–69.

177. Hürzeler M, Strub J. Guided bone regeneration around exposed implants: a new bioresorbable device and bioresorbable membrane pins. Pract Periodontics Aesthet Dent. 1994;7(9):37–47; quiz 50.

178. Lundgren D, et al. The use of a new bioresorbable barrier for guided bone regeneration in connection with implant installation. Case reports. Clin Oral Implants Res. 1994;5(3):177–84.

179. Nobréus N, Attström R, Linde A. Guided bone regeneration in dental implant treatment using a bioabsorbable membrane. Clin Oral Implants Res. 1997;8(1):10–7.

180. Ratner BD. Biomaterials science: an introduction to materials in medicine. Boston: Academic; 2004.

181. Simion M, et al. Guided bone regeneration using resorbable and nonresorbable membranes: a comparative histologic study in humans. Int J Oral Maxillofac Implants. 1996;11(6):735–42.

182. Parodi R, Santarelli G, Carusi G. Application of slow-resorbing collagen membrane to periodontal and peri-implant guided tissue regeneration. Int J Periodontics Restorative Dent. 1996;16(2):174–85.

183. Avera SP, Stampley WA, McAllister BS. Histologic and clinical observations of resorbable and nonresorbable barrier membranes used in maxillary sinus graft containment. Int J Oral Maxillofac Implants. 1996;12(1):88–94.

184. Gotfredsen K, Nimb L, Hjørting-hansen E. Immediate implant placement using a biodegradable barrier, polyhydroxybutyrate-hydroxyvalerate reinforced with polyglactin 910. An experimental study in dogs. Clin Oral Implants Res. 1994;5(2):83–91.

185. Bunyaratavej P, Wang H-L. Collagen membranes: a review. J Periodontol. 2001;72(2):215–29.

186. Behring J, et al. Toward guided tissue and bone regeneration: morphology, attachment, proliferation, and migration of cells cultured on collagen barrier membranes. A systematic review. Odontology. 2008;96(1):1–11.

187. Lee C, Grodzinsky A, Spector M. The effects of cross-linking of collagen-glycosaminoglycan scaffolds on compressive stiffness, chondrocyte-

mediated contraction, proliferation and biosynthesis. Biomaterials. 2001;22(23):3145–54.

188. Oh TJ, et al. Comparative analysis of collagen membranes for the treatment of implant dehiscence defects. Clin Oral Implants Res. 2003;14(1):80–90.

189. Lee S-W, Kim S-G. Membranes for the guided bone regeneration. Korean Assoc Maxillofac Plast Reconstr Surg. 2014;36(6):239–46.

190. Magnusson I, Batich C, Collins B. New attachment formation following controlled tissue regeneration using biodegradable membranes*. J Periodontol. 1988;59(1):1–6.

191. Tanner MG, Solt CW, Vuddhakanok S. An evaluation of new attachment formation using a microfibhllar collagen barrier*. J Periodontol. 1988;59(8):524–30.

192. Schliephake H, et al. Enhancement of bone ingrowth into a porous hydroxylapatite-matrix using a resorbable polylactic membrane: an experimental pilot study. J Oral Maxillofac Surg. 1994;52(1):57–63.

193. Wang H-L, Carroll M. Guided bone regeneration using bone grafts and collagen membranes. Quintessence Int (Berlin, Germany: 1985). 2000;32(7):504–15.

194. Vert M. Bioresorbable polymers for temporary therapeutic applications. Die Angew Makromol Chem. 1989;166(1):155–68.

195. Vert M, et al. Bioresorbability and biocompatibility of aliphatic polyesters. J Mater Sci Mater Med. 1992;3(6):432–46.

196. Minabe M. A critical review of the biologic rationale for guided tissue regeneration*. J Periodontol. 1991;62(3):171–9.

197. Jepsen S, et al. A systematic review of guided tissue regeneration for periodontal furcation defects. What is the effect of guided tissue regeneration compared with surgical debridement in the treatment of furcation defects? J Clin Periodontol. 2002;29(s3):103–16.

198. Caton J, Greenstein G, Zappa U. Synthetic bioabsorbable barrier for regeneration in human periodontal defects. J Periodontol. 1994;65(11):1037–45.

199. Israelachvili J, Wennerström H. Role of hydration and water structure in biological and colloidal interactions. Nature. 1996;379(6562):219–25.

200. Milella E, et al. Physicochemical, mechanical, and biological properties of commercial membranes for GTR. J Biomed Mater Res. 2001;58(4):427–35.

201. Simion M, et al. Treatment of dehiscences and fenestrations around dental implants using resorbable and nonresorbable membranes associated with bone autografts: a comparative clinical study. Int J Oral Maxillofac Implants. 1996;12(2):159–67.

202. Aurer A, Jorgie-Srdjak K. Membranes for periodontal regeneration. Acta Stomatol Croat. 2005;39:107–12.

203. Rapiey J, et al. The use of biodegradable polylactic acid barrier materials in the treatment of grade II periodontal furcation defects in humans—part II: a multi-center investigative surgical study. Int J Periodontics Restorative Dent. 1999;19:57–65.

204. Araujo M, Berglundh T, Lindhe J. GTR treatment of degree III furcation defects with 2 different resorbable barriers. An experimental study in dogs. J Clin Periodontol. 1998;25(3):253–9.

205. Taddei P, Monti P, Simoni R. Vibrational and thermal study on the in vitro and in vivo degradation of a bioabsorbable periodontal membrane: Vicryl® Periodontal Mesh (Polyglactin 910). J Mater Sci Mater Med. 2002;13(1):59–64.

206. Park YJ, et al. Porous poly (L-lactide) membranes for guided tissue regeneration and controlled drug delivery: membrane fabrication and characterization. J Control Release. 1997;43(2):151–60.

207. Dörfer CE, et al. Regenerative periodontal surgery in interproximal intrabony defects with biodegradable barriers. J Clin Periodontol. 2000;27(3):162–8.

208. Singh AK. GTR membranes: the barriers for periodontal regeneration. DHR Int J Med Sci 2013;4:31–8.

209. Ouanounou A, Hassanpour S, Glogauer M. The influence of systemic medications on osseointegration of dental implants. J Can Dent Assoc. 2016;82(g7):1488–2159.

210. Hwang D, Wang H-L. Medical contraindications to implant therapy: part II: relative contraindications. Implant Dent. 2007;16(1):13–23.

211. Beikler T, Flemmig TF. Implants in the medically compromised patient. Crit Rev Oral Biol Med. 2003;14(4):305–16.

212. Mortensen M, Lawson W, Montazem A. Osteonecrosis of the jaw associated with bisphosphonate use: presentation of seven cases and literature review. Laryngoscope. 2007;117(1):30–4.

213. Mavrokokki T, et al. Nature and frequency of bisphosphonate-associated osteonecrosis of the jaws in Australia. J Oral Maxillofac Surg. 2007;65(3):415–23.

214. Wang H-L, Weber D, McCauley LK. Effect of long-term oral bisphosphonates on implant wound healing: literature review and a case report. J Periodontol. 2007;78(3):584–94.

215. Stanford CM. Dental implants: a role in geriatric dentistry for the general practice? J Am Dent Assoc. 2007;138:S34–40.

216. Duygu G, et al. Dental implant complications. Int J Oral Maxillofac Surg. 2007;36(11):1092–3.

217. Taba M Jr, et al. Current concepts in periodontal bioengineering. Orthod Craniofac Res. 2005;8(4):292–302.

218. Becker W, et al. A comparison of ePTFE membranes alone or in combination with platelet-derived growth factors and insulin-like growth factor-I or demineralized freeze-dried bone in promoting bone formation around immediate extraction socket implants. J Periodontol. 1992;63(11):929–40.

219. Simion M, et al. Vertical ridge augmentation by means of deproteinized bovine bone block and recombinant human platelet-derived growth factor-BB: a histologic study in a dog model. Int J Periodontics Restorative Dent. 2006;26(5):415–23.

220. Kammerer PW, et al. Influence of a collagen membrane and recombinant platelet-derived growth factor on vertical bone augmentation in implant-fixed deproteinized bovine bone—animal pilot study. Clin Oral Implants Res. 2013;24(11):1222–30.
221. Tsuchiya N, et al. Effect of a chitosan sponge impregnated with platelet-derived growth factor on bone augmentation beyond the skeletal envelope in rat calvaria. J Oral Sci. 2014;56(1):23–8.
222. Cabbar F, et al. The effect of bovine bone graft with or without platelet-rich plasma on maxillary sinus floor augmentation. J Oral Maxillofac Surg. 2011;69(10):2537–47.
223. Eskan MA, et al. Platelet-rich plasma-assisted guided bone regeneration for ridge augmentation: a randomized, controlled clinical trial. J Periodontol. 2014;85(5):661–8.
224. Khairy NM, et al. Effect of platelet rich plasma on bone regeneration in maxillary sinus augmentation (randomized clinical trial). Int J Oral Maxillofac Surg. 2013;42(2):249–55.
225. Marx RE, et al. Platelet-rich plasma: growth factor enhancement for bone grafts. Oral Surg Oral Med Oral Pathol Oral Radiol Endod. 1998;85(6):638–46.
226. Wallace SS, Froum SJ. Effect of maxillary sinus augmentation on the survival of endosseous dental implants. A systematic review. Ann Periodontol. 2003;8(1):328–43.
227. Sanchez AR, Sheridan PJ, Kupp LI. Is platelet-rich plasma the perfect enhancement factor? A current review. Int J Oral Maxillofac Implants. 2003;18(1):93–103.
228. Sheikh Z, et al. Bone regeneration using bone morphogenetic proteins and various biomaterial carriers. Materials. 2015;8(4):1778–816.
229. Edmunds RK, et al. Maxillary anterior ridge augmentation with recombinant human bone morphogenetic protein 2. Int J Periodontics Restorative Dent. 2014;34(4):551–7.
230. Katanec D, et al. Use of recombinant human bone morphogenetic protein (rhBMP2) in bilateral alveolar ridge augmentation: case report. Coll Antropol. 2014;38(1):325–30.
231. Kim YJ, et al. Ridge preservation using demineralized bone matrix gel with recombinant human bone morphogenetic protein-2 after tooth extraction: a randomized controlled clinical trial. J Oral Maxillofac Surg. 2014;72(7):1281–90.
232. Shweikeh F, et al. Assessment of outcome following the use of recombinant human bone morphogenetic protein-2 for spinal fusion in the elderly population. J Neurosurg Sci. 2016;60(2):256–71.
233. Zhang H, et al. A meta analysis of lumbar spinal fusion surgery using bone morphogenetic proteins and autologous iliac crest bone graft. PLoS One. 2014;9(6):e97049.
234. Lieberman JR, et al. The effect of regional gene therapy with bone morphogenetic protein-2-producing bone-marrow cells on the repair of segmental femoral defects in rats. J Bone Joint Surg Am. 1999;81(7):905–17.
235. Breitbart AS, et al. Gene-enhanced tissue engineering: applications for bone healing using cultured periosteal cells transduced retrovirally with the BMP-7 gene. Ann Plast Surg. 1999;42(5):488–95.
236. Ishaug SL, et al. Osteoblast function on synthetic biodegradable polymers. J Biomed Mater Res. 1994;28(12):1445–53.
237. Malekzadeh R, et al. Isolation of human osteoblast-like cells and in vitro amplification for tissue engineering. J Periodontol. 1998;69(11):1256–62.
238. Freed LE, et al. Neocartilage formation in vitro and in vivo using cells cultured on synthetic biodegradable polymers. J Biomed Mater Res. 1993;27(1):11–23.
239. De Kok IJ, et al. Evaluation of mesenchymal stem cells following implantation in alveolar sockets: a canine safety study. Int J Oral Maxillofac Implants. 2005;20(4):511–8.
240. Bruder SP, et al. The effect of implants loaded with autologous mesenchymal stem cells on the healing of canine segmental bone defects. J Bone Joint Surg Am. 1998;80(7):985–96.

Loading Strategies 

10

Mélanie Menassa and Thomas T. Nguyen

Abstract

Implantology has offered an alternative to the conventional denture providing much more stability and retention. This alternative is referred to as an implant overdenture. According to *The McGill Consensus Statement on Overdentures* (Romanos, Advanced immediate loading, Quintessence Books, 2012, p. 179), the minimum standard of care for an edentulous mandible is a two-implant overdenture. Therefore, in the case of an edentulous mandible, conventional dentures should be considered an alternative treatment. In fact, there are several advantages of two-implant overdentures as they improve support, retention, and stability. Consequently, they improve the patients' ability to chew food. Patients found implant overdentures more comfortable, and an ease of speech was noted in comparison with a conventional denture (Romanos, Advanced immediate loading, Quintessence Books, 2012, p. 179). Implant overdentures should also be considered for their benefits from a bone-conservation point of view. Implants stimulate the bone and help maintain its level (Davarpanah and Szmukler-Moncler, Manuel d'implantologie clinique: concepts, protocoles et innovations récentes, Paris, 2008).

The timing suggested for implant loading after placement of the implant, which also refers to the delivery of the prostheses, varies. Traditionally, there was a wait period of 3–6 months prior to implant loading in the mandible which is referred to as the conventional loading protocol, introduced initially by Brånemark (Javed and Romanos, J Dent 38:612–20, 2010). In order to reduce this wait period, other protocols have been introduced: immediate loading (under 1 week) and early loading (1 week to 2 months). Additionally, due to improved implant surfaces and techniques, conventional loading is now acceptable as of 2 months (Misch, Contemporary implant dentistry, Elsevier Health Sciences, 2007; Misch et al., J Oral Maxillofac Surg 57:700–6, 1999). There are numerous factors that come into play when determining the appropriate loading protocol.

M. Menassa
Clin. dent. Hôpital Juif, Montréal, QC, Canada
e-mail: m.menassa@umontreal.ca

T. T. Nguyen, DMD, MSc, Cert Perio, Dip ABP (✉)
Department of Oral Health, Faculty of Dentistry,
University of Montreal, Montreal, QC, Canada
e-mail: thomas.thong.nguyen@umontreal.ca

10.1 Introduction

In the last decade, immediate loading has been introduced as a viable option to reduce the wait period and accelerate implant treatment.

© Springer International Publishing AG, part of Springer Nature 2018
E. Emami, J. Feine (eds.), *Mandibular Implant Prostheses*,
https://doi.org/10.1007/978-3-319-71181-2_10

However, the success of this concept relies mainly on implant stability and adequate osseointegration. Several factors have been identified as playing a key role in osseointegration: initial implant stability, implant surface characteristics, bone metabolism, interim prosthesis design, and occlusion pattern during the healing phase [1]. Ideally, all these factors should be considered in the selection of an appropriate loading protocol for the edentulous patient.

This chapter will explore the different factors affecting the osseointegration of an implant. It will describe various methods of evaluating the stability of the implant in the bone. Finally, conventional, early and immediate loading protocols will be defined and discussed.

10.2 Osseointegration

10.2.1 Concept of Primary Stability

In order to have a long-term success with dental implants, the surrounding bone has to be mechanically stable, bearing the occlusal loading forces. Initial mechanical stability of the implant with the surrounding lamellar bone is necessary during implant insertion. The gentle osteotomy, without overheating or significant mechanical trauma, is necessary to get good primary contact between the implant and bone. This is clinically determined as primary implant stability [1].

Primary stability is defined as the mechanical anchorage immediately after implant insertion. It is obtained by surface of contact between the implant and bone [2, 3]. It is an important factor in the establishment of osseointegration and contributes to determining the prognosis of the implant and, in consequence, to the choice of the appropriate loading protocol [2].

Primary stability is obtained through the quality and quantity of the contact area between the implant and the bone [2]. The measure of this contact area is given by the bone-implant contact (BIC) measured in percentage [4]. Several factors related to the bone (bone quality and quantity) and implant type (implant length, diameter, surface type, and macrogeometry) influence the BIC.

The quality of bone density has been classified into four categories by Lekholm and Zarb [2, 4]. Quality 1 bone consists of homogenous compact bone, quality 2 consists of a thick layer of cortical bone surrounding a think layer of compact trabecular bone, quality 3 consists of resistant trabecular bone surrounded by a thin layer of cortical bone, and lastly quality 4 consists of low-density trabecular bone surrounded by a thin cortical bone layer [4]. Low-density trabecular bone, being more porous than cortical bone, offers a reduced BIC and leads to uneven and concentrated force distribution from implant to bone. The increased forces on the implant-bone interface can lead to excessive microstrain and in some cases implant mobility and failure [4, 5]. In general, higher bone density has a higher BIC, and consequently, the greater the bone density, the greater the primary stability [4]. However, it is to be noted that this does not automatically translate to a higher implant success rate.

Next, the implant length plays an important role in increasing the bone-implant contact area. A longer implant can increase the bone-implant contact area and further engage the cortical bone [6–8]. Ideally the length should vary between 10 and 15 mm. An implant length above 15 mm is deemed unnecessary. The risk of implant failure increases if the implant length is under 10 mm [8]. In the case of poor bone quality, an increase in implant length has a more significant increase on primary stability [7]. In fact, every 3 mm increase of length of the implant can increase the bone-implant interface (or contact area) by approximately 20–30% [5]. However, placement of short dental implants could be a predictable alternative to longer implants to reduce surgical complications and patient morbidity in situations where vertical augmentation procedures are needed. The 1-year and 5-year cumulative survival rates for short implants were reported to be 98.7% and 93.6%, respectively [9].

It is found that the larger the diameter, the greater the primary stability due to the increased contact area [8]. This is limited by the width of the alveolar ridges. Increased diameter implants allow for a greater distribution of forces by further engaging the cortical bone, thus increasing primary stability and reducing micromotions [4]. This effect is more prominent in the cortical bone already absorbing a greater proportion of forces due to its larger contact area [2]. However, it should be noted that several studies on wide-diameter implants have reported an increased failure rate, which was linked with over-instrumentation and heat generation [10]. More recent studies believe the failure rate is mainly associated with operators' learning curves, poor bone density, implant design, and site preparation [11]. Hultin-Mordenfeld et al. reported a higher implant failure rate with wide-diameter implants but better results in the mandible (94.5%) than the maxilla (78.3%).

Next, macrogeometry and morphology can influence the BIC as well. Primary stability was found to be more positively affected by a slightly tapered implant in comparison to a cylindrical one [12]. With regard to the macrogeometry of the implant, the form of the neck is important as it engages the cortical, and in a lower-density bone, smaller treads promote a better primary stability [5].

Additionally, the surface topography of the implant is an important factor in the process of osseointegration. However, surface topography does not affect primary stability and will be discussed in the next section regarding secondary stability [13].

After taking into consideration and maximizing all these variables, it is important to assess the implant's primary stability. To do so, it is recommended to evaluate the implant's torque. A torque is a measure of the force applied to the implant causing it to rotate and is expressed in newton centimeters (Ncm). There are different ways of assessing it, such as cutting torque resistance analysis and insertion torque value (ITV). For cutting torque resistance analysis, a torque gauge is incorporated into the drill used to cut into the bone. This measures the energy required to cut the bone. This value correlates with bone density types which contribute to the primary stability [3]. Cutting resistance during insertion is commonly used to determine primary stability. In this case, a sudden stop while seating the implant indicates better primary stability [14]. However,

one of the preferred techniques of assessing primary stability is the ITV, a measure of the highest insertion torque obtained by the motor during placement of the implant. ITV of 32, 35, and 40 Ncm and higher have been suggested as indicating adequate stability for an immediate loading protocol [3, 15, 16]. Studies demonstrate a high failure rate at 20 Ncm or less with an immediate loading protocol (ILP) [17], and so many studies exclude ILP when the ITV is low. Additionally, it is to be noted that several studies found that there was no statistically significant difference in insertion torque and cutting resistance in failed versus successful implants with a conventional loading protocol [18, 19].

Above, the graph (Fig. 10.1) represents a generalized overview of early wound healing after implant placement: showing the implant stability in function of time. It is suggested that implant stability is at its maximum immediately following the surgery; this is known as primary stability. In the beginning, osteoclastic activity causes the implant stability to decrease, which causes a micromotion of the implant. It was found that micromovements between 50 and 150 μm could jeopardize the osseointegration of the implant [21]. This period marked by a drop in primary stability is shown until week 4, at which time secondary stability gradually takes over, provid-

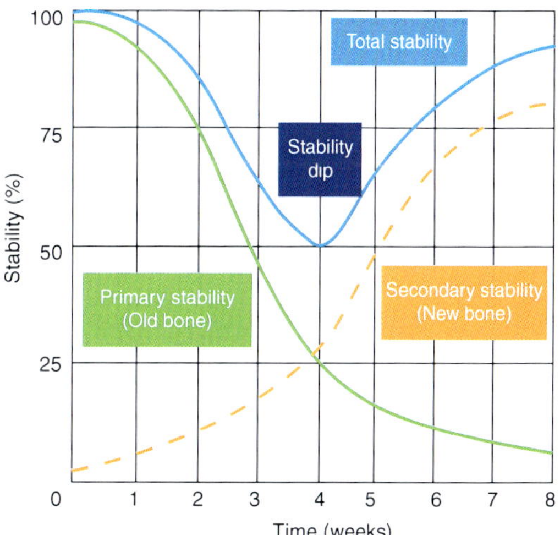

Fig. 10.1 Primary and secondary stability in function of time [20]

ing the main source of stability (Fig. 10.1). Secondary stability refers to the formation of new bone around the implant.

10.2.2 Concept of Secondary Stability

Secondary stability refers to the formation of new bone around the implant. After implant placement, the bone surrounding the newly placed implant is reorganized, and during this process, primary stability is gradually replaced by secondary stability. Secondary stability is given by the level of osseointegration. This refers to the concept of an anatomical and functional junction formed directly between the living bone and implant without the presence of fibrous matter.

Depending on temperature during preparation of the implant bed and placement of the implant, there is a certain amount of necrosis of the adjacent bone, generally up to 1 mm. For osteogenesis to take place, there must be a stable surface; adequate cells, either from the bone marrow or from undifferentiated mesenchymal cells; nutrition for these cells; and an appropriate biomechanical environment. Although some mechanical stimulation is necessary for osteogenesis, too much (50–150 μm) has the undesirable effect of stimulating differentiation through the fibroblast lineage [21]. This leads to the formation of a fibrous mass parallel to the vertical axis of the implant known as fibrointegration, as opposed to osseointegration [2].

In the trabecular bone, secondary stability begins with the formation of a blood clot, filling the gap between the implant and remaining bone. The fibrinogen in the blood attaches to the implant, allowing for preferential adsorption of platelets to the implant surface, and their immediate degranulation, releasing factors attracting undifferentiated cells to the site [2].

A network of fibrin is then formed followed by angiogenesis, which allows the undifferentiated mesenchymal cells to arrive to the site, providing both the adequate cells and cell nutrition necessary for osteogenesis. Ideally, these cells would then differentiate following the osteoblast lineage.

As these cells migrate toward the implant surface, they exert a certain amount of tension on the fibers causing a retraction. At this point, the osteogenesis can be divided into two types. Depending on whether or not the fibers manage to resist this force, the osteogenesis will be in contact or in distance [22]. Therefore, it is important to limit micromovements as discussed above [2].

In contact osteogenesis, the cells arrive directly to the implant surface, recognizing it as stable, and begin to differentiate into osteoblasts producing trabecular bone. Bone apposition occurs simultaneously from the implant to the bone and from the bone to the implant, thus creating a trabecula that is perpendicular to the vertical axis of the implant [2]. On the other hand, in osteogenesis at distance cells begin apposition from the most stable surface away from the implant, the walls of the socket, and move toward the implant. This type of osteogenesis is a slower process and creates an osseous shell (corticolization) [2].

The type of osteogenesis can be influenced by the type of surface modification used. The first category is topographic modification. Implants with a rough and/or etched surface offer more retention for the fibers compared to smooth surface implants, allowing for contact osteogenesis rather than osteogenesis at a distance. The second category is surface coating. It has been reported that hydrophilic implant surfaces, such as Straumann's SLActive®, can reduce the risks during the critical early treatment by accelerating implant integration. The bone formation process is initiated at an earlier stage, resulting in improved implant stability in the "critical dip" period (Fig. 10.2). The improved and optimized secondary stability process leads to a higher implant stability between week 2 and 4. While healing showed similar characteristics with bone resorptive and appositional events for both regular and hydrophilic surfaces between 7 and 42 days, the degree of osseointegration after 2 and 4 weeks was superior for the SLActive® compared with the regular implant surface [23].

In cortical bone, the process of osteogenesis is much slower due to the reduced vascularization. The effects of the implant surface are also less apparent than in the trabecular bone. These fac-

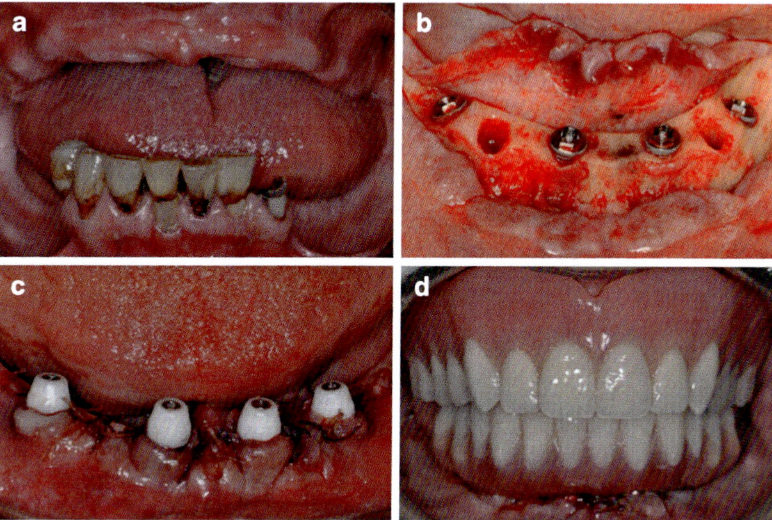

Fig. 10.2 Edentulous patient with lower worn dentition (**a**). Extraction of lower teeth, alveoloplasty, and placement of four mandibular dental implants (**b**). Placement of multiunit abutments and closure of the surgical site (**c**). Immediate loading of the four implants with an acrylic fixed provisional prosthesis

tors can explain the lower degree of osseointegration seen in quality 1 bone. In fact, the quickest degree of osteogenesis is usually seen in quality 3 or 4 trabecular bone with rough surface implants. However, overall, qualities 2 and 3 tend to yield better results for implant success [2].

10.2.3 Evaluation of Osseointegration

In order to evaluate implant success, several criteria have been established. The most recognized criteria were established by Albrektsson et al. [24]. Initially, accepted vertical bone loss was set at 1.5 mm during the first year and 0.1 mm for the following years. These criteria were later revised, and the accepted vertical bone loss was changed to 0.2 mm annually after the first year of service [25].

Criteria for implant success [26]:

- An individual unattached implant is immobile when tested clinically.
- The radiograph does not demonstrate any evidence of periimplant radiolucency.
- Vertical bone loss is less than 0.2 mm annually after the first year of service of the implant.
- Individual implant performance is characterized by an absence of persistent or irreversible signs and symptoms such as pain, infections,

neuropathies, paresthesia, or violation of the mandibular canal.
- Success rates of 85% at the end of a 5-year observation period and 80% at the end of a 10-year period are minimum criteria for success.

There are also several techniques used to evaluate osseointegration. To begin, it is important to perform a clinical examination of the implant. This exam should determine if the implant is mobile, if there is sensitivity to percussion, and eventually if there is presence of infection, as these can be signs of implant failure. Radiographs are essential to assess bone height as well as any radiotranslucency surrounding the implant. The implant threads are commonly used as a reference of dimension [27, 28]. It is also important to take a periapical X-ray, in particular when implant presents mobility. If a radiotranslucent border appears around the implant in the X-ray, this is a sign that the implant did not osseointegrate [8].

There are also other methods to evaluate osseointegration that are available to clinicians. These include the Periotest® and the Osstell™ method.

10.2.3.1 Periotest®

The Periotest® is an electromechanical instrument consisting of a metallic rod and handpiece. The rod percusses the implant 16 times, while a sensor records the length of time of contact. The greater the time, the more mobile the implant and the greater the Periotest value. The lower the value, the greater the stability and damping effects of the measured implant or tooth. Values of −8 to 0 indicate that the implant may be loaded, and +1 to 9 indicate that further clinical examination is needed prior to loading [28]. Superior values indicate that the osseointegration is insufficient. This test has proven to be a reliable method to evaluate primary stability [28, 29].

10.2.3.2   Osstell™

Osstell™ is an indirect measure of osseointegration. This instrument measures the frequency at which the sensor on the implant vibrates, which is known as the resonance frequency analysis (RFA). This value is converted into an implant stability quotient (ISQ). Values on this scale range from 1 to 100, with greater values indicating greater stability. According to Osstell™, an ISQ of 70 and greater represents high stability, 60–69 represents medium stability, and below 60 is low stability. According to another source, a resonance frequency of at least 60 was required from ILP; however, the evidence base is lacking in this area [30]. Although this test gives information regarding failure to osseointegrate, single readings offer limited clinical value [31].

10.3   Implant Loading Protocols

There are three recognized loading protocols for implants: conventional loading, immediate loading, and early loading. A conventional loading protocol is when the restoration is delivered 2 months after implant placement. Immediate loading refers to a restoration delivered within 1 week following implant placement. Finally, early loading implies that the restoration is delivered between 1 week and 2 months after implant placement [32].

10.3.1   Definitions

Loading protocols	New definitions
Conventional	Restoration delivered after 2 months following implant placement
Immediate	Restoration delivered within 1 week following implant placement
Early	Restoration delivered between 1 week and 2 months following implant placement

10.3.2   Conventional Loading Protocol

During the 1960s, Dr. Brånemark established the first surgical protocol for implants. This was a two-stage conventional loading protocol. For this protocol there is a first surgery to place the implants, followed by a 4–6-month waiting period to allow the implants to become osseointegrated, thereby ensuring a certain secondary stability regardless of primary stability [33]. This is particularly important in low-density bone. Next is a second surgery to uncover the implants and place healing caps, followed by a 4–8-week waiting period to allow soft tissue to heal prior to taking an impression for the two-implant overdenture and loading of the implants [2].

The multiple surgeries suggested by this protocol demand time from both the patient and the dentist, as well as recovery periods during each of which the patient experiences some discomfort. Additionally, during the combined wait periods prior to loading, the completely edentate patient must function with either a conventional denture or no denture. Consequently, the patient must deal with unsatisfactory function and aesthetics for several months before receiving their final treatment (two-implant overdenture) [2].

In order to reduce the inconveniences of waiting for the final restoration, without compromising osseointegration, a one-stage conventional protocol was established. With this protocol, healing caps are placed during the first surgery immediately following implant placement, thus eliminating the specific wait period for soft tissue healing by merging it with the osseointegration wait period [34]. Nonetheless, with this protocol, there is still a wait period [2]. Today implant surfaces have been improved, lessening the time necessary for osseointegration and decreasing the wait period for the conventional loading protocol to 2 months.

To this day, the conventional loading protocol remains the option of choice. However, for those with good primary stability, there are more possibilities that may be of greater interest to the patient.

10.3.3 Immediate Loading Protocol

In fact, an immediate loading protocol was suggested in order to answer to the demand to shorten this wait period. Following the immediate loading protocol, the overdenture is delivered within 1 week of implant placement, meaning prior to osseointegration [35]. Through several studies, it has been proven that the immediate loading protocol is an effective treatment option yielding a success rate comparable with that of the conventional loading protocol and offering greater patient satisfaction than the later [36]. That said, it is necessary to mention that there are some requirements prior to adopting an immediate loading protocol and that it is only indicated in cases involving good primary stability, otherwise the success rate plummets [17]. Indeed, when the overdenture is delivered and put into occlusion, it exerts certain forces on the implants, and without adequate primary stability to immobilize these, they are more susceptible to micromotion. When this micromotion exceeds 50–150 µm, it will prevent osseointegration by causing fibrointegration instead, which will lead to implant failure. Hence, the importance of primary stability when subjecting implants to a load prior to osseointegration, such as in the immediate loading protocol. In order to prevent implant failure, primary stability must be gauged prior to selecting a loading protocol. There are many methods and values suggested to deem whether or not primary stability is sufficient for the use of the immediate loading protocol, but one of the best and most commonly used is the insertion torque value (ITV). ITV takes into account bone density, which should be of quality 1, 2, or 3 for immediate loading, as the lower the bone density, the less torque is necessary to cut through it and place the implant [2]. Again, as ITV is a good indicator of primary stability, it is suggested to have a minimum ITV of 32 Ncm to proceed with an immediate loading [3, 16].

Additionally, with immediate loading, it is particularly important to minimize forces that may cause micromotion. For instance, splinting of the implants allows the occlusal forces to be more evenly distributed on the implants and diminishes the stress placed on each of them, allowing the horizontal forces to be minimized at the bone-implant interface [4]. Moreover, it is recommended to place the implant(s) in nonfunctional occlusion in order to minimize stress and optimize primary stability [8]. In fact, a study has shown that immediate nonfunctional loading increased the implant survival rate when compared with immediate functional loading [37]. The implant surface is also important in the ILP, and a rough surface implant is found to yield the best result [8]. It is also important to mention that the patient adhering to a liquid and soft diet for 6–8 weeks after implant placement decreases the risk of overload failure [8].

10.3.4 Early Loading Protocol

Finally, an early loading protocol, where the restoration is delivered between 1 week and 2 months of implant placement, has also been suggested as an alternative to conventional loading. This protocol, however, is not ideal as it has a higher failure rate [35]. Referring back to Fig. 10.1 (page 4), necrosis of the bone adjacent to the implant occurs gradually in the weeks following placement of the implant bringing primary stability from 100% the day of implant placement to 75% in the first

2 weeks and then to 25% by the fourth week and continuing to diminish. At this time, the process of osseointegration has begun to offer some secondary stability but is still only at 25% by the fourth week and takes another 4 weeks to provide an adequate total stability as primary stability continues to diminish. Consequently, this process of acquiring stability spans the entire window of restoration delivery of the early loading protocol. That said adopting the early loading protocol means subjecting implants to forces when stability is at its lowest and putting osseointegration at risk. This explains the higher failure rate associated with this particular loading protocol [2].

10.4　Patient Perception of Immediate Loading

Another important factor in determining whether a particular treatment or loading protocol could be advised is patient perception and satisfaction with this option. As these are subjective, they vary from person to person and do not rest entirely upon the degree of fulfillment of the patient's functional needs (reestablishment of phonetic and masticatory capacity). In fact, the patient's expectations, preferences, and knowledge, as well as their sociocultural background, level of education, and even personality, can influence their level of satisfaction [38–40]. That being said, it can be noted that patients were generally more satisfied and had an improved oral health quality of life (OHQoL) with two-implant mandibular overdentures in comparison with conventional mandibular dentures [39, 41]. Additionally, it has been suggested that the use of an immediate loading protocol could further increase said patient satisfaction and OHQoL [42]. Although studies on this subject are scarce and can refer to fixed prostheses, bar, or other attachments [41–44], some including one pilot trial referring to immediate loading of two-implant overdentures seem to indicate a high satisfaction rate (94.4% with 100% of patients recommending this treatment option) [41, 45–47]. The high patient satisfaction rate for the ILP is due to the decreased wait period prior to achieving the following: satisfactory aesthetic results, positive impact on social life, decrease in discomfort, improved stability and masticatory ability, no additional surgeries, and reduced number of visits [45, 48]. It is also interesting to note that the pain experienced during the longer appointment associated with ILPs did not negatively impact patients' opinion of this loading protocol. However, more research must be done on immediate loading of mandibular two-implant overdentures to confirm this information.

References

1. Romanos GE. Advanced immediate loading. Hanover Park, IL: Quintessence Books; 2012. p. 179.
2. Davarpanah M, Szmukler-Moncler S. Manuel d'implantologie clinique: concepts, protocoles et innovations récentes. Paris: Wolters Kluwer France; 2008.
3. Javed F, Romanos GE. The role of primary stability for successful immediate loading of dental implants. A literature review. J Dent. 2010;38(8):612–20.
4. Misch CE. Contemporary implant dentistry. Elsevier Health Sciences; 2007.
5. Misch CE, Qu Z, Bidez MW. Mechanical properties of trabecular bone in the human mandible: implications for dental implant treatment planning and surgical placement. J Oral Maxillofac Surg. 1999;57(6):700–6; discussion 706.
6. Chatzigianni A, et al. Effect of mini-implant length and diameter on primary stability under loading with two force levels. Eur J Orthod. 2011;33(4):381–7.
7. Barikani H, et al. The effect of implant length and diameter on the primary stability in different bone types. J Dent (Tehran, Iran). 2013;10(5):449–55.
8. Davarpanah M, Szmukler-Moncler S, Molloy S. Théorie et pratique de la mise en charge immédiate. Paris: Quintessence International; 2007.
9. Lee SA, et al. Systematic review and meta-analysis of randomized controlled trials for the management of limited vertical height in the posterior region: short implants (5 to 8 mm) vs longer implants (>8 mm) in vertically augmented sites. Int J Oral Maxillofac Implants. 2014;29(5):1085–97.
10. English C, et al. What are the clinical limitations of wide-diameter (4 mm or greater) root-form endosseous implants? Int J Oral Maxillofac Implants. 2000;15(2):293–6.
11. Renouard F, Nisand D. Impact of implant length and diameter on survival rates. Clin Oral Implants Res. 2006;17(Suppl 2):35–51.
12. O'Sullivan D, et al. A comparison of two methods of enhancing implant primary stability. Clin Implant Dent Relat Res. 2004;6(1):48–57.

13. O'Sullivan D, Sennerby L, Meredith N. Measurements comparing the initial stability of five designs of dental implants: a human cadaver study. Clin Implant Dent Relat Res. 2000;2(2):85–92.

14. Sennerby L, Meredith N. Implant stability measurements using resonance frequency analysis: biological and biomechanical aspects and clinical implications. Periodontology 2000. 2008;47(1):51–66.

15. Degidi M, Piattelli A. 7-year follow-up of 93 immediately loaded titanium dental implants. J Oral Implantol. 2005;31(1):25–31.

16. Lorenzoni M, et al. Immediate loading of single-tooth implants in the anterior maxilla. Preliminary results after one year. Clin Oral Implants Res. 2003;14(2):180–7.

17. Barewal RM, Stanford C, Weesner TC. A randomized controlled clinical trial comparing the effects of three loading protocols on dental implant stability. Int J Oral Maxillofac Implants. 2012;27(4):945–56.

18. Friberg B, et al. On cutting torque measurements during implant placement: a 3-year clinical prospective study. Clin Implant Dent Relat Res. 1999;1(2):75–83.

19. Johansson B, Back T, Hirsch JM. Cutting torque measurements in conjunction with implant placement in grafted and nongrafted maxillas as an objective evaluation of bone density: a possible method for identifying early implant failures? Clin Implant Dent Relat Res. 2004;6(1):9–15.

20. Froum S. Dental implant complications: etiology, prevention, and treatment. Hoboken, NJ: Wiley; 2011.

21. Szmukler Moncler S, et al. Timing of loading and effect of micromotion on bone-dental implant interface: review of experimental literature. J Biomed Mater Res. 1998;43(2):192–203.

22. Davies JE. Understanding peri-implant endosseous healing. J Dent Educ. 2003;67(8):932–49.

23. Lang NP, et al. Early osseointegration to hydrophilic and hydrophobic implant surfaces in humans. Clin Oral Implants Res. 2011;22(4):349–56.

24. Albrektsson T, et al. The long-term efficacy of currently used dental implants: a review and proposed criteria of success. Int J Oral Maxillofac Implants. 1986;1(1):11–25.

25. Smith DE, Zarb GA. Criteria for success of osseointegrated endosseous implants. J Prosthet Dent. 1989;62(5):567–72.

26. Karthik K, et al. Evaluation of implant success: a review of past and present concepts. J Pharm Bioallied Sci. 2013;5(Suppl 1):S117–9.

27. Meredith N. Assessment of implant stability as a prognostic determinant. Int J Prosthodont. 1998;11(5):491–501.

28. Romanos GE, Nentwig GH. Immediate functional loading in the maxilla using implants with platform switching: five-year results. Int J Oral Maxillofac Implants. 2009;24(6):1106–12.

29. Romanos GE, Nentwig GH. Immediate versus delayed functional loading of implants in the posterior mandible: a 2-year prospective clinical study of 12 consecutive cases. Int J Periodontics Restorative Dent. 2006;26(5):459–69.

30. Henry PJ, Liddelow GJ. Immediate loading of dental implants. Aust Dent J. 2008;53(Suppl 1):S69–81.

31. Aparicio C, Lang NP, Rangert B. Validity and clinical significance of biomechanical testing of implant/bone interface. Clin Oral Implants Res. 2006;17(Suppl 2):2–7.

32. Esposito M, et al. Interventions for replacing missing teeth: horizontal and vertical bone augmentation techniques for dental implant treatment. Cochrane Database Syst Rev. 2009;(4):Cd003607.

33. Adell R, et al. A 15-year study of osseointegrated implants in the treatment of the edentulous jaw. Int J Oral Surg. 1981;10(6):387–416.

34. Becker W, et al. One-step surgical placement of Branemark implants: a prospective multicenter clinical study. Int J Oral Maxillofac Implants. 1997;12(4):454–62.

35. Esposito M, et al. Interventions for replacing missing teeth: different times for loading dental implants. Cochrane Database Syst Rev. 2013;(3):CD003878.

36. Schimmel M, et al. Loading protocols for implant-supported overdentures in the edentulous jaw: a systematic review and meta-analysis. Int J Oral Maxillofac Implants. 2014;29(Suppl):271–86.

37. Degidi M, Piattelli A. Immediate functional and non-functional loading of dental implants: a 2- to 60-month follow-up study of 646 titanium implants. J Periodontol. 2003;74(2):225–41.

38. Awad MA, Feine JS. Measuring patient satisfaction with mandibular prostheses. Community Dent Oral Epidemiol. 1998;26(6):400–5.

39. Heydecke G, et al. Do mandibular implant overdentures and conventional complete dentures meet the expectations of edentulous patients? Quintessence Int. 2008;39(10):803–9.

40. Awad MA, et al. Determinants of patients' treatment preferences in a clinical trial. Community Dent Oral Epidemiol. 2000;28(2):119–25.

41. Buttel AE, et al. Immediate loading of two unsplinted mandibular implants in edentulous patients with an implant-retained overdenture: an observational study over two years. Schweiz Monatsschr Zahnmed. 2012;122(5):392–7.

42. Alfadda SA, Attard NJ, David LA. Five-year clinical results of immediately loaded dental implants using mandibular overdentures. Int J Prosthodont. 2009;22(4):368–73.

43. Liddelow G, Henry P. The immediately loaded single implant-retained mandibular overdenture: a 36-month prospective study. Int J Prosthodont. 2010;23(1):13–21.

44. Schnitman PA, et al. Ten-year results for Branemark implants immediately loaded with fixed prostheses at implant placement. Int J Oral Maxillofac Implants. 1997;12(4):495–503.

45. Menassa M, et al. Patients' expectations, satisfaction, and quality of life with immediate loading protocol. Clin Oral Implants Res. 2016;27(1):83–9.

46. Liddelow GJ, Henry PJ. A prospective study of immediately loaded single implant-retained mandibular overdentures: preliminary one-year results. J Prosthet Dent. 2007;97(6 Suppl):S126–37.
47. Emami E, et al. Does immediate loading affect clinical and patient-centered outcomes of mandibular 2-unsplinted-implant overdenture? A 2-year within-case analysis. J Dent. 2016;50:30–6.
48. Avila G, et al. Immediate implant loading: current status from available literature. Implant Dent. 2007;16(3):235–45.

Part III

Prosthetic Phase

Fundamental Surgical and Prosthetic Principles of Mandibular Implant Assisted Prostheses

11

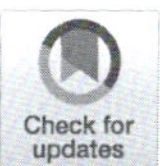

Samer Abi Nader and Samer Mesmar

Abstract

The introduction of dental implants has dramatically changed the lives of many edentulous patients by providing a mechanism of anchorage that contributes to stabilizing the mandibular denture during function. This has provided a variety of new options for the treatment of complete upper and lower edentulism (Emami et al., Periodontol 66:119–31, 2014).

This chapter will discuss the fundamental principles and differences between the implant-retained and implant-supported mandibular dentures. The implant-retained overdenture presents a unique clinical situation that requires distinct surgical and prosthetic considerations to help optimize the clinical outcome (Kimoto et al., Clin Oral Implants Res 20:838–43, 2009). A multitude of stud-type attachment systems are available today to provide retention and stability for the mandibular complete implant-retained denture. A description of the various morphological characteristics and the impact that they have on the retention and wear behavior of stud attachments will be reviewed.

This chapter will also cover the basic surgical and prosthetic principles that underline the planning of implant-supported removable and fixed mandibular prosthesis.

11.1 Introduction

The loss of natural dentition is inevitably accompanied by anatomic and physiological changes, which result in the resorption of the alveolar bone [1, 2]. These changes affect the mandibular lower denture as they manifest clinically with a loss of retention and stability of the prosthesis and a possible reduction in the functional capacity of the patient. The introduction of dental implants has dramatically changed the lives of many edentulous patients by providing a mechanism of anchorage that assists in stabilizing the mandibular denture. They also have been shown to slow down the detrimental loss of the residual ridge over time.

Historically, fixed implant-supported prostheses were considered the ideal treatment modality for the completely edentulous patient. The survival rates of dental implants supporting a fixed mandibular prosthesis are well documented [3]. Overdentures were considered as a secondary option in cases of anatomical and financial limitations. They were often regarded as a lesser treatment. However, in the past few years, the efficacy of overdentures for the treatment of

S. A. Nader, BSc, DMD, MSc, FRCD(C) (✉)
Department of Restorative Dentistry, Faculty of Dentistry, McGill University, Montreal, QC, Canada
e-mail: samer.abinader@mcgill.ca

S. Mesmar, DMD., MSc, FRCD(C)
Division of Prosthodontics, McGill University Health Centre, Montreal, QC, Canada

© Springer International Publishing AG, part of Springer Nature 2018
E. Emami, J. Feine (eds.), *Mandibular Implant Prostheses*,
https://doi.org/10.1007/978-3-319-71181-2_11

edentulous patients has been clearly recognized. In fact, in 2002 at the McGill Consensus Conference, this treatment modality was considered as the first choice of treatment for the edentulous mandible and is currently regarded by the scientific community as a standard of care [4]. This was further reinforced by the York Consensus in 2009 [5, 6].

Multiple prospective, randomized clinical trials were carried out to determine the survival rates of un-splinted dental implants [7]. The assessment criteria used by different authors are based primarily on implant survival. The high implant survival rates reported in these studies reflect the success of this treatment approach and are comparable to the survival of implants supporting a fixed prosthesis [3].

Mandibular two-implant overdentures have been recognized as the standard of care for the treatment of edentulous patients [4]. When compared with conventional complete dentures, they provide higher patient satisfaction [8] and better masticatory ability [9] and preserve residual ridge height over time [10]. Furthermore, two-implant overdentures are more cost-effective when compared with implant-supported prostheses [11]. Indeed, they are characterized by a reduced cost [4, 12] and a simpler technique of fabrication [12]. Also, hygiene is generally facilitated by the removable nature of the prosthesis, the limited number of dental implants, and the absence of a metal bar. Therefore, for all the abovementioned reasons, this option of treatment presents a considerable amount of advantages, particularly to the elderly patients.

11.2 Implant-Retained Mandibular Dentures

11.2.1 Definitions

Implant overdentures can be categorized according to the support offered by dental implants as implant-supported or implant-retained prosthesis. Implant-supported prostheses are generally fully sustained by dental implants. They are characterized by a higher number of implants ensuring the majority of support of the lower denture (Fig. 11.1). In contrast, implant-retained prosthesis depends mainly on the posterior edentulous ridges for their support. The dental implants in the anterior region of the mandible participate only partially in supporting the lower prosthesis (Fig. 11.2). These implants, however, offer adequate anterior anchorage and a significant improvement in prosthetic retention.

11.2.2 Movement Pattern of Implant-Retained Overdentures

The implant-retained overdenture presents a unique clinical situation that is distinct from the implant-supported prosthesis. In fact, overdentures retained by two implants in the inter-canine region

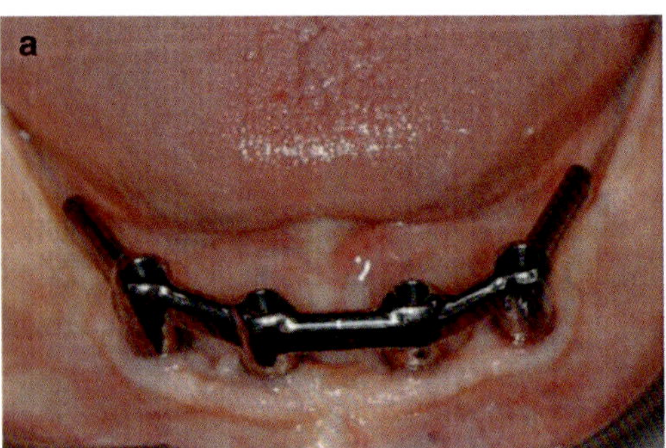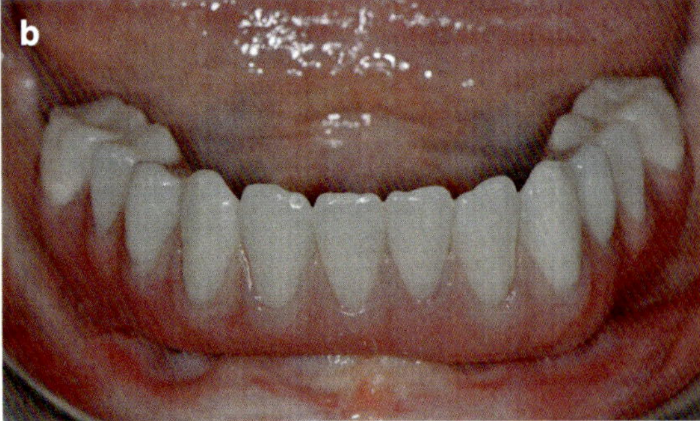

Fig. 11.1 Implant-supported mandibular prosthesis (**a**) Removable prosthesis supported by a Dolder bar (**b**) Fixed prosthesis supported by four dental implants

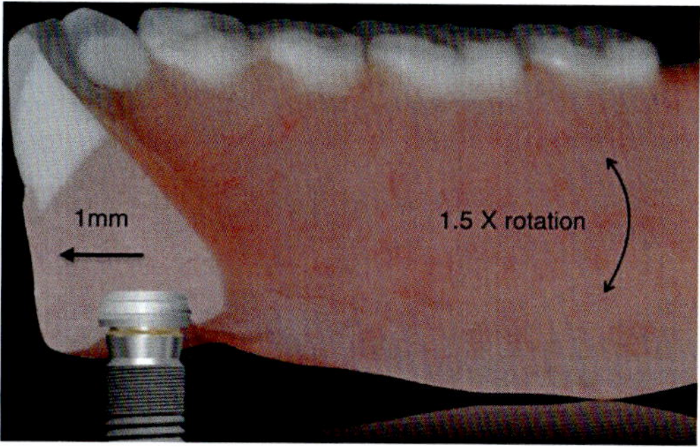

Fig. 11.3 Increase in rotational movement of the lower implant-retained mandibular denture as the distance between the incisal edge of the anterior prosthetic teeth and the denture border increases

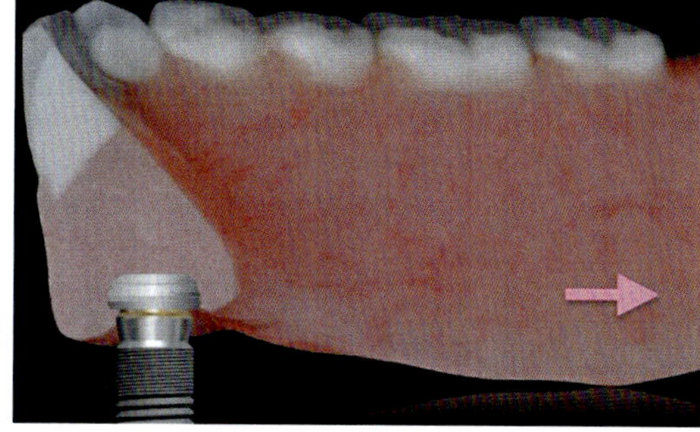

Fig. 11.4 Decrease in rotational movement of the implant-retained mandibular denture as the length of the denture base increases

of the mandible are subject to a series of complex movements during mastication. The denture often exhibits an occluso-gingival movement during chewing. This rotational movement is centered on an imaginary axis that is drawn between the two anterior implants. The amplitude of this movement has been historically associated to the thickness and the compressibility of the supporting tissues, the resiliency of the attachment system, the distance of the application of force relative to the axis of rotation, and the magnitude of the applied force. It is very similar in its behavior to the Kennedy class 2 removable partial dentures.

Recently, certain prosthetic parameters have been associated with an increase in rotational displacement of the denture during function. In a cross-sectional study, Kimoto et al. assessed a variety of prosthetic factors in order to determine their involvement on implant overdenture rotation and the influence of rotation on general satisfaction and chewing ability. They reported that participants were more likely to detect rotational movement when the distance between the tip of the anterior teeth and the anterior denture border increased (Fig. 11.3). In fact, the horizontal position of the anterior teeth was considered to be the most important factor in rotational movements. Conversely, increasing the length of the denture base was associated with a decrease in the perception of this displacement (Fig. 11.4). Patients that were aware of rotational movements of their denture reported a reduced ability to chew compared to the ones that were unaware of the rotation [13].

It has been historically postulated that the condition of the alveolar ridge is very important for the success of denture treatments [14]. Kimoto et al. also assessed the relationship between bone height and perceived rotation. They were able to establish that the percentage of the participants who complained about rotation increased as bone resorption increased [13]. This suggests that implant-retained prosthesis may more easily rotate as resorption of the residual alveolar ridge becomes more severe which will have an impact on the patient's functional capacity. However, no relationship has been established between this resorption and the satisfaction of patients with the treatment outcome. Nevertheless, in these cases, the attachment system is subjected to an increased functional stress. Consequently, wear of the attachments is accelerated because of greater dependence on the soft tissue support.

Rotational awareness may have a negative impact on the perceived functional capacity of patients with implant-retained prosthesis. However, when compared to complete dentures, patients will still often rate their implant overdentures higher in terms of functional capacity, general satisfaction, and prosthesis stability regardless of the residual bone height [15].

11.2.3 Surgical Considerations

A considerable amount of surgical and restorative concepts currently used in designing implant overdentures are derived from the experience of clinicians with tooth-borne overdentures. Historically, the canine sites were selected as the first choice for implant placement in the case of implant-retained overdentures (Fig. 11.5). This is often due to the common retention of canine teeth for tooth-borne overdentures. As we discussed previously, the placement of implants in the canine position will establish for the most part an anteroposterior cantilever. This is highly dependent on the shape of the edentulous ridge and the position of the prosthetic teeth. In fact, "V-shaped" jaw forms will be more prone to establishing an anterior cantilever when compared to a "U-shaped" ridge.

The occluso-gingival displacement of the denture in the posterior quadrants is generally better tolerated by patients due to the support provided by the primary and secondary bearing areas. However, the anterior displacement that may result as we push on the lower incisors will create a tipping effect that is poorly resisted by the vestibular tissues. The posterior lifting will be amplified, as the rotation axis established by the two implants is located further from the anterior teeth. This situation can be improved by the addition of a third implant that will act as an indirect retainer. This implant should be placed most anteriorly to create a tripod in the anterior quadrant that would improve denture stability as well as retention [16] (Fig. 11.6). Moreover, the accelerated wear of the attachment is prevented with the previous parameters improved.

An alternative to the placement of a third implant would be to consider the lateral sites instead of the canines (Fig. 11.7). This will be favorable for patients with a V-shaped jaw, as it would limit the anterior cantilever. Positioning implants in the most anterior position will also open the possibility of adding two implants in

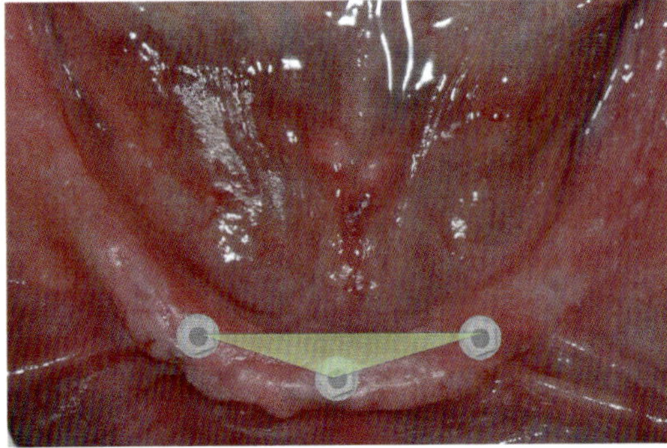

Fig. 11.6 Implant placement in canine sites with the addition of an anterior implant creating a tripod and acting as an indirect retainer

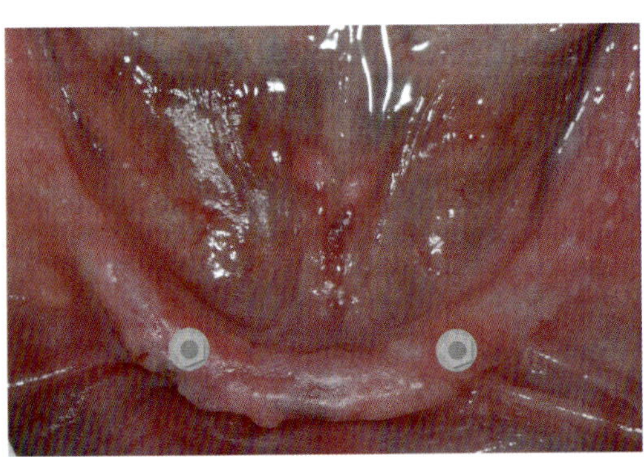

Fig. 11.5 Implant placement in canine sites for implant-retained mandibular dentures

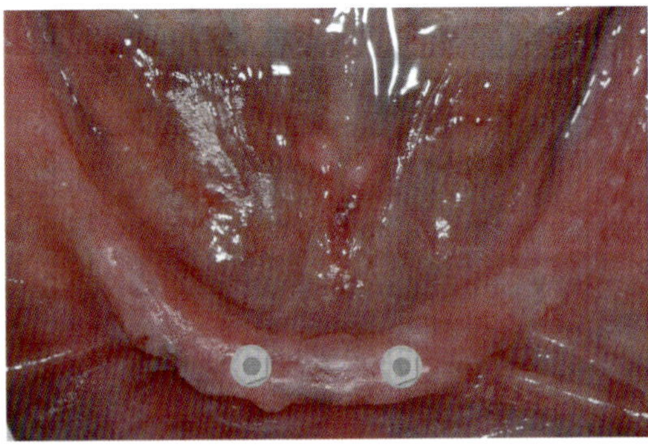

Fig. 11.7 Implant placement in lateral sites for implant-retained mandibular dentures

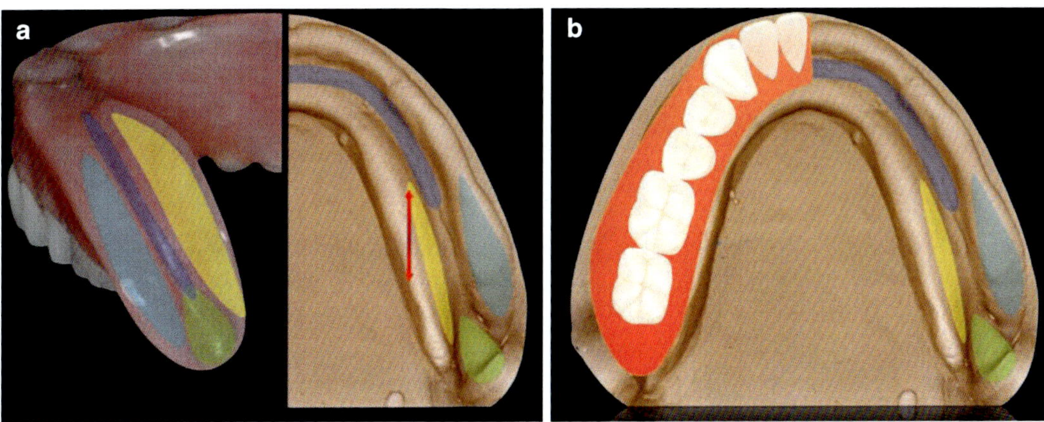

Fig. 11.8 (**a, b**) Design principles of complete dentures for the mandible illustrating key anatomical factors involved in establishing appropriate extensions for support, retention, and stability of the prosthesis

the premolar sites that would allow patients to change the prosthetic design to implant-supported prosthesis should they want to improve the retention and stability of their denture at a later date.

Emami et al. reviewed these surgical principles in 2015 by evaluating a group of 135 participants that received three implants and single-unit attachments. Only 20% of participants were aware of rotational movement of their overdentures. For these patients, awareness of rotational movements was correlated to a decrease in stability, comfort, ability to chew, and general satisfaction. The results were independent of the type of attachments and implants used [17].

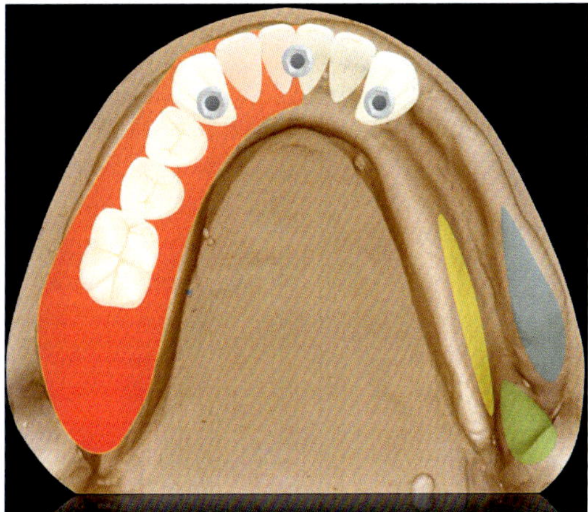

Fig. 11.9 Design principles of implant-retained mandibular dentures, the addition of an implant in the anterior sextant acting as an indirect retainer

11.2.4 Prosthetic Considerations

A significant amount of design concepts for implant overdentures have been historically derived from the complete denture philosophies (Fig. 11.8). The importance of proper denture extensions and coverage in order to optimize the support, stability, and retention of lower dentures has been reported [14].

Denture teeth are generally positioned in a similar location as the patients' natural teeth. Often, this will result with the anterior teeth positioned anterior to the alveolar ridge and closer to the vestibular area, which is located

anterior to the fulcrum line formed between the two mandibular implants. Based on findings by Kimoto et al., this will create a rotational movement of the implant overdenture when incising on the anterior teeth. This movement will increase as the distance between the tip of the anterior teeth and the anterior denture border increases [13]. The presence of a third implant providing added support can minimize this movement by acting as an indirect retainer as described earlier (Fig. 11.9).

Alternatively, contrary to the prosthodontic rationale mentioned above, limiting the position of the anterior teeth to the area above the ridge is

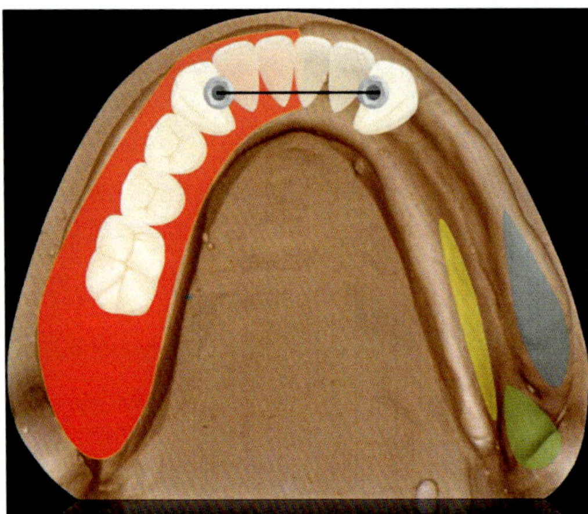

Fig. 11.10 Placement of the anterior teeth above the ridge will help diminish the anterior cantilever in cases where two implants are placed for mandibular implant-retained prosthesis

recommended to minimize the magnitude of the forward rotation when foods are incised. Moreover, limiting the posterior dentition to the first molar for implant-retained prosthesis can further assist in restricting the lifting motion of the denture during the consumption of sticky foods (Fig. 11.10). This can be challenging in certain conditions, particularly for patients with a class II skeletal relationship.

Denture rotation has been reported to negatively affect the perceived chewing ability of patients. Although patients who experience rotation may still be generally satisfied with their prosthesis, the reduction in their ability to chew is important, because they may not be benefiting from the full potential of this treatment.

11.2.5 Attachment Mechanism

11.2.5.1 Definitions

Attachments are manufactured in a large variety of designs and are compatible with most of the implant systems commercially available today. The attachment systems for implant-retained overdentures can be classified as bar or stud types. The first type employs plastic or metal clips in the denture base engaging a metal bar connected to the implants. Stud types include ball-socket or magnetic mechanisms.

11.2.5.2 Bar-Type Attachments

The majority of bar-type attachment systems consist of a metallic bar connected to the implant and a clip mechanism nested in the denture base. Most of the retentive bars are often distinguished by the morphological characteristics of their walls and their composition. Based on the latter, bars can be characterized as resilient or non-resilient. Resilient (round) bars are designed to allow movement around their axis and are often recommended for the restoration of implant-retained prosthesis in order to accommodate the movement of the denture during mastication. The non-resilient designs are often recommended for implant-supported prosthesis. They are characterized by parallel walls that once engaged by the clip assembly, limit significantly the movement of the dentures (Fig. 11.1a).

11.2.5.3 Stud-Type Attachments

A multitude of stud-type attachment systems are available today to provide retention and stability for the mandibular complete denture. The majority of attachment systems consist of a male part connected to the implant and a female part nested in the denture base. Most of these attachments are often distinguished by the morphological differences between their male and female components.

The male parts often show variations in their morphology and composition. Some attachments have a spherical shape with extracoronal retentive portion (Fig. 11.11). Other attachments rely solely on the internal retentive cavity in which the retention element is inserted. Recent systems comprise of both extra- and intracoronal retentive characteristics (Fig. 11.12).

The female parts are often categorized according to their retention mechanism. Three different types are generally recognized:

1. O-ring anchors: These female attachments include a metal housing containing a rubber band that engages the male component.
2. Metallic anchors: These female attachments include a metal housing often containing a

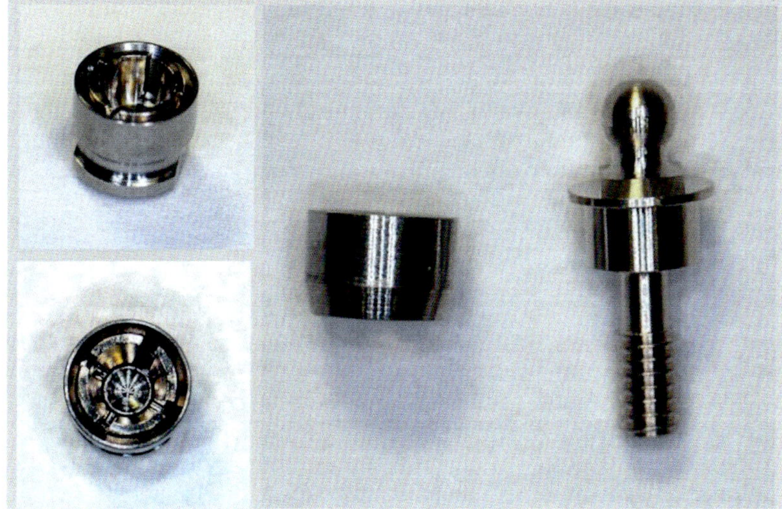

Fig. 11.11 Stud-type attachment system with a spherical-shaped extracoronal male component and a female part comprised of a metal retentive mechanism in a metallic housing

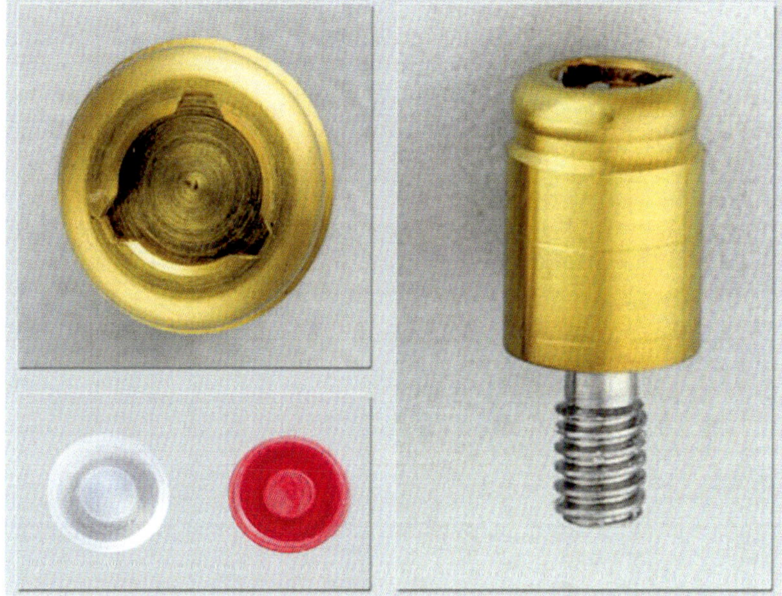

Fig. 11.12 Stud-type attachment system with a cylindrical-shaped male component displaying both extra- and intracoronal retentive characteristics and a female part comprised of nylon inserts in a metallic housing

metallic mechanism that engages the male component. The retention is often due to the friction between the two elements. Companies that offer this design often provide a key to adjust the level of the retention provided by female component (Fig. 11.11).

3. Nonmetallic anchors: These female attachments may or may not include a metal housing containing a nonmetallic insert that engages the male component. The retention is often the result of the friction between the insert and the retentive surfaces of the attachment (Fig. 11.12).

11.2.5.4 Retention Characteristics

The retention of stud-type attachments can be defined as the maximum amount of force required to separate the male component from the female component [18]. Retention forces of most attachment systems have been reported to be in the range of 17–30 N for bars, 7–28 N for stud attachments, and 1–9 N for magnets [19–22]. The values of the initial retention not only vary significantly between attachment systems but also within the same system. This variability is often associated with a host of morphological characteristics. Physical features such as the parallelism of the walls, number of resistive surfaces, and presence of undercuts have been related to the variation in retentive capabilities of an attachment system [23, 24].

The resiliency of the female retentive element also plays a role in the final value of the retention of the prosthetic attachment assembly. Several systems provide a variety of inserts with different retention forces. These inserts vary in their ability to deform upon removal. Essentialy, a stiffer insert will often provide more resistance to dislodgment during removal.

Lehmann et al. reported that a value of only 7 newton is needed to retain prosthesis during function [25]. However, patients seem to prefer prostheses that offer a degree of greater retention and stability [22]. A positive correlation between retentive values and stability, patient preference, quality of life has been established by several authors [7, 19, 26].

11.2.5.5 Wear Behavior of Attachments

In the oral cavity, attachment systems are exposed to continuous mechanical stimuli and thermal variations, which may ultimately lead to a loss of their retentive capacity. This degradation can be the result of the manipulation of the prosthesis by the patient, including insertion and retraction, distortion related to mastication [27], and deterioration following the cleaning of the prosthetic elements [28, 29].

Different angulations of the implants could also influence the wear behavior of attachments. Attachments placed on parallel implants are less suscetible to retention loss when compared to those on fixtures with excessive angulations. Jabbour et al. reported that implant angulations influenced the loss of retention of the Locator after 1 year of clinical use [30].

Several studies have attempted to explain the wear characteristics of attachment systems. Stud-type attachments tend to exhibit gradual and continuous loss of retention associated with repeated insertion-removal of the prosthesis [31, 32].

Depending on the morphological characteristics of the system, the loss is often abrupt and can sometimes reach 60–80% of their initial value [32]. This is often the result of structural changes in both the patrix and matrix over time [33, 34]. In contrast, it was found that bar attachments are less susceptible to this type of wear [35].

Implant-retained overdentures are also exposed to wear due to the movement of the denture during mastication. Only a limited amount of studies assessed the wear behavior of single unsplinted attachments simulating the movement patterns of the mandibular prosthesis during mastication. Abi Nader et al. assessed in vitro the effect of simulated mastication on the retention of two stud attachment systems for two-implant overdentures. The loss of retention after approximately 1 year of simulated function was reported to reach up to 60% of the initial value of the tested attachments [27].

11.3 Implant-Supported Mandibular Dentures

11.3.1 Definitions

Implant-supported prostheses are generally fully sustained by dental implants. They are frequently classified as fixed (Fig. 11.13) or removable (Fig. 11.14) appliances [36]. They are generally characterized by a higher number of implants that ensure the majority of the support for the lower denture. The number and location of the implants are highly dependent on the type of

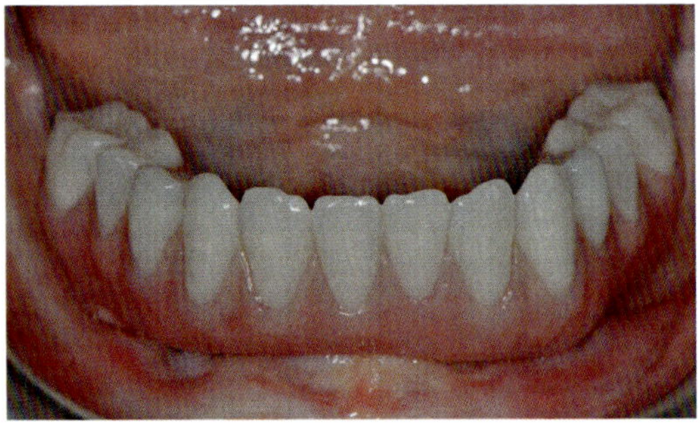

Fig. 11.13 Implant-supported fixed mandibular denture

prosthesis as well as the available bone volume. Implants can be distributed equally in the mandibular arch (Fig. 11.15) or located in the anterior region of the mandible (Fig. 11.15). The latter is often a common occurrence due to the alveolar resorption and the anatomical limitations present in the posterior quadrants. This prosthetic design offers superior anchorage and an improvement in retention when compared to the implant-retained overdentures.

11.3.2 Surgical Considerations

A minimum of four implants is generally recommended for implant-supported mandibular dentures. Some studies suggest that the placement of three implants may be sufficient [37, 38]. However, more favorable results have been reported with the use of four dental implants for this prosthetic design [39]. In fact, as a general guideline, it is often agreed that the length of the prosthetic distal cantilever should not exceed 1.5 times the anterior-posterior (A-P) distance between the corresponding implants. Therefore, a proper distribution in the anterior zone maximizing the anterior-posterior spread of the implants (Fig. 11.16) is essential to allow for an appropriate design.

This may be challenging in certain conditions due to the presence of an anterior loop of the inferior alveolar nerve, as it exists the mental foramen. In fact, Apostolakis and Brown in 2012 [40] reported the presence of a 3-mm (or smaller) anterior loop in 95% of the 93 cases assessed. Some clinical reports suggest that in certain situations, distally tilting the two posterior implants may allow to increase the anterior-posterior spread as well as avoid the nerve (Fig. 11.17). This will optimize the distribution of the implants and minimize the distal cantilever when designing this type of prosthesis [41].

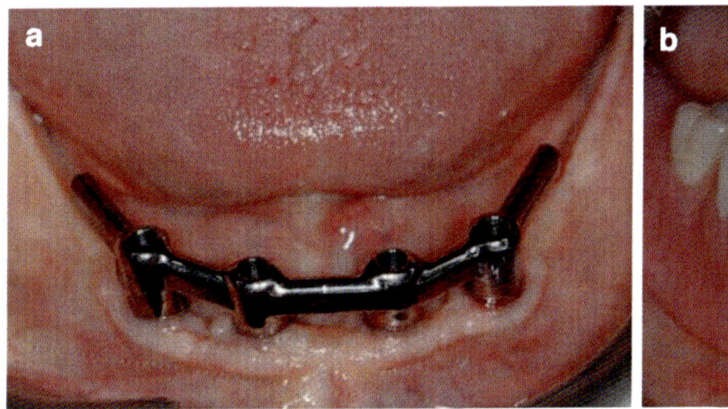
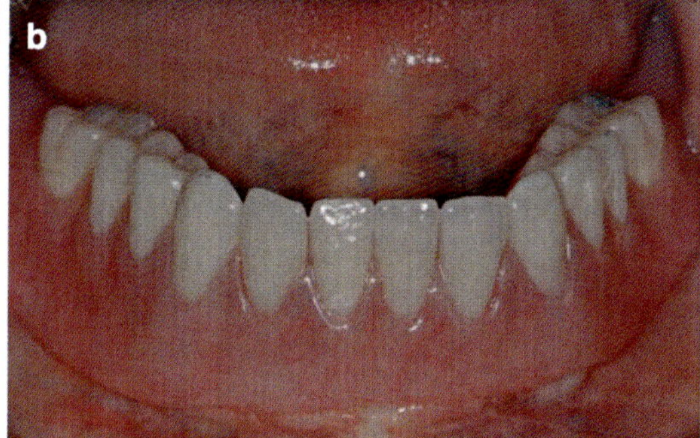

Fig. 11.14 Implant-supported removable mandibular denture (**a**) Dolder bar secured to the mandibular implants (**b**) Removable mandibular denture connected to the Dolder bar

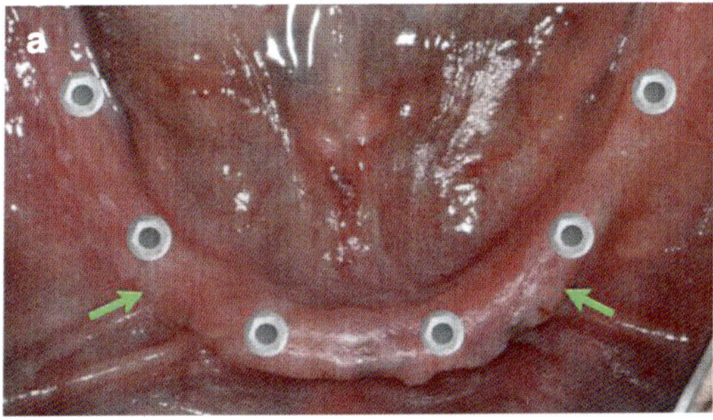
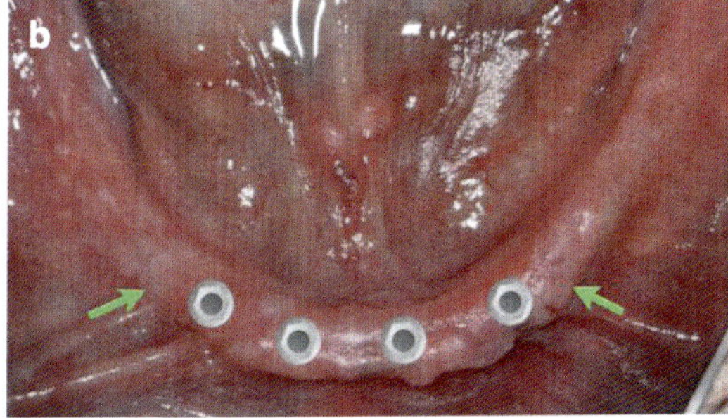

Fig. 11.15 Surgical strategies for implant-supported mandibular prostheses (**a**) Six implants evenly distributed (**b**) Four implants limited to the anterior sextant

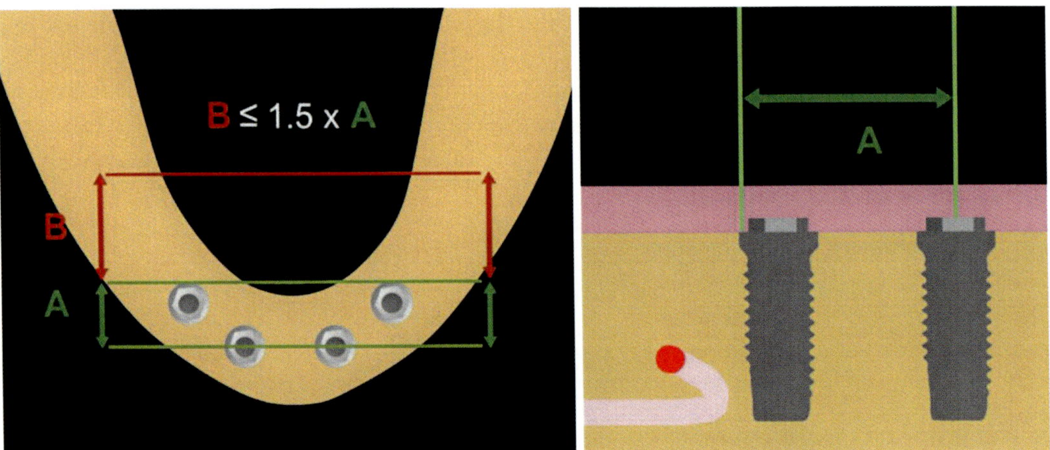

Fig. 11.16 Anterior-posterior spread of the mandibular implants for an implant-supported fixed mandibular denture and the corresponding prosthetic design characteristics

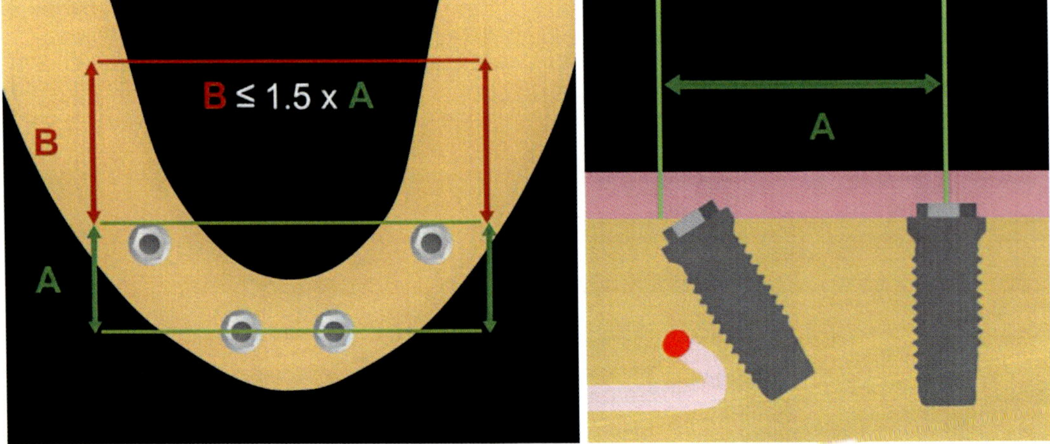

Fig. 11.17 Inclining the distal implants increases the anterior-posterior spread allowing to extend the distal cantilever

11.3.3 Prosthetic Considerations

The design principles of the implant-supported removable and fixed prosthesis are centered on creating a singular prosthesis that is sustained in the anterior area by four implants and suspended over the posterior ridges by a cantilever. This is often the case due to the anatomical limitations discussed earlier. Therefore, cantilevers serve an important role as an adjunct treatment in helping to overcome these anatomical restrictions and maintain a functional occlusal table. There are several design rules in relation to the geometry of this prosthetic restoration and the implant locations that have been reported in the literature. Rangert et al. have defined most of the guidelines in 1989 regarding implant positions and their anterior-posterior (A-P) spread [42]. A-P spread is defined as the distance measured from the center of the most anterior implant to the distal aspect of the most distal implant (Figs. 11.16 and 11.17). It was concluded that implants should have a spread of at least 10 mm along the curve of the arch and that the bone quality of the mandible would allow a cantilever of about 15–20 mm. In fact, as a general guideline, it is often agreed that the length of the prosthetic distal cantilever should not exceed 1.5 times the anterior-posterior (A-P) distance between the corresponding implants. These biomechanical principles for the lower implant-supported prosthesis have been recommended in order to prevent biological and prosthetic complications. A systematic review conducted by Romeo and Storelli in 2012 concluded that there was no increase in complication rate due to the presence of a cantilever extension. The cumulative survival rate of implants supporting cantilevered prosthesis is 98.9%, and the prosthesis itself had a survival estimated at 97.1% after 5 years [43].

Fixed and removable implant-supported complete dentures provide several advantages in comparison to an implant-retained removable prosthesis. They offer better retention by having the prosthesis fully secured in place resulting in higher biting forces and better chewing efficiency [44]. They also provide minimal tissue coverage and no movement during function. This can be very benefiting for patients suffering from a reduced salivary flow. The absence of contact with tissues and the stability of these prostheses minimize the rubbing effect of the resin that may cause ulceration and discomfort.

For the elderly patient, fixed implant supported prostheses can be less appealing for a variety of reasons. Implant-supported prostheses are generally more costly to fabricate when compared to implant-retained prosthesis [11]. Technical complications occur continuously over time as a result of fatigue [45] and can represent a significant source of cost in terms of after care and maintenance when compared to the implant-retained prosthesis [46]. The hygienic maintenance of this type of prosthesis is also considered more challenging. Plaque often accumulates on the fitting surface of the denture in proximity to the soft tissues [47] and would require a daily maintenance routine. This could be challenging for elderly patients with limited manual dexterities. Moreover, from an esthetic perspective, it is more difficult to restore atrophied ridges with the absence of prosthetic flanges due to the possible compromise that this may have on their lip support. Phonetics presents an additional concern with airway leakage. However, these concerns are more relevant for the maxillary prosthesis and are often well managed in the mandibular arch.

11.4 Space Requirements for Implant Prosthesis

Implant-assisted prostheses have different restorative space requirements. This can often vary widely depending on the type of prosthesis planned as well as the type of attachments utilized. Several authors have reported on the different space requirements. The interocclusal space required is generally measured from the soft tissue ridge to the opposing dentition or surface of occlusion. Swadosky and Hansen [48] reported that implant prostheses retained by Locator attachments require 8–9 mm, bar overdentures require from 10 to 12 mm, and fixed complete dental prostheses require 12–15 mm. These are general guidelines and may vary depending on the height of the stud attachments used, the design of the retentive bar, and the materials selected for the fixed implant-supported prosthesis. In order to properly assess the restorative space available, a prosthetically driven treatment plan should be performed. A definitive denture or denture-teeth setup is critical to measure the available space and avoid diagnostic errors. Moreover, implant position should be planned based on the selected definitive prosthetic plan and anticipated design of the final prosthesis (Fig. 11.18).

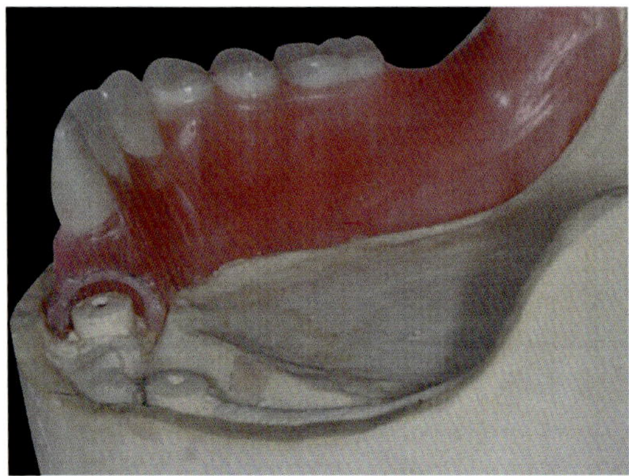

Fig. 11.18 A sagittal view of a denture-teeth setup for a planned implant-retained mandibular denture illustrating the available restorative space as well as the implant position

Conclusion

Mandibular implant-assisted prostheses can offer tremendous advantages to the denture wearer. Appropriate case selection and planning, strategic implant positioning as well as suitable prosthetic designs are some of the essential parameters required to ensure the successful outcome of these treatments. The next three chapters will detail the surgical and prosthetic guidelines recommended for the fabrication of implant-retained as well as implant-supported fixed and removable prostheses.

References

1. Atwood DA. Reduction of residual ridges: a major oral disease entity. J Prosthet Dent. 1971;26(3):266–79.
2. Tallgren A. Alveolar bone loss in denture wearers as related to facial morphology. Acta Odontol Scand. 1970;28(2):251–70.
3. Attard NJ, Zarb GA. Long-term treatment outcomes in edentulous patients with implant-fixed prostheses: the Toronto study. Int J Prosthodont. 2004;17(4):417–24.
4. Feine JS, Carlsson GE, Awad MA, Chehade A, Duncan WJ, Gizani S, et al. The McGill consensus statement on overdentures. Mandibular two-implant overdentures as first choice standard of care for edentulous patients. Gerodontology. 2002;19:3–4.
5. Thomason JM, Feine J, Exley C, Moynihan P, MEuller F, Naert I, Ellis JS, Barclay C, Butterworth C, Scott B, Lynch C, Stewardson D, Smith P, Welfare R, Hyde P, McAndrew R, Fenlon M, Barclay S, Barker
6. D. Mandibular two implant-supported overdentures as the first choice standard of care for edentulous patients–the York consensus statement. Br Dent J. 2009;207:185–6.
7. Thomason JM, Kelly SA, Bendkowski A, Ellis JS. Two implant retained overdentures—a review of the literature supporting the McGill and York consensus statements. J Dent. 2012;40:22–34.
8. Naert I, Alsaadi G, van Steenberghe D, Quirynen M. A 10-year randomized clinical trial on the influence of splinted and unsplinted oral implants retaining mandibular overdentures: peri-implant outcome. Int J Oral Maxillofac Implants. 2004;19(5):695–702.
9. Thomason JM, Lund JP, Chehade A, Feine JS. Patient satisfaction with mandibular implant overdentures and conventional dentures 6 months after delivery. Int J Prosthodont. 2003;16:467–73.
10. Raghoebar GM, Meijer HJ, Stegenga B, van't Hof MA, van Oort RP, Vissink A. Effectiveness of three treatment modalities for the edentulous mandible. A five-year randomized clinical trial. Clin Oral Implants Res. 2000;11:195–201.
11. Kordatzis K, Wright PS, Meijer HJ. Posterior mandibular residual ridge resorption in patients with conventional dentures and implant overdentures. Int J Oral Maxillofac Implants. 2003;18:447–52.
12. Attard N, Wei X, Laporte A, Zarb GA, Ungar WJ. A cost minimization analysis of implant treatment in mandibular edentulous patients. Int J Prosthodont. 2003;16(3):271–6.
13. Naert I, Quirynen M, Theuniers G, van Steenberghe D. Prosthetic aspects of osseointegrated fixtures supporting overdentures. A 4-year report. J Prosthet Dent. 1991;65(5):671–80.
14. Kimoto S, Pan S, Drolet N, Feine JS. Rotational movements of mandibular two-implant overdentures. Clin Oral Implants Res. 2009;20(8):838–43.
15. Critchlow SB, Ellis JS. Prognostic indicators for conventional complete denture therapy: a review of the literature. J Dent. 2010;38(1):2–9.
16. Awad MA, Lund JP, Dufresne E, Feine JS. Comparing the efficacy of mandibular implant retained overdentures and conventional dentures among middle-aged edentulous patients: satisfaction and functional assessment. Int J Prosthodont. 2003;16(2):117–22.
17. Oda K, Kanazawa M, Takeshita S, Minakuchi S. Influence of implant number on the movement of mandibular implant overdentures. J Prosthet Dent. 2017;117(3):380–5.
18. Emami E, de Souza RF, Bernier J, Rompré P, Feine JS. Patient perceptions of the mandibular three-implant overdenture: a practice-based study. Clin Oral Implants Res. 2015;26(6):639–43.
19. Petropoulos VC, Smith W. Maximum dislodging forces of implant overdenture stud attachments. Int J Oral Maxillofac Implants. 2002;17:526–35.
20. Burns DR, Unger JW, Elswick RK Jr, Beck DA. Prospective clinical evaluation of mandibular implant overdentures: Part I: retention, stability, and tissue response. J Prosthet Dent. 1995;73(4):354–63.

20. Petropoulos VC, Smith W, Kousvelari E. Comparison of retention and release periods for implant overdenture attachments. Int J Oral Maxillofac Implants. 1997;12(2):176–85.
21. Van Kampen F, Cune M, van der Bilt A, Bosman F. Retention and postinsertion maintenance of bar-clip, ball and magnet attachments in mandibular implant overdenture treatment: an in vivo comparison after 3 months of function. Clin Oral Implants Res. 2003;14(6):720–6.
22. Naert I, Gizani S, Vuylsteke M, Van Steenberghe D. A 5-year prospective randomized clinical trial on the influence of splinted and unsplinted oral implants retaining a mandibular overdenture: prosthetic aspects and patient satisfaction. J Oral Rehabil. 1999;26(3):195–202.
23. Chung KH, Chung CY, Cagna DR, Cronin RJ Jr. Retention characteristics of attachment systems for implant overdentures. J Prosthodont. 2004;13:221–6.
24. Leung T, Preiskel HW. Retention profiles of stud-type precision attachments. Int J Prosthodont. 1991;4(2):175–9.
25. Lehmann KM, Arnim FV. Studies on the retention forces of snap-on attachments. Quintessence Dent Technol. 1978;7:45–8.
26. Geckili O, Cilingir A, Erdogan O, Kesoglu AC, Bilmenoglu C, Ozdiler A, Bilhan H. The influence of momentary retention forces on patient satisfaction and quality of life of two-implant-retained mandibular overdenture wearers. Int J Oral Maxillofac Implants. 2015;30(2):397–402.
27. Abi Nader S, de Souza RF, Fortin D, De Koninck L, Fromentin O, Albuquerque Junior RF. Effect of simulated masticatory loading on the retention of stud attachments for implant overdentures. J Oral Rehabil. 2011;38(3):157–64.
28. Nguyen CT, Masri R, Driscoll CF, Romberg E. The effect of denture cleansing solutions on the retention of pink locator attachments: an in vitro study. J Prosthodont. 2010;19(3):226–30.
29. You W, Masri R, Romberg E, Driscoll CF, You T. The effect of denture cleansing solutions on the retention of pink locator attachments after multiple pulls: an in vitro study. J Prosthodont. 2011;20(6):464–9.
30. Jabbour Z, Fromentin O, Lassauzay C, Abi Nader S, Correa JA, Feine J, de Albuquerque Junior RF. Effect of implant angulation on attachment retention in mandibular two-implant overdentures: a clinical study. Clin Implant Dent Relat Res. 2014;16(4):565–71.
31. Fromentin O, Picard B, Tavernier B. In vitro study of the retention and mechanical fatigue behavior of four implant overdenture stud-type attachments. Pract Periodontics Aesthet Dent. 1999;11:391–7.
32. Gamborena JI, Hazelton LR, NaBadalung D, Brudvik J. Retention of ERA direct overdenture attachments before and after fatigue loading. Int J Prosthodont. 1997;10:123–30.
33. Fromentin O, Lassauzay C, Nader SA, Feine J, de Albuquerque RF Jr. Wear of matrix overdenture attachments after one to eight years of clinical use. J Prosthet Dent. 2012;107(3):191–8.
34. Fromentin O, Lassauzay C, Nader SA, Feine J, de Albuquerque RF Jr. Wear of ball attachments after 1 to 8 years of clinical use: a qualitative analysis. Int J Prosthodont. 2011;24(3):270–2.
35. Pigozzo MN, Mesquita MF, Henriques GE, Vaz LG. The service life of implant-retained overdenture attachment systems. J Prosthet Dent. 2009;102(2):74–80.
36. Emami E, Michaud PL, Sallaleh I, Feine JS. Implant-assisted complete prostheses. Periodontol 2000. 2014;66(1):119–31.
37. Brånemark PI, Engstrand P, Ohrnell LO, Gröndahl K, Nilsson P, Hagberg K, Darle C, Lekholm U. Brånemark Novum: a new treatment concept for rehabilitation of the edentulous mandible. Preliminary results from a prospective clinical follow-up study. Clin Implant Dent Relat Res. 1999;1(1):2–16.
38. De Kok IJ, Chang KH, Lu TS, Cooper LF. Comparison of three-implant-supported fixed dentures and two-implant-retained overdentures in the edentulous mandible: a pilot study of treatment efficacy and patient satisfaction. Int J Oral Maxillofac Implants. 2011;26(2):415–26.
39. De Bruyn H, Kisch J, Collaert B, Lindén U, Nilner K, Dvärsäter L. Fixed mandibular restorations on three early-loaded regular platform Brånemark implants. Clin Implant Dent Relat Res. 2001;3(4):176–84.
40. Apostolakis D, Brown JE. The anterior loop of the inferior alveolar nerve: prevalence, measurement of its length and a recommendation for interforaminal implant installation based on cone beam CT imaging. Clin Oral Implants Res. 2012;23(9):1022–30.
41. Maló P, de Araújo Nobre M, Lopes A, Ferro A, Gravito I. All-on-4® treatment concept for the rehabilitation of the completely edentulous mandible: a 7-year clinical and 5-year radiographic retrospective case series with risk assessment for implant failure and marginal bone level. Clin Implant Dent Relat Res. 2015;(17 Suppl 2):e531–41.
42. Rangert B, Jemt T, Jörneus L. Forces and moments on Branemark implants. Int J Oral Maxillofac Implants. 1989;4(3):241–7.
43. Romeo E, Storelli S. Systematic review of the survival rate and the biological, technical, and aesthetic complications of fixed dental prostheses with cantilevers on implants reported in longitudinal studies with a mean of 5 years follow-up. Clin Oral Implants Res. 2012;(23 Suppl 6):39–49.
44. Elsyad MA, Hegazy SA, Hammouda NI, Al-Tonbary GY, Habib AA. Chewing efficiency and electromyographic activity of masseter muscle with three designs of implant-supported mandibular overdentures. A cross-over study. Clin Oral Implants Res. 2014;25(6):742–8.

45. Papaspyridakos P, Chen CJ, Chuang SK, Weber HP, Gallucci GO. A systematic review of biologic and technical complications with fixed implant rehabilitations for edentulous patients. Int J Oral Maxillofac Implants. 2012;27(1):102–10.
46. Attard NJ, Zarb GA, Laporte A. Long-term treatment costs associated with implant-supported mandibular prostheses in edentulous patients. Int J Prosthodont. 2005;18(2):117–23.
47. Abi Nader S, Eimar H, Momani M, Shang K, Daniel NG, Tamimi F. Plaque accumulation beneath maxillary All-on-4™ implant-supported prostheses. Clin Implant Dent Relat Res. 2015;17(5):932–7.
48. Sadowsky SJ, Hansen PW. Evidence-based criteria for differential treatment planning of implant restorations for the mandibular edentulous patient. J Prosthodont. 2014;23(2):104–11.

Case Presentation: Implant Retained Mandibular Prostheses

12

Samer Abi Nader and Samer Mesmar

Abstract

This chapter will present a clinical case describing the treatment of a lower edentulous patient with an implant-retained prosthesis. The surgical strategies underlining the placement and the distribution of the dental implants to optimize the prosthetic outcome will be highlighted and discussed. The various clinical and laboratory steps starting from the planning to the completion of the prostheses will be presented as well as the criteria for the selection of single attachments for this prosthetic design. This also includes the description and review of the various techniques available to connect the matrix component of the attachment to the denture base. The advantages of each technique will be discussed and their inconveniences highlighted.

Digital dentistry can present tremendous advantages for the elderly patient. This chapter will also present the various clinical steps and digital workflow involved in the fabrication of implant-retained mandibular complete dentures for the edentulous patient. The advantages and inconveniences related to the use of computer-aided design and manufacturing (CAD/CAM) in complete denture will be underlined.

12.1 Patient History and Background

A 62-year-old male patient presented with the following chief complaint: "I want new dentures, my lower denture is very loose and I can't eat properly." The patient's maxillary and mandibular teeth were extracted when he was in his early 30s because he was unable to afford replacement restorations. He was rendered completely edentulous by the age of 33.

He presented with a moderately resorbed mandible (Fig. 12.1) and is interested in improving the stability and retention of his lower prosthesis. He is content with the general performance of his maxillary removable complete denture but would like to improve the appearance. The maxillary arch presents with a mild alveolar ridge resorption (Fig. 12.2).

12.1.1 Medical History

- Hypertension: controlled with medication
- Allergic to penicillin
- No history of smoking or drug abuse

S. A. Nader, BSc, DMD, MSc, FRCD(C) (✉)
Department of Restorative Dentistry, Faculty of
Dentistry, McGill University, Montreal, QC, Canada
e-mail: samer.abinader@mcgill.ca

S. Mesmar, DMD, MSc, FRCD(C)
Division of Prosthodontics, McGill University Health
Centre, Montreal, QC, Canada

© Springer International Publishing AG, part of Springer Nature 2018
E. Emami, J. Feine (eds.), *Mandibular Implant Prostheses*,
https://doi.org/10.1007/978-3-319-71181-2_12

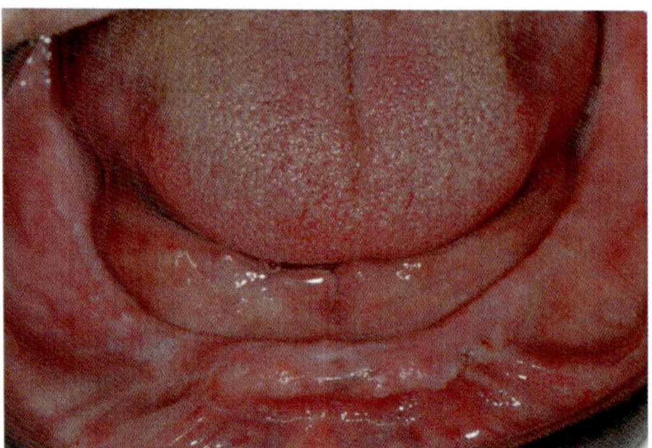

Fig. 12.1 Mandibular residual ridge

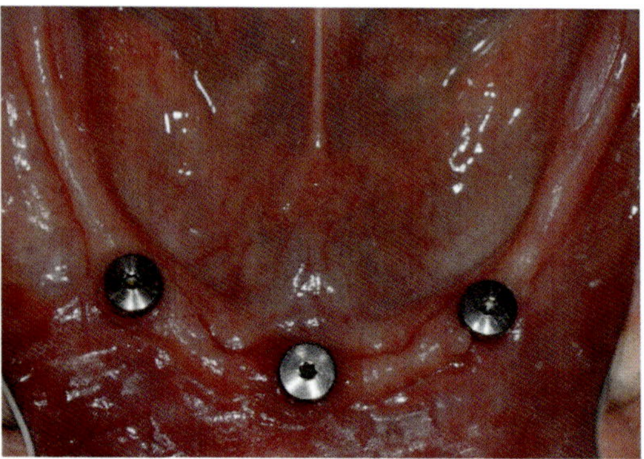

Fig. 12.3 Mandibular residual ridge following implant placement. Surgery: Dr. Veronique Benhamou, Periodontist

12.2 Implant Placement Strategy

Clinical assessment of the edentulous mandible reveals a wide U-shaped jaw with moderate resorption of the posterior ridges. A preliminary assessment was completed, and an implant-retained mandibular denture was recommended. Three dental implants (Straumann Soft Tissue Level Implants) were planned for placement in the anterior sextant to improve the support, retention, and stability of his lower prosthesis. The two posterior implants were placed in the most retruded position considering the anatomy and location of the alveolar nerve. The third implant was placed most anteriorly to optimize the distribution. This placement strategy was discussed in the previous chapter and should enhance the effect of the indirect retainer provided by the anterior implant. This will minimize the rotation of the lower denture during function and improve denture stability as well as retention (Fig. 12.3).

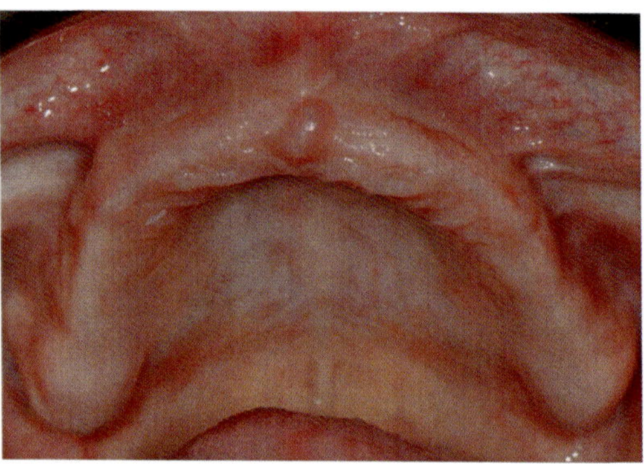

Fig. 12.2 Maxillary residual ridge

12.1.2 Dental History

– Multiple extractions
– Complete upper and lower dentures

12.1.3 Clinical Findings

– Complete edentulism
– Inadequate existing complete dentures
– Compromised chewing function
– "U-shaped" mandibular arch form

12.1.4 Diagnosis

– Complete upper and lower edentulism
– Moderate mandibular residual ridge resorption
– Moderate maxillary residual ridge resorption

12.3 Clinical Procedures

12.3.1 Preliminary Impressions of the Upper and Lower Arch

The clinical procedure starts with preliminary impressions of the maxillary and mandibular arches following implant placement and an adequate healing period to ensure proper osteo-integration. An irreversible hydrocolloid material (*Jeltrate Alginate, Dentsply Caulk, Canada*)

placed in stock edentulous metal trays *(Patterson Dental Supply, Canada)* is generally used for this step (Fig. 12.4a, b). Impressions are poured using type III dental stone *(GC America Inc., USA)* to produce preliminary casts (Fig. 12.5a, b) which will be used for custom tray fabrication.

12.3.2 Custom Tray Fabrication and Design

Customized trays are fabricated using a light cured acrylic material *(Triad TruTray, Dentsply, Canada)* following the basic principles of flange height reduction to allow room for border molding procedures (Fig. 12.6a, b). Custom trays are then tried intra-orally to verify extensions and fit (Fig. 12.7). Bolder

molding of the periphery is performed using dental compounds *(Kerr Dental, Canada)* (Fig. 12.8) and the manipulation of the patient's tissue to capture the muscles and soft tissue attachments.

12.3.3 Final Impressions of the Upper and Lower Arches

Final impressions are completed for the maxillary and mandibular arches by capturing the anatomical structure including the functional periphery, using polysulfide material *(Permlastic™, Kerr Dental)* (Fig. 12.9). Definitive casts are produced, and baseplates with wax rims are fabricated to register the appropriate clinical parameters.

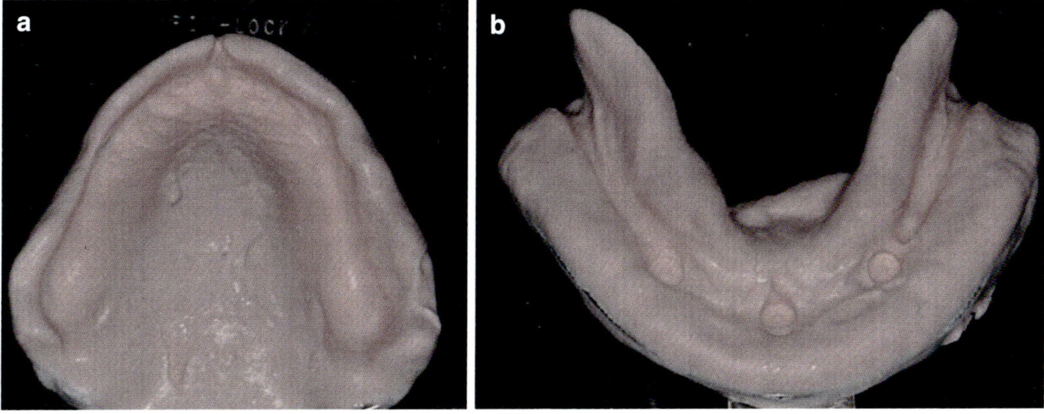

Fig. 12.4 (**a**) Irreversible hydrocolloid impressions of the maxillary and (**b**) mandibular arches

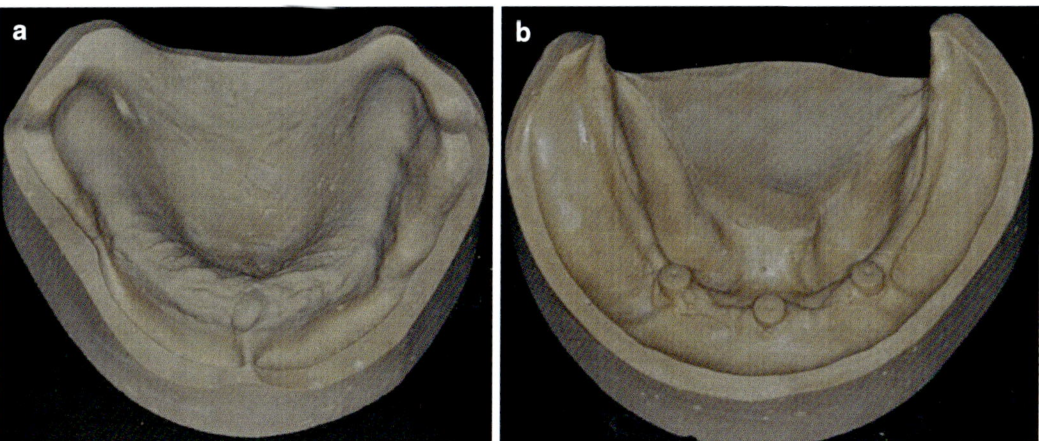

Fig. 12.5 (**a**) Preliminary cast of maxillary and (**b**) mandibular arches

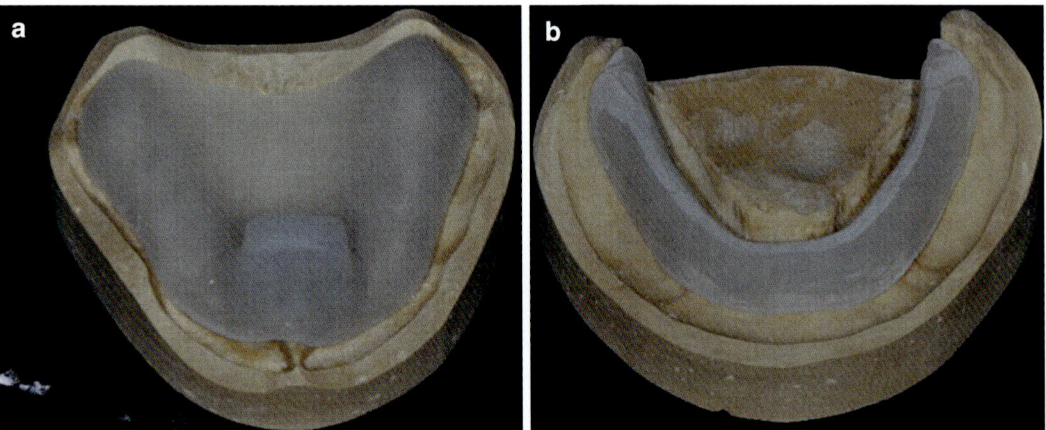

Fig. 12.6 (**a** and **b**) Design of the custom trays for final impressions

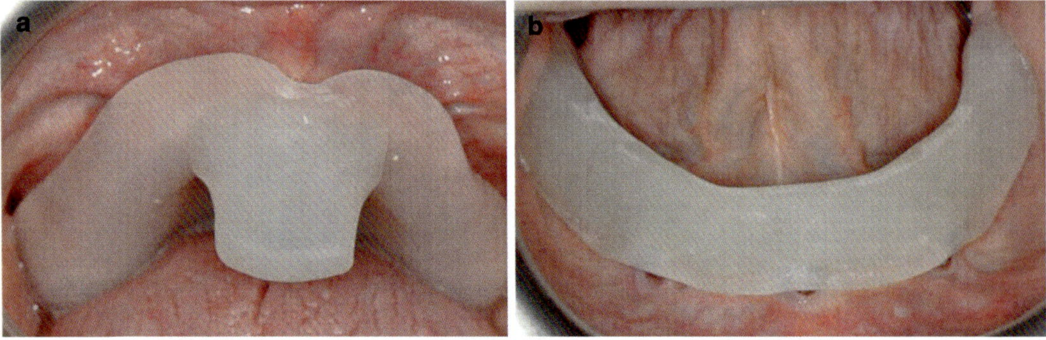

Fig. 12.7 (**a** and **b**) Try-in of the maxillary and mandibular custom trays prior to the border molding procedures

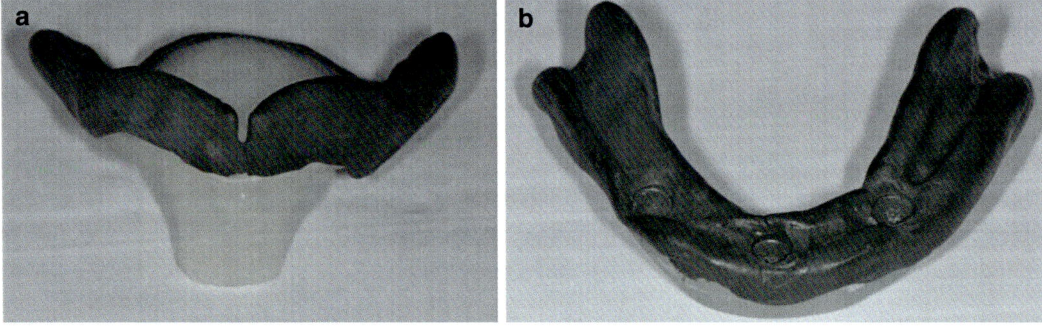

Fig. 12.8 (**a** and **b**) Border molding of the maxillary and mandibular arches using dental compound

12.3.4 Wax Rim Adjustments

Adjustments of occlusal wax rims start by determining the lip support, incisal display, and occlusal plane of the maxillary wax rim. Incisal display is determined by considering the age, gender, and preference of the patient. With age, the maxillary incisal teeth tend to be less apparent; this is more significant for men when compared to women [1]. Lip activity should also be taken into consideration. Some patients have a hypermobile lip that could result in excessive display during smile.

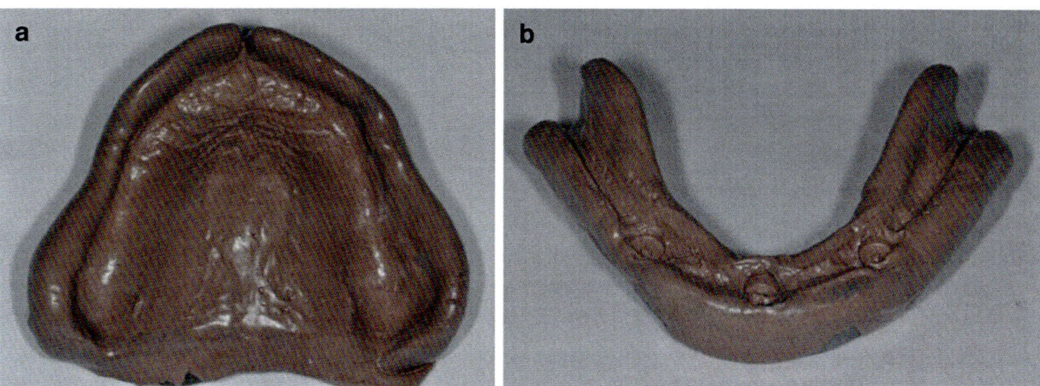

Fig. 12.9 (**a** and **b**) Final impression using polysulfide of the maxillary and mandibular arches

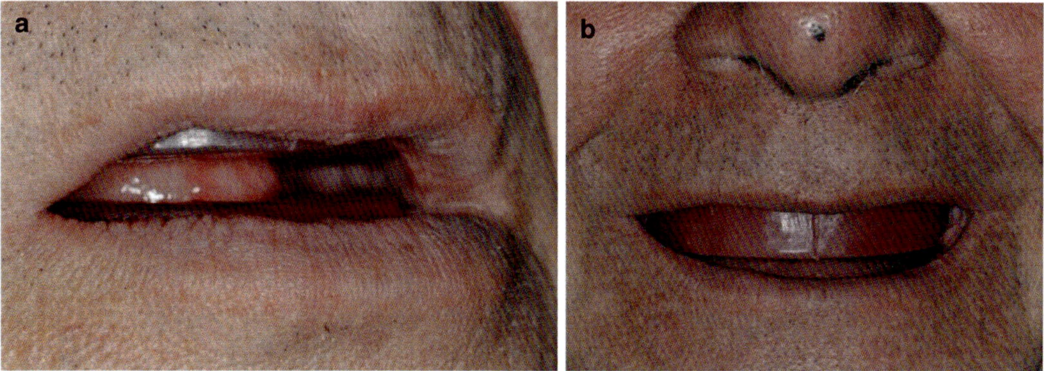

Fig. 12.10 Wax rim adjustments: (**a**) lip support and (**b**) esthetic and occlusal plane alignment

Once the display is determined, the midline and smile line are marked on the wax rim (Fig. 12.10).

The occlusal plane is adjusted to be parallel with the bi-pupillary and bi-commissural lines using the Fox Plane. In the posterior region, it should be parallel to camper plane joining the inferior border of the tragus of the ear to the infra-nasal angle.

Different methods have been described in the literature to determine the occlusal vertical dimension [2]. At this stage, the physiological rest position was used. This method starts by marking two reference points, one on the nose tip and the chin, in order to perform some measurements. The physiological rest position is then recorded using the phonetics approach by having the patient pronounce the labial *m* sound [3].

Once the physiological rest position measure is recorded, the occlusal vertical dimension is obtained by subtracting the interocclusal space. The interocclusal space can vary depending on numerous factors including gender, age, and Angle classification. Several authors estimate an average value of 2–4 mm being acceptable for most of patients [3, 4].

Maxillomandibular relationship is then recorded in centric relation using a fast-set bite registration material *(Jet Blue Bite registration material, Coltene Whaledent)*. The mandible can be guided into centric relation using patient- or dentist-mediated techniques. The recorded position is then verified for reproducibility (Fig. 12.11).

Finally, a facebow record is performed to position the maxillary cast and facilitate mounting on a semi-adjustable articulator. A maxillary positioning jig can also be used to mount the maxillary model within an average setting. This will often position the model within the triangle of Bonwill. All records are sent to the dental laboratory to have the casts mounted and denture teeth set per the determined clinical and anatomical parameters (Fig. 12.12). Balanced occlusion is often recommended for complete denture therapy, although very little clinical evidence is available to support the use of this occlusal scheme for complete dentures and implant-retained/implant-supported prosthesis.

12.3.5 The Trial Denture

As described previously, anterior denture teeth for implant-retained overdentures are generally placed over the attachments as much as possible to decrease cantilevering effect and rotational movement anterior to the fulcrum line drawn

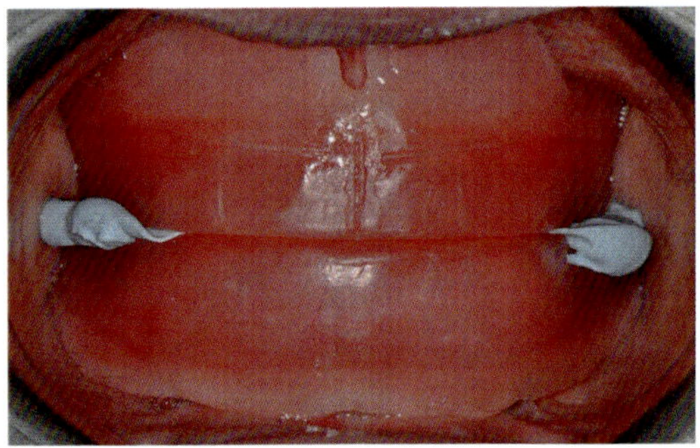

Fig. 12.11 Intermaxillary relationship recorded in centric relation using patient-mediated technique and bite registration material

between the implants [5] (Fig. 12.13). The addition of a third implant acting as an indirect retainer in this case greatly diminishes the rotational effect. Consequently, the stability of the denture is increased, and the accelerated wear of the nylon-retentive elements of the Locator attachment system is diminished.

The denture teeth setup is then tried clinically in order to evaluate the esthetics, phonetics, and occlusal stability (Figs. 12.14 and 12.15). Once all esthetic and occlusal parameters are verified and the patient is satisfied with the anticipated outcome, the case is sent back to the dental laboratory to start the acrylization process (Figs. 12.16 and 12.17).

12.3.6 Delivery of the Final Prostheses

12.3.6.1 Locator Attachment

The Locator is a resilient attachment that has a self-aligning feature with dual retention provided by both external and internal mating surfaces. The nylon component is resilient and provides the ability to pivot in any direction over the matrix, which accommodates for the natural movements of the denture base during occlusion and the pliancy of the supporting soft tissue. It provides a multitude of nylon inserts with a varying degree of retention and angulation versatility. In fact, the extended range matrices allow for insertion of the overdenture with up to 40° of divergence between implants.

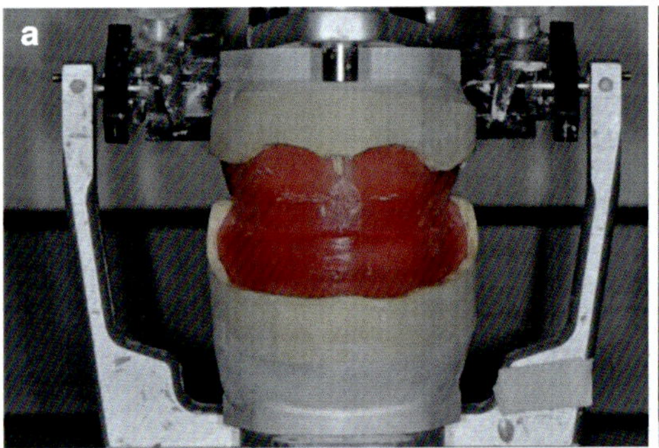
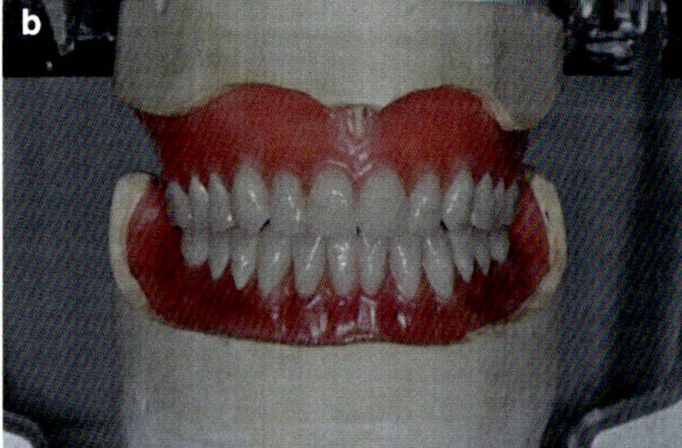

Fig. 12.12 (**a** and **b**) Mounting on semi-adjustable articulator and setting of denture teeth according to the determined parameters

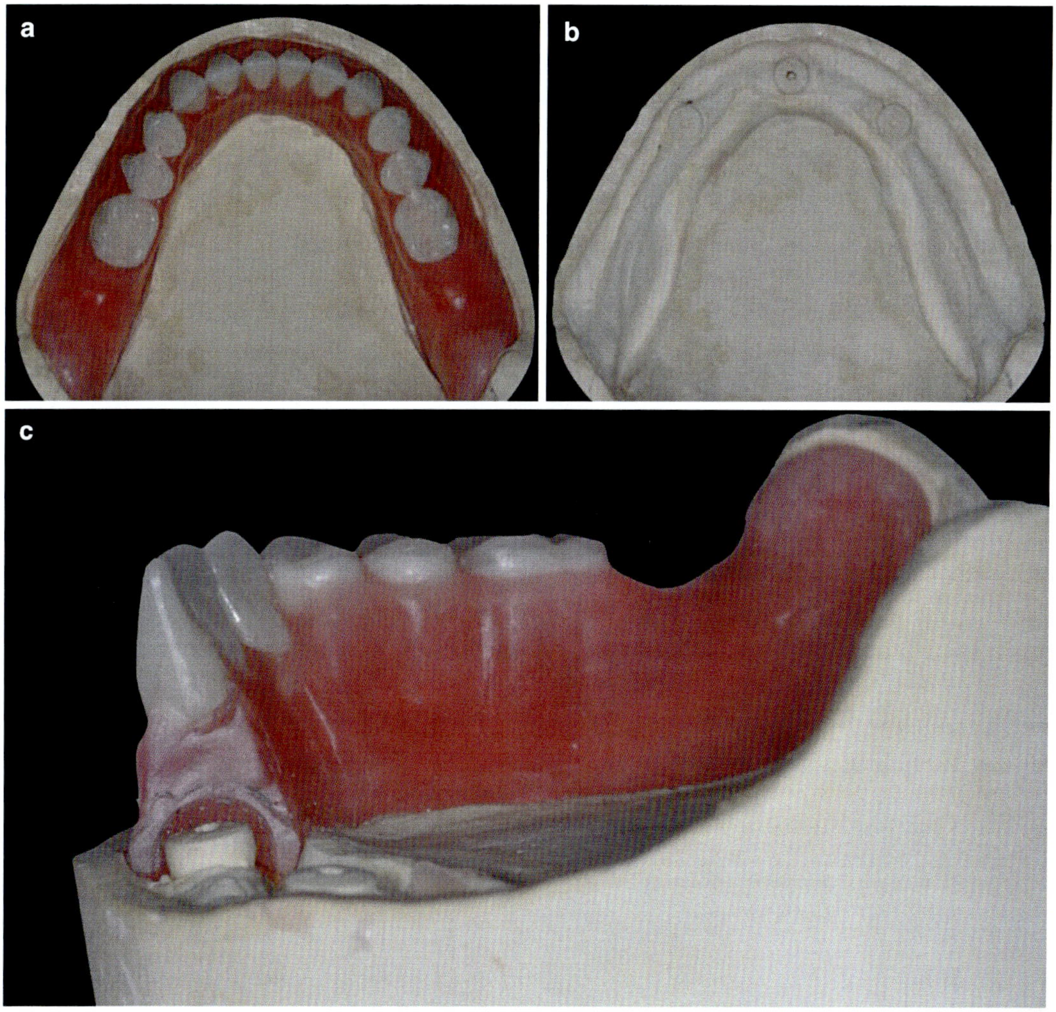

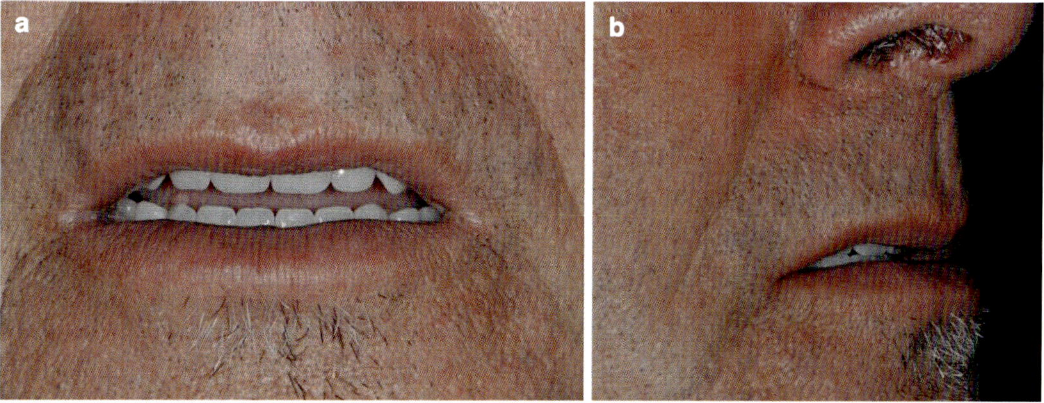

Fig. 12.13 (**a, b**) Occlusal view illustrating the denture teeth position. (**c**) Cross-sectional and lateral view demonstrating the position of anterior prosthetic teeth over the attachments as well as the effect of the third implant in minimizing the anterior cantilever

Fig. 12.14 (**a** and **b**) Denture teeth try-in to evaluate esthetics, phonetics, function, stability, and occlusal contacts during mandibular movements

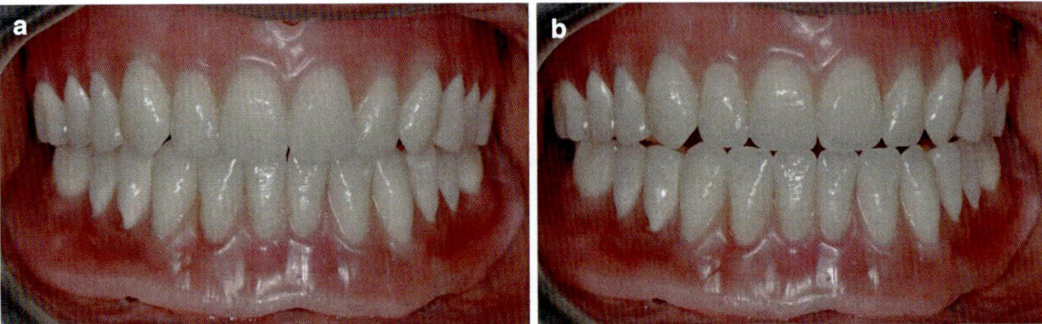

Fig. 12.15 (**a** and **b**) Verification of centric and occlusal scheme

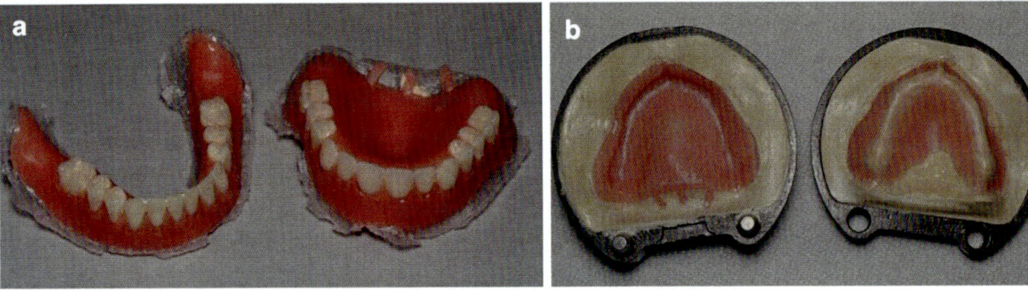

Fig. 12.16 (**a** and **b**) Conventional acrylization process

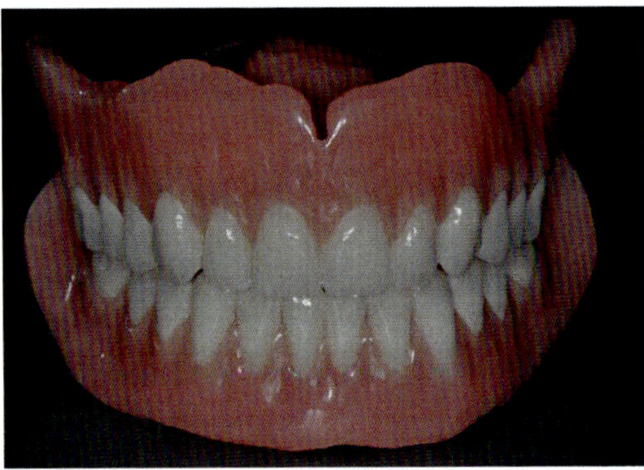

Fig. 12.17 Acrylized dentures ready for delivery

The Locator consists of a metal patrix made from a titanium alloy with TiN coating attached to the implant. The engaging component of the patrix is approximately 1.5 mm in length. The transmucosal cuff height varies depending on the soft tissue thickness. The total vertical height of the Locator attachment including the matrix and the engaging component of the patrix is only 3.17 mm (Fig. 12.18). Therefore, it requires minimal interocclusal space. It is a relatively durable system that has been widely and commonly used.

12.3.6.2 Selection Process

The selection process for the Locator attachment starts by determining the type of implant and diameter being used. Secondly, the soft tissue thickness is measured from the apical rim of the implant body to the highest contour of the gingiva (Fig. 12.19). The required height of the Locator abutment corresponds exactly to the soft tissue measurement described previously or is the next closest higher size available. The working engaging part of the attachment will be positioned supragingivally. Once the abutment is selected, it is attached to the implant using an abutment driver that engages the inside diameter of the Locator abutment. Final torque tightening of the abutment is performed using a torque wrench. To prevent screw loosening, follow the torque value recommended by the implant manufacturer according to the implant specifications.

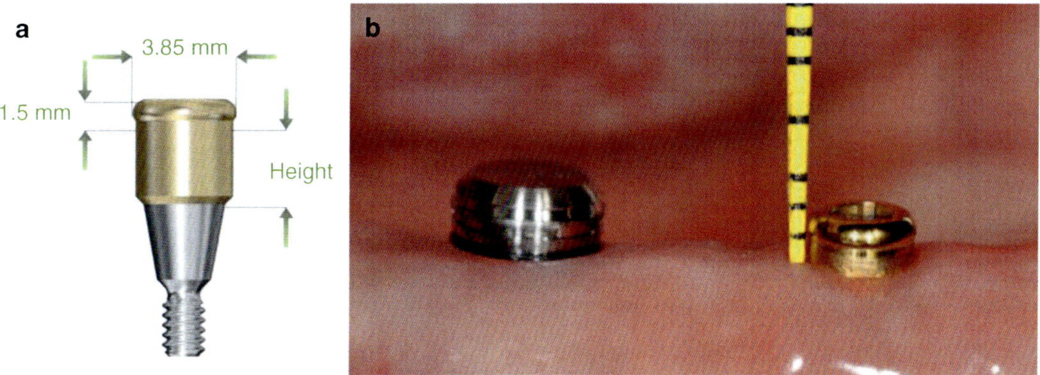

Fig. 12.18 (**a**) The Locator attachment and (**b**) height measurement of the patrix and the matrix

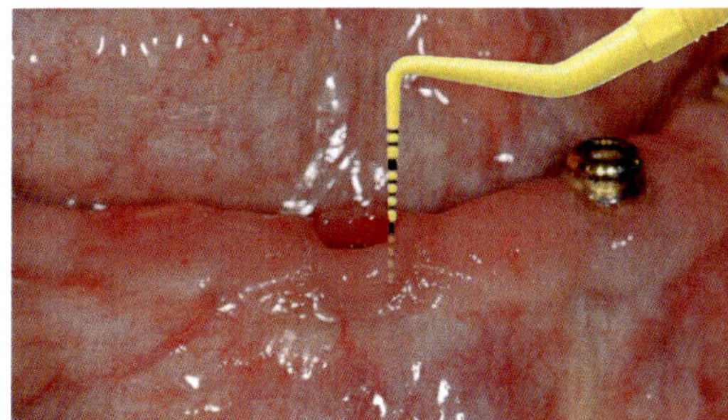

Fig. 12.19 Soft tissue measurement for Locator attachment height selection

Various techniques are available to attach the matrix component of the attachment to the denture base. They are classified as direct, indirect, or a combination of both. Several factors should be considered when selecting the technique for incorporating attachments for overdenture. The angulation of implants, complexity of maxillo mandibular relationships, operatory preference, availability of inventory of prosthetic components, and cost are some of these factors [6].

12.3.6.3 The Direct Method

The direct method involves the connection of the inserts and the housing to the abutment intraorally using a resinous or acrylic material. This requires an additional clinical step when compared to the indirect method. However, it offers the advantage of minimizing errors during the acrylization process of the matrix component in the denture base.

It is important to consider that all attachments should engage and be passively seated with the denture base adequately supported by the soft tissue in areas of primary and secondary support. This will prevent any movements of the denture and/or wear of the attachment. Considering that the direct method is done intraorally with the denture seated and occluding properly with the opposing denture, errors in the acrylization process of the matrix components leading to improper seating are minimized.

However, the direct method requires additional clinical steps to be performed at the delivery appointment. Moreover, this method is technique sensitive and requires proper isolation and saliva control to ensure the success of the bonding procedure. Furthermore, it is imperative that all surfaces in an undercut area around the Locator attachment are blocked to prevent any flow of acrylic which could lock the denture in place and prevent its removal following the connection procedure.

Description of the Direct Technique

Once the patrix is torqued in place, it should be prepared for the pickup process. The first step is to verify if the denture is properly relieved to accommodate the addition of the matrix as well as the connection material (Figs. 12.20 and 12.21). The use of a disclosing medium such as a fast-set impression material (*Fit Test, Quick Up, VOCO, Germany*) syringed into the created space can alert to the presence of a contact between the matrices and the resinous base (Fig. 12.21a, b).

This should be done by placing the denture intra-orally and in occlusion (Fig. 12.21c). In that case, the denture is adjusted further by selective grinding at the implant location to accommodate for the attachment complex. It is important to eliminate any contact between the denture base and the metal matrix and to have enough thickness for the material to function properly and prevent any excess pressure on the implant.

The pickup process starts by attaching the Locator matrix to the abutment using the black processing nylons that will maintain the overdenture in the upper limit of its vertical resiliency during the acrylization process (Fig. 12.22). This is followed by placing a prepunched piece of rubber dam over each Locator attachment. The addition

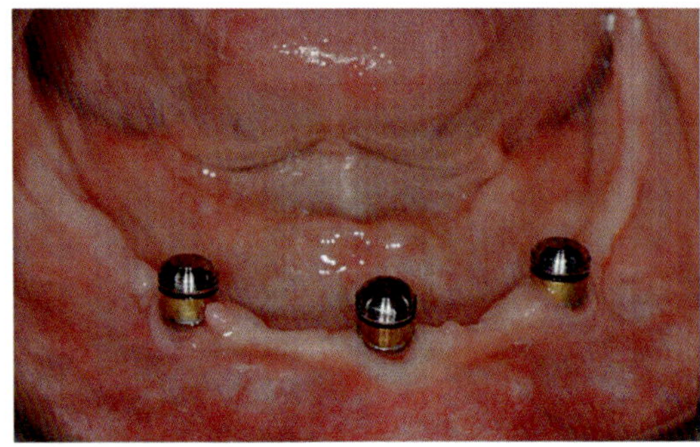

Fig. 12.20 Mandibular denture adjusted to accommodate enough space for the matrices, the Locator abutments, and the material used for the connection

Fig. 12.22 Metal matrices with black processing inserts attached to Locator abutments

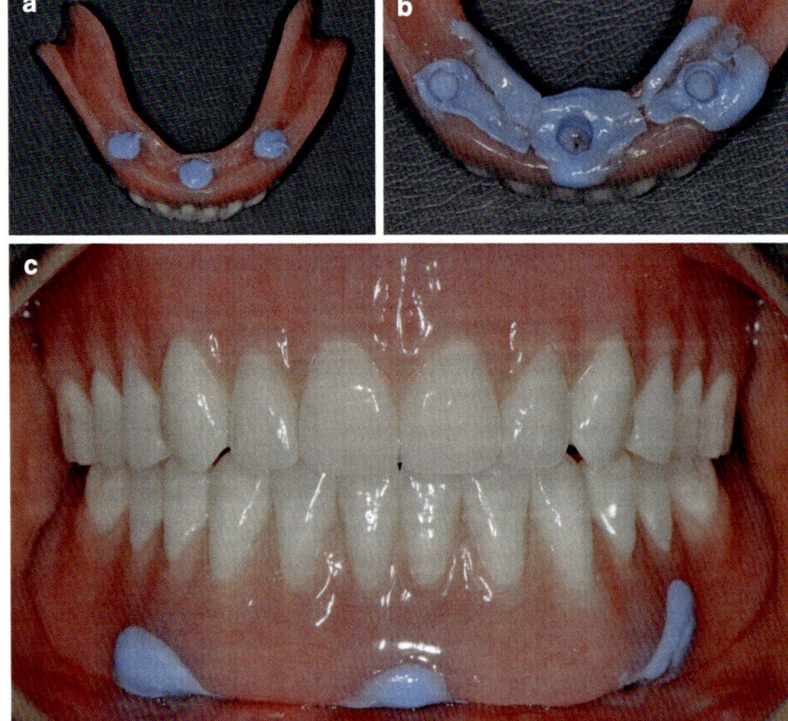

Fig. 12.21 (**a**) Disclosing medium placed inside prepared spaces of mandibular denture. (**b**) Anterior implant showing contact between the matrix and the resinous base; further adjustments are then done to relieve the area. (**c**) Mandibular denture placed over the metal matrices to detect any contact between the resinous base and the attachment complex

of the rubber dam will minimize the flowing of material in the undercuts of the male attachment and prevent the locking of the denture during the procedure. Secondly, a white blockout spacer is placed over the head of each Locator abutment. It is used to block out the area immediately surrounding the abutment and will provide the space required to allow for the resilient function of the matrix without traumatizing the tissue (Fig. 12.23).

The surface is then cleaned and a bonding agent placed (Fig. 12.24). The pickup procedure is done by placing a small amount of the auto-polymerizing resin *(Quick Up, VOCO, Germany)* around each cap as well as in the relief areas (Figs. 12.25 and 12.26). Intraoral saliva control is important for this technique. Any contamination during this procedure may cause the material to dissociate from the denture base. The denture is then positioned properly onto the soft tissues, and

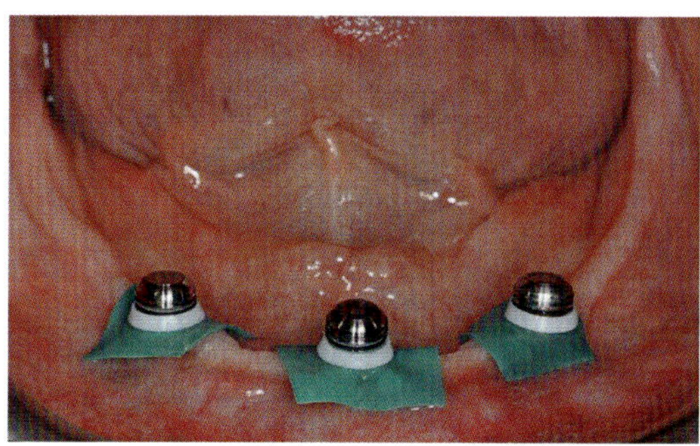

Fig. 12.23 Isolating rubber dam and white blockout spacer placed under metal matrices

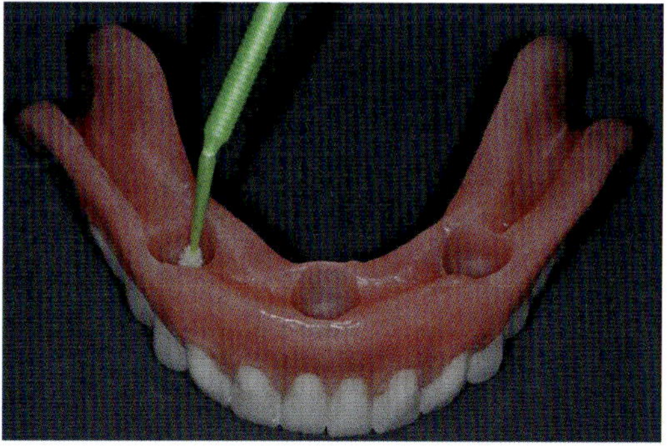

Fig. 12.24 The inner surface of the denture is cleaned prior to the application of the bonding agent into the prepared spaces

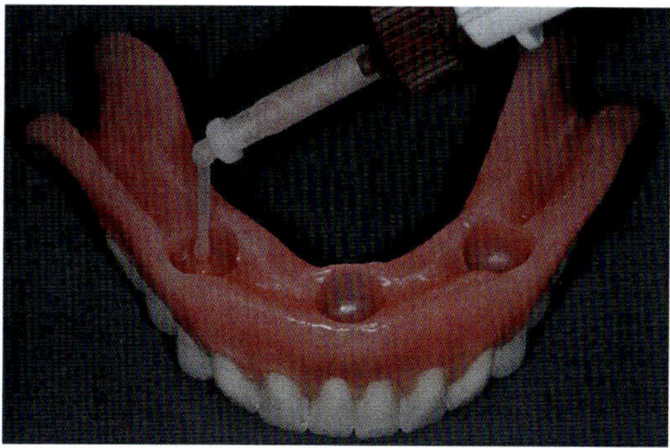

Fig. 12.25 Application of auto-polymerizing resin into the prepared spaces

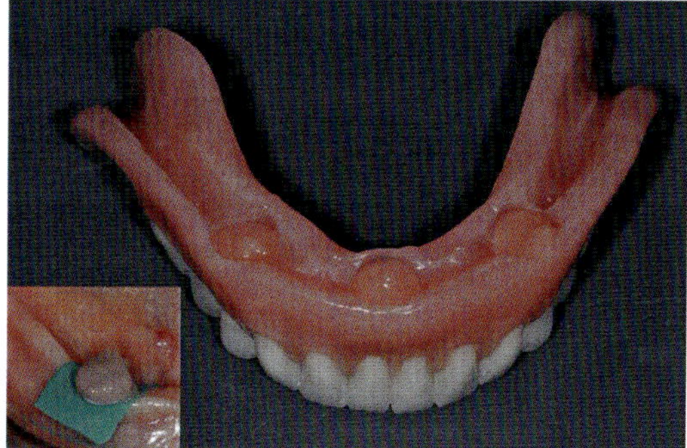

Fig. 12.26 Prepared spaces filled with auto-polymerizing resin and application of auto-polymerizing resin directly onto the metal matrices intraorally

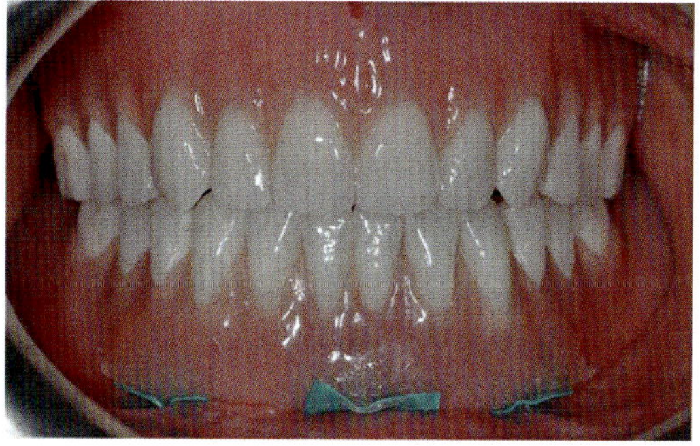

Fig. 12.27 Mandibular denture in occlusion during the setting phase

the patient is guided into occlusion (Fig. 12.27). It is important to have the patient hold the position without excessive compression of the soft tissue which could cause tissue recoil against the denture base and potentially cause dislodging and wear of the nylon inserts.

Once the polymerizing is completed, the denture is removed (Fig. 12.28). Any excess of material around the matrix should be removed with care, not to damage any of the components; the area is then cleaned and polished.

Using the Locator removal tool, the black processing nylons are replaced with the desired inserts (Fig. 12.29). Inserts are categorized based on their design characteristics and retentive capabilities. Selecting the appropriate ones is dependent on the desired retention, the angulation of the implants and the dexterity of the patient. To remove the nylons, the circular edge on the end of the removal tool is wedged down into the nylon and pulled at an angle out of the metal housing. The replacing nylon is placed using the Locator seating tool and firmly pushed in place while supporting the denture (Figs. 12.30 and 12.31).

12.3.6.4 The Indirect Method

The indirect method is less time-consuming and requires no clinical time to attach the matrices into the denture base. This technique requires an implant impression to be made at the level of the implant or abutment with the appropriate impression copings in order to produce an accurate cast of the abutment or implant position. This cast is subsequently used by the laboratory technician to incorporate the metal housings into the mandibular denture during the acrylization process. This facilitates the connection procedure and ensures a more predictable outcome. However, any error during the impression-taking procedure, the connection of analogs into the impression copings, as well as pouring the impression could result in difficulty with seating the denture onto the attachments clinically. In a case where all attachments are not engaging passively, accelerated wearing of the nylon component could occur [6].

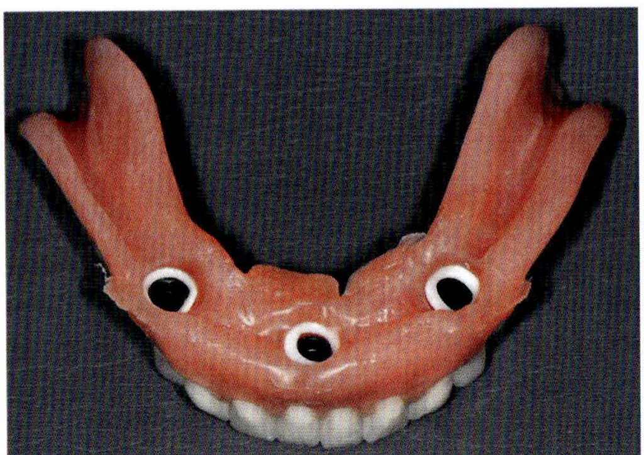

Fig. 12.28 Mandibular denture removed showing excess resinous material

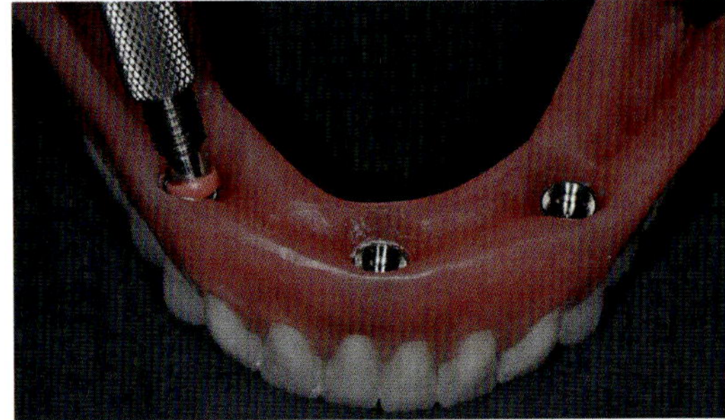

Fig. 12.30 Insertion of pink nylons into metal housing using the Locator core tool

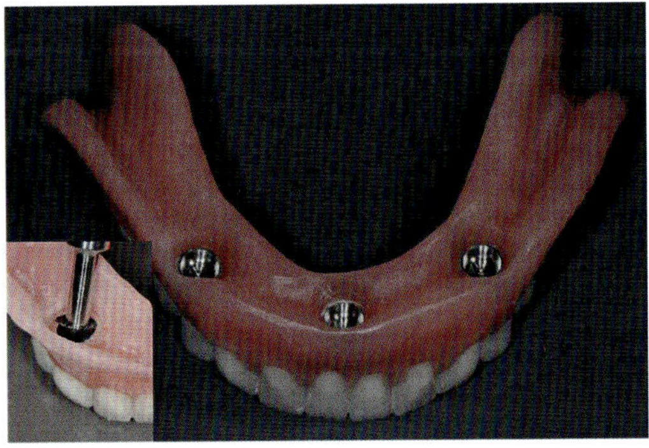

Fig. 12.29 Trimming of the resinous excess and removal of black processing nylon

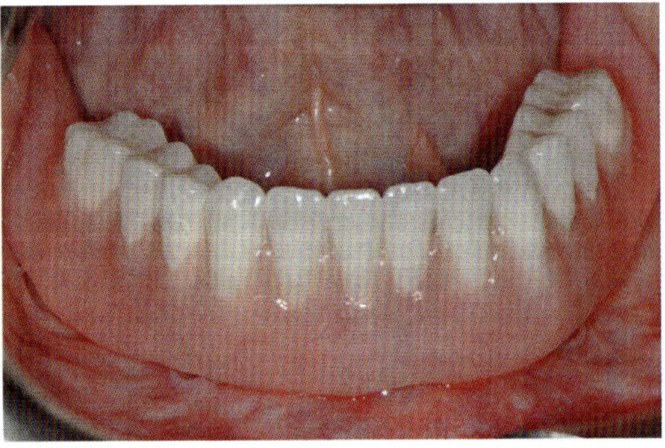

Fig. 12.31 Mandibular denture in place with Locator attachments engaged and passively seated

Description of the Indirect Technique

The indirect technique starts by taking an impression of the implant position and edentulous ridge. The impression can be made at implant shoulder level or abutment level.

The Implant Level Impression Method

The implant shoulder impression registers the implant angulation and position as well as the soft tissue height around each implant. Impression copings are attached to the implants, and seating can be confirmed radiographically. Open-tray or closed-tray technique can be used (Fig. 12.32). The remaining clinical steps such as border molding, wax-rim adjustments, try-in and delivery are similar to conventional denture procedures. The Locator abutment selection is then made on the cast using the same method described earlier. The abutments are ordered with the specific soft tissue height for each implant and delivered to the

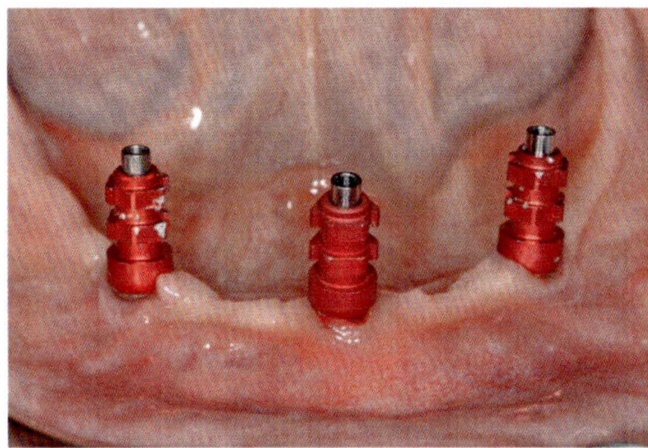

Fig. 12.32 Indirect technique: open-tray implant level final impression

patient during the delivery appointment. This method has the advantage of decreasing the inventory required of different heights and diameters of Locator abutments.

The Abutment Level Impression Method

This method requires the selection of the Locator abutments by measuring the soft tissue height intraorally. Once the abutments are inserted intraorally onto the implants, an abutment level impression is completed using Locator impression copings (Fig. 12.33a). The remaining clinical steps are similar to the conventional denture techniques described earlier (Fig. 12.33b).

When performing an abutment level impression, are must be taken to properly stabilize the impression copings during the procedure (Fig. 12.34). Improperly designing the tray may lead to a premature contact and possible displacement of the impression copings during the impression (Fig. 12.34b). A premature contact with the tray may cause the displacement of the impression coping, therefore creating an imprecise working model. This can be difficult to verify clinically during the impression procedure and would only be picked up at a later stage. Locator analogs are then placed onto the impression copings, and a cast is poured reproducing the Locator abutment inserted clinically (Fig. 12.35a).

The indirect method has the added advantage of allowing for the fabrication of a baseplate into which the Locator metal matrices can be incorporated and used during the different denture fabri-

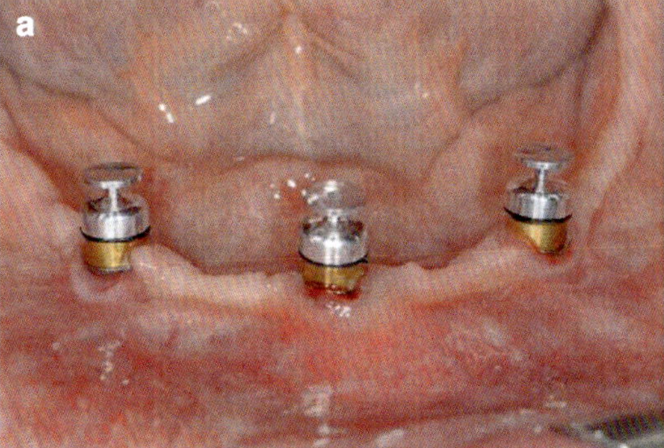
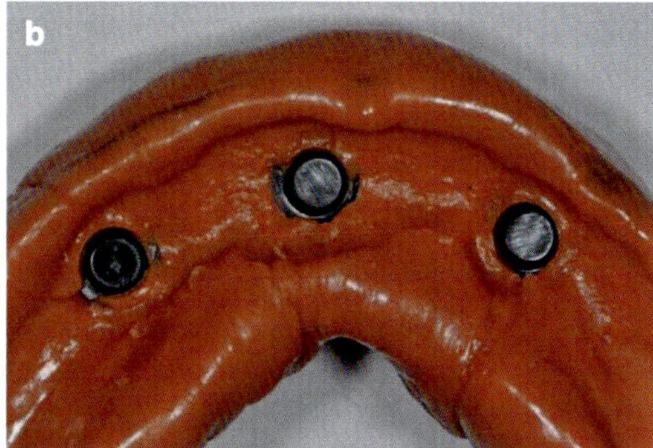

Fig. 12.33 (**a**) Locator impression copings placed on Locator abutments (**b**) abutment level final impression

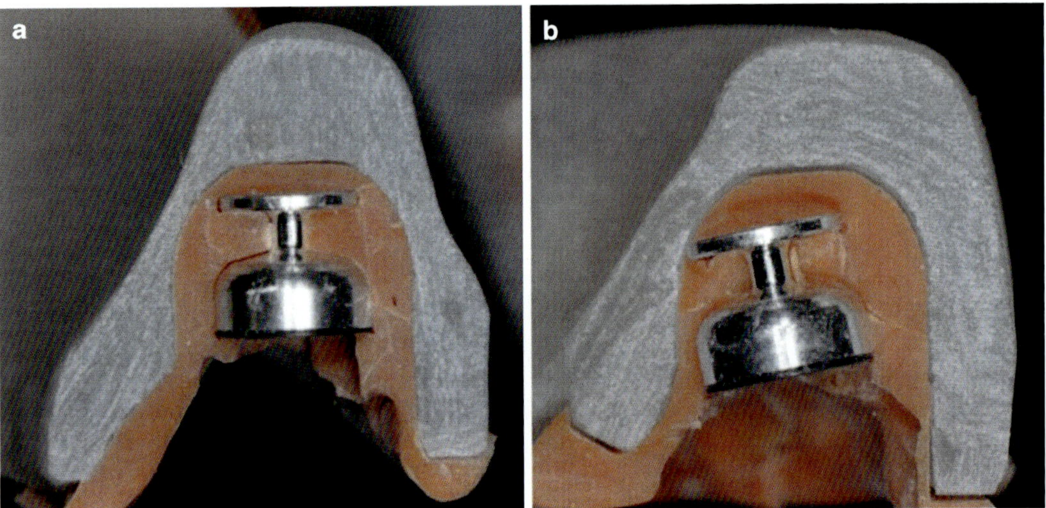

Fig. 12.34 (**a**) Proper seating of the abutment impression coping (**b**) displacement of the impression coping during the impression procedure

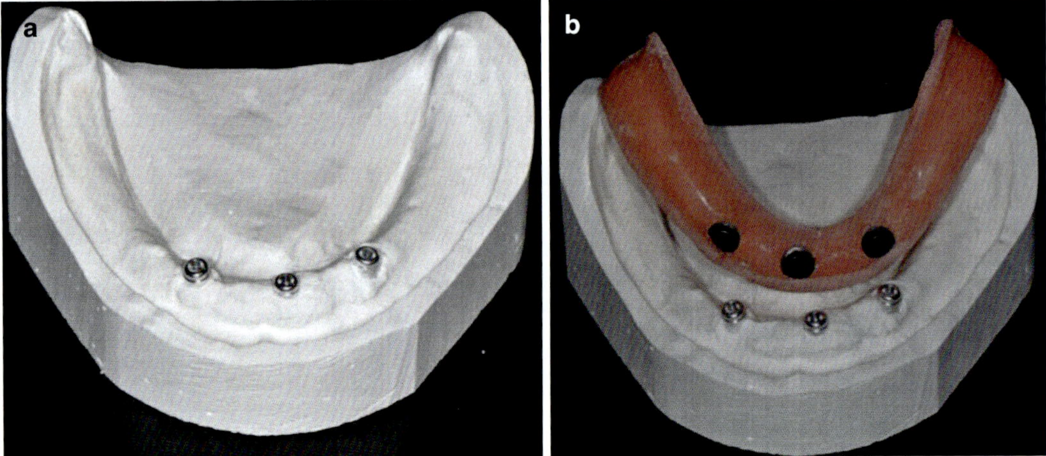

Fig. 12.35 (**a**) Mandibular cast with Locator analogs (**b**) wax-rim fabrication incorporating the metal matrices

cation procedures (Fig. 12.35b). It provides stability for the mandibular occlusion rims by having it engage onto the Locator abutments, which facilitates the adjustments of the wax rims and the registration of centric relation.

Both the direct and indirect techniques have been described and are widely used by clinicians today. The main advantage of the direct method is its simplicity and limited cost. However, this approach requires care not to cause binding of the prosthesis due to implant misalignment or to resin flowing into undercuts. There is also the added difficulties in finishing and polishing the resinous material; in fact, porosities can often be observed in the vicinity of the metal housing (Fig. 12.36a, b). Benefits of the indirect technique include reduced chair time and optimal polishing of the resin in proximity to the matrices; however, the added technical steps may introduce certain discrepancies, which can create imprecisions in the final outcome.

Limited information is available when comparing the two techniques of connecting attachments to dentures. Nissan et al. in 2011 [7]

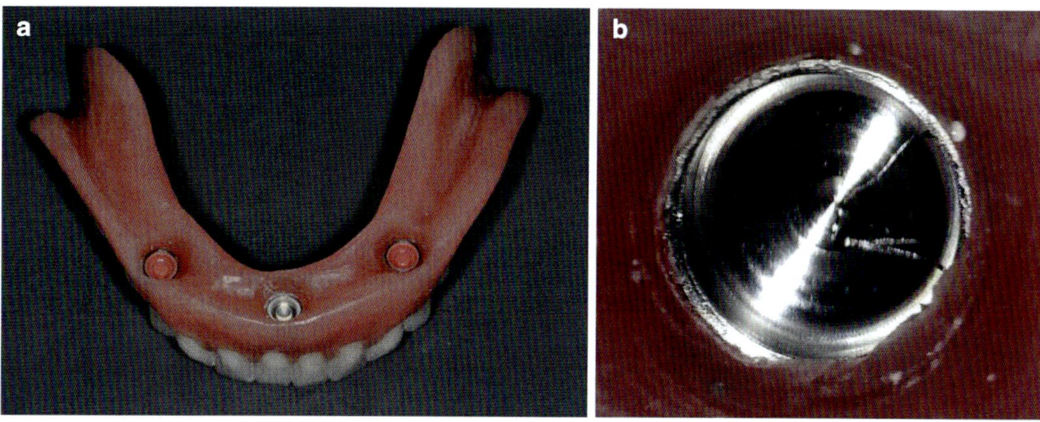

Fig. 12.36 (**a**) The incorporated Locator matrix housings using the direct method (**b**) showing porosities and excess material under a microscopic image

reported on the long-term prosthetic aftercare of direct vs. indirect techniques for mandibular implant-retained overdenture on ball abutments. A group of 45 patients were followed for a period of 20 years. The patients were randomly assigned to two groups based on the connection technique used. Prosthetic complications were significantly higher when indirect method was used. Interestingly, attachment replacement due to wear occurred mainly in the indirect technique group.

one of the main advantages of the digital environment is the preservation of all the parameters registered clinically. In fact, a significant portion of the patients' anatomical features as well as the image of the final dentures remains available in the software. Therefore, in case of lost or damaged dentures, the remake procedure is greatly facilitated. For this chapter, we proceeded to fabricate a set of digital dentures for the patient; the steps and procedures are detailed below.

12.4 CAD/CAM Complete Denture Fabrication

Complete denture rehabilitation is the most traditional prosthodontic treatment for edentulous patients. The methods of fabrication have remained relatively unchanged for many years. The conventional approach involves a sequence of multiple clinical and laboratory steps. An accelerated method of denture fabrication has been described by Kawai et al. in 2005 [8] and was shown to have comparable clinical outcomes to the more complex procedure. However, in both instances, the acquired clinical parameters are lost once the dentures are processed and delivered to the patient.

Digital dentistry can present a tremendous amount of advantages for the elderly patient. It is often presented to the clinicians by the manufactures as a timesaving procedure. However,

12.5 Clinical Procedures

The clinical procedure starts with impressions of maxillary and mandibular arches (Fig. 12.37a, b) using an irreversible hydrocolloid material *(Jeltrate Alginate, Dentsply Caulk, Canada)* placed in stock edentulous metal trays *(Patterson Dental Supply, Canada)*. Impressions are poured using type III dental stone *(GC America Inc., USA)* in order to produce preliminary casts (Fig. 12.38a, b).

The preliminary casts are used to fabricate custom occlusion rims for the upper and lower jaws (Fig. 12.39). If the existing dentures of the patients are acceptable or require minor changes, they can be utilized as a guideline for the fabrications of the rims. If there are changes necessary, these can be incorporated during the clinical procedures. The rims are then tried and adjusted intraorally as described earlier. The lip support,

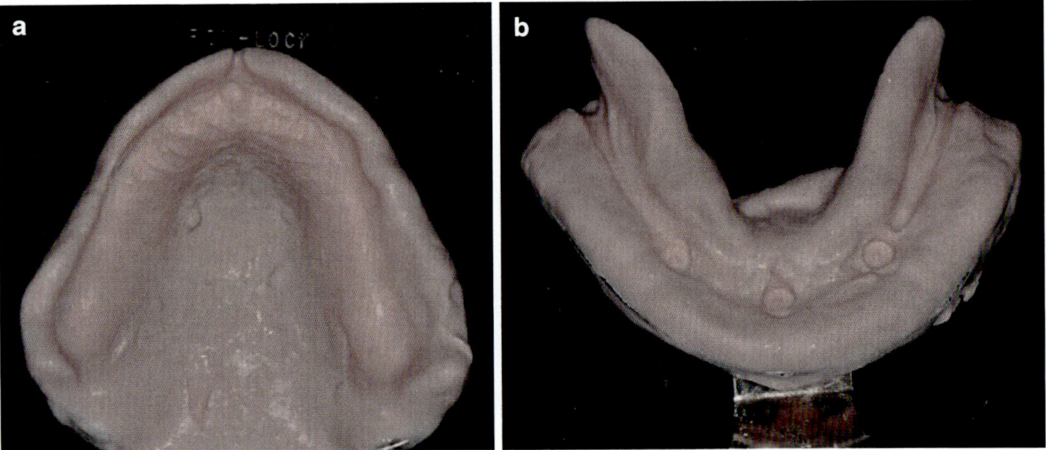

Fig. 12.37 (**a** and **b**) Alginate impression of the maxillary and mandibular arches using stock metal trays

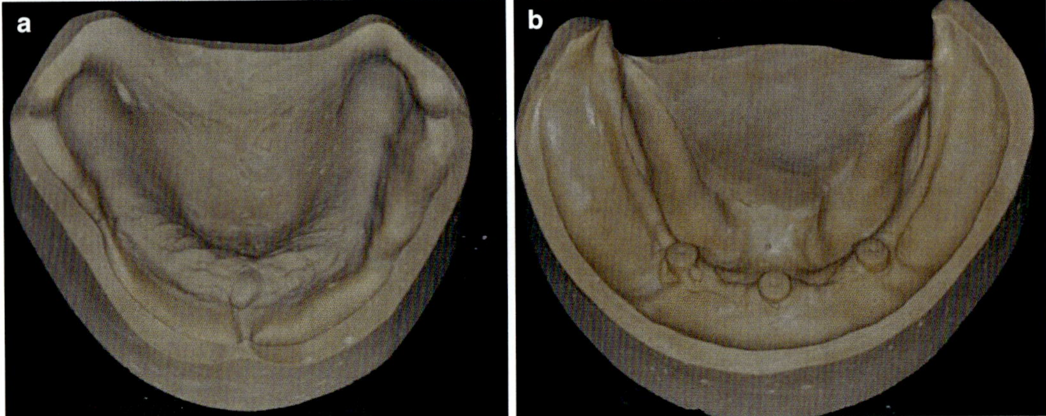

Fig. 12.38 (**a** and **b**) Preliminary cast of the maxillary and mandibular arches

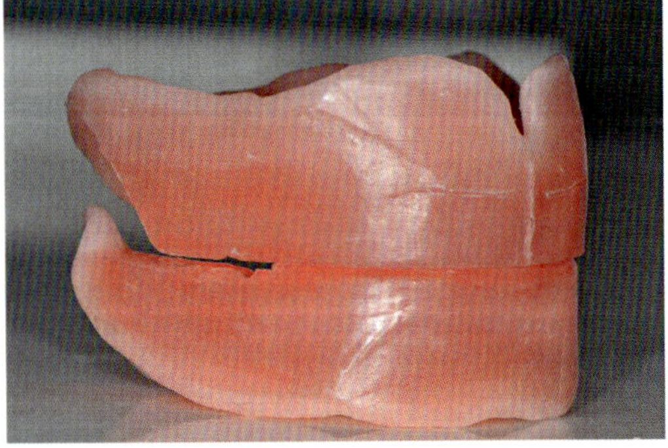

Fig. 12.39 Upper and lower occlusion rims

incisal display, midline, occlusal plane, and vertical dimension of occlusion are recorded following the conventional complete denture protocols (Fig. 12.40a). The rims are then used to capture the details of the soft tissues, the border of the muscular attachment, as well as the interocclusal registration (Fig. 12.40b).

This setup provides all the necessary information to the laboratory to progress into the digital medium (Fig. 12.41a, b). This sequence is one of multiple ways to transfer clinical information into the digital environment.

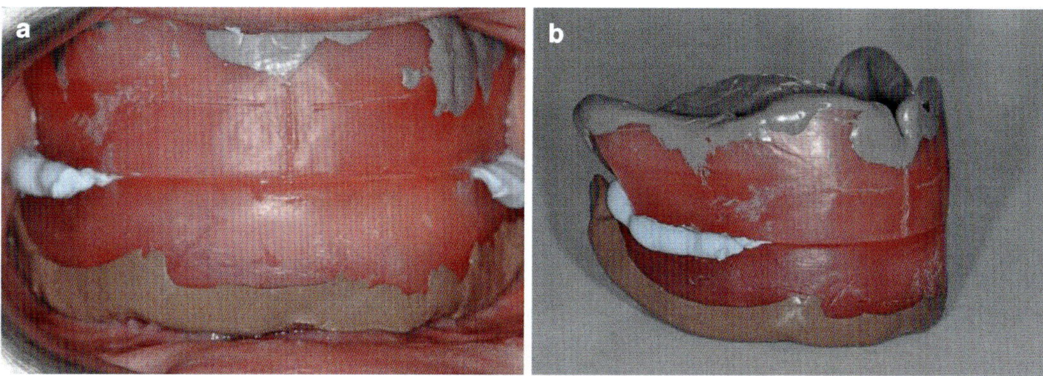

Fig. 12.40 (**a**) Final impressions of the upper and lower arches (**b**) bite registrations using the occlusion rims

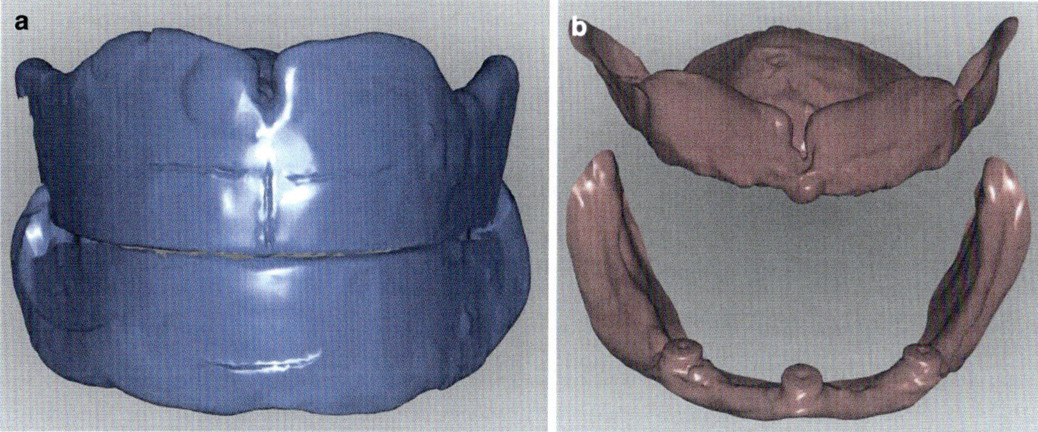

Fig. 12.41 (**a** and **b**) Digitized upper and lower wax rims with all the relevant clinical parameters

Once the clinical features are digitized, the tooth setup can be started on the software (AvaDent Digital Dental Solution, USA) by selecting the appropriate tooth mold and color. The placement of the teeth is guided by the parameters provided by the rims (Fig. 12.41a). It is important to provide the technician with all the information and guidelines to allow the placement of the prosthetic teeth (Fig. 12.42). Anatomic features such as the residual ridge and the retromolar pad can also be used to facilitate the setup procedure (Fig. 12.41b). Once the procedure of placing the teeth on the software is completed, the restorative dentist will generally have to validate the final setup. Adjustments can

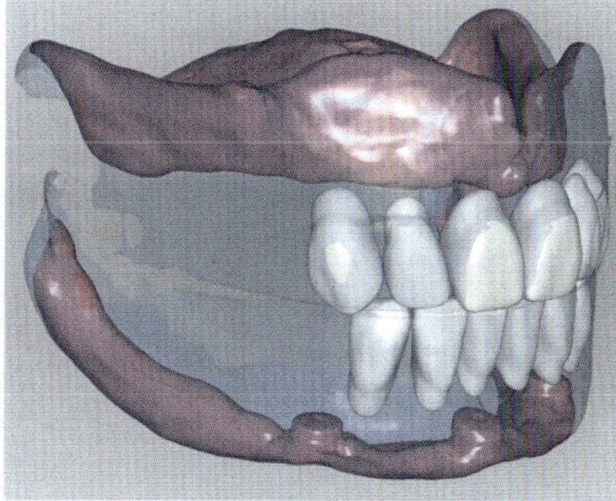

Fig. 12.42 Placement of the prosthetic teeth is facilitated by the clinical guidelines provided as well as some anatomical features

be made easily before the fabrication process. Working in the digital environment allows for a clearer unhindered view of the design process specifically for implant-retained overdentures. A clear image of the prosthetic teeth in relation to the residual ridges as well as to the implants can be obtained (Fig. 12.43a, b). Thus, an evaluation of the anterior tooth positioning in relation to the anticipated axis of rotation around the implants can be assessed, and alterations can be done accordingly.

Once the tooth setup is approved, the laboratory can generate a try-in denture that would allow to properly visualize the clinical outcomes. In fact, the try-in denture can assess certain esthetic parameters (midline, lip support, and tooth shape) as well as functional ones (centric relation and occlusal contacts). The try-in denture is generally machined from a singular block of polymethyl methacrylate (Fig. 12.44a, b). If adjustments are required, they can be done directly on the try-in denture and sent back to the laboratory in order to modify the digital setup. This process may be limiting for patients with high esthetic demands that may have difficulty assessing the end result prior to the fabrication of the definitive prosthesis. For these cases a wax try-in may be indicated. Moreover, in cases where significant adjustments must be made to the try-in denture, it may require a digital modification with fabrication of an additional try-in denture to properly assess the modifications and allow for the patient to evaluate the result [9]. An additional appointment is required with an increase in the laboratory fees. Understanding the digital workflow is critical for the success of these cases.

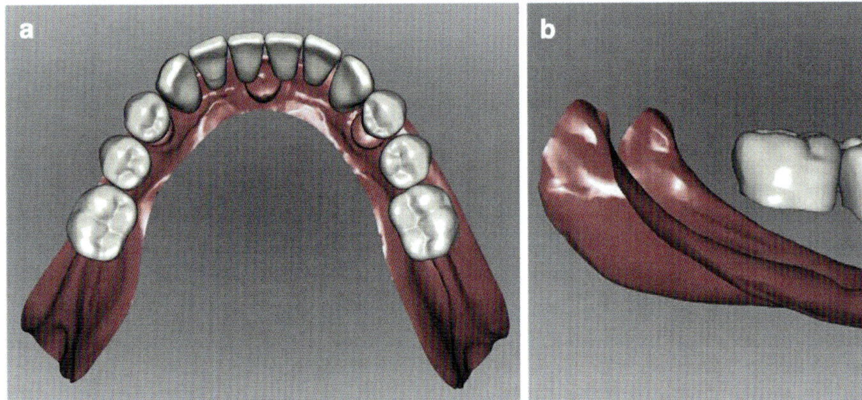

Fig. 12.43 (**a**) Occlusal view of the prosthetic teeth in relation to the mandibular ridges and implants (**b**) Sagittal view of the final tooth position for implant-retained mandibular denture

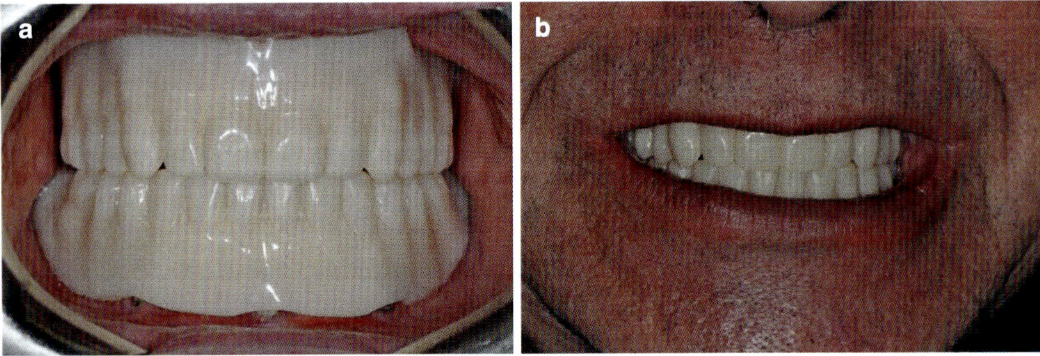

Fig. 12.44 (**a** and **b**) Trial upper and lower dentures to assess all the relevant clinical parameters

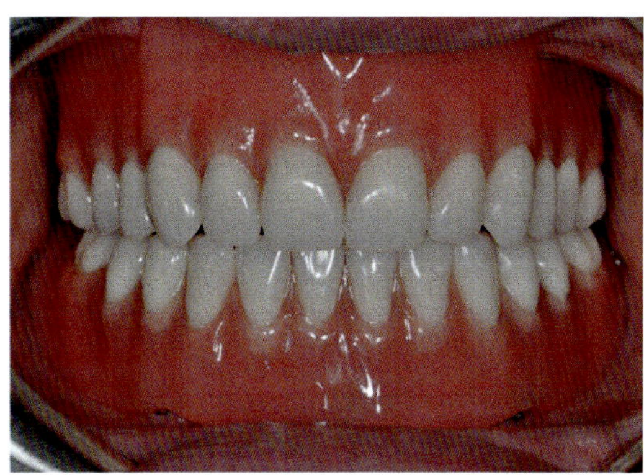

Fig. 12.45 Delivery of upper and lower CAD/CAM dentures

Once the changes are completed, the dentures can be machined for delivery to the patient (Fig. 12.45). This process requires that the female component be picked up directly in the oral cavity as described earlier.

The technique presented incorporates digital technology (CAD/CAM) without disregarding the fundamentals of complete denture fabrication. The main advantage of this technique is focused on providing the patient with complete dentures without losing the clinical information in the process. Therefore, in cases of lost or damaged dentures, the remake procedure is greatly facilitated. Most manufactures can regenerate a new set of dentures within a few working days. These can be provided to the patient or re-adapted to the oral condition depending on the changes in the residual ridges. In cases where significant intraoral changes have occurred, new impressions may have to be taken followed by the same steps described.

The fabrication process is also unique to the digital setting. All the bases are generally machined from a solid block of pink polymethyl methacrylate. Therefore, this process is not susceptible to any contraction due to conventional processing, material properties, or human errors [9]. Goodacre et al. [10] compared the denture base adaptation between CAD/CAM and conventional fabrication techniques to determine which process produces the most accurate and reproducible adaptation. They compared the conventional pack, press, pour,

and injection techniques to the CAD/CAM process. They concluded that the CAD/CAM fabrication process was the most accurate and reproducible denture fabrication technique. The dentures are also denser and less porous. This feature may have an impact on the wear behavior of the prosthetic teeth, the strength of the denture, as well as the plaque retention [11]. More research is needed to validate the importance of these parameters on the longevity and clinical outcomes of digitally generated removable prosthesis vs. conventional techniques.

References

1. Tjan AHL, Miller GD, The JGP. Some esthetic factors in a smile. J Prosthet Dent. 1984;51(1):24–8.
2. Mesmar S, Nguyen TC, Wyatt C. Occlusal vertical dimension for complete removable dental prostheses. Can J Restor Dent Prosthodont. 2015;8(3):28–38.
3. Turrell AJ. Clinical assessment of vertical dimension. J Prosthet Dent. 1972;28(3):238–46.
4. Millet C, Leterme A, Jeannin C, Jaudoin P. [Vertical dimension in the treatment of the edentulous patient]. Rev Stomatol Chir Maxillofac. 2010;111(5–6):315–30.
5. Kimoto S, Pan S, Drolet N, Feine JS. Rotational movements of mandibular two-implant overdentures. Clin Oral Implants Res. 2009;20(8):838–43.
6. Bidra AS, et al. Techniques for incorporation of attachments in implant-retained overdentures with unsplinted abutments. J Prosthet Dent. 2012;107(5): 288–99.
7. Nissan J, Oz-Ari B, Gross O, Ghelfan O, Chaushu G. Long-term prosthetic aftercare of direct vs. indirect attachment incorporation techniques to mandibular implant-supported overdenture. Clin Oral Implants Res. 2011;22(6):627–30.
8. Kawai Y, Murakami H, Shariati B, Klemetti E, Blomfield JV, Billette L, Lund JP, Feine JS. Do traditional techniques produce better conventional complete dentures than simplified techniques? J Dent. 2005;33(8):659–68.
9. Wimmer T, Gallus K, Eichberger M, Stawarczyk B. Complete denture fabrication supported by CAD/CAM. J Prosthet Dent. 2016;115(5):541–6.
10. Goodacre BJ, Goodacre CJ, Baba NZ, Kattadiyil MT. Comparison of denture base adaptation between CAD-CAM and conventional fabrication techniques. J Prosthet Dent. 2016;116(2):249–25.
11. Bidra AS, et al. Computer-aided technology for fabricating complete dentures: systematic review of historical background, current status, and future perspectives. J Prosthet Dent. 2016;109(6):361–6.

Case Presentation: Implant-Supported Removable Mandibular Prostheses

13

Samer Abi Nader and Meng François Seng

Abstract

Uses of modern dental implants are providing new options for the treatment of complete upper and lower edentulism. Implant-supported removable overdentures have proven to be an effective treatment option, especially for the treatment of patients with severely atrophied residual ridges.

This clinical report describes the treatment of a completely edentulous patient complaining of a lack of retention and stability of her existing mandibular conventional complete denture. Clinical steps and laboratory procedures involved in the fabrication of a removable mandibular overdenture supported by a milled Dolder bar will be described in detail in this chapter.

13.1 Patient History and Background

The patient, a 60-year-old female patient, was referred for prosthodontics evaluation by her general dentist. Her chief complaint at the time of presentation was "My lower denture is becoming very loose and I sometimes feel pain on my left side when I eat." The patient explains that she has been edentulous since a very young age and has been wearing complete dentures since. Her most recent dentures were fabricated approximately 10 years ago, and recently she has been having discomfort described as a tingling sensation when she eats, specifically on the left side.

The patient presents clinically with a severely atrophied mandibular residual ridge with poor soft tissue quality and loading capacity. Due to the extensive resorption, her left mental nerve is now located on top of her residual ridge which may explain her discomfort. In addition, the floor of the mouth is very mobile. She is content with the overall performance of her maxillary complete denture but has noticed that it is starting to "feel loose." She is interested in improving the stability and function of her prostheses.

13.1.1 Medical History

- Hypertension: controlled with medication
- Type II diabetes: controlled with medication
- Medication: Metformin
- No known drug allergy
- No history of smoking or drug abuse

13.1.2 Dental History

- Full mouth extraction at age 24

S. A. Nader, BSc, DMD, MSc, FRCD(C) (✉)
M. F. Seng, DMD, FRCD(C)
Department of Restorative Dentistry, Faculty of Dentistry, McGill University, Montreal, QC, Canada
e-mail: samer.abinader@mcgill.ca

© Springer International Publishing AG, part of Springer Nature 2018
E. Emami, J. Feine (eds.), *Mandibular Implant Prostheses*,
https://doi.org/10.1007/978-3-319-71181-2_13

13.1.3 Clinical Findings

- Complete edentulism
- Inadequate existing complete dentures
- "U-shaped" arch form
- Mobile floor of mouth
- Left mental nerve located on crest of alveolar ridge

13.1.4 Diagnosis

- Maxillary and mandibular complete edentulism
- Severely atrophied mandibular residual ridge
- Moderately atrophied maxillary residual ridge

Following a preliminary assessment, the fabrication of a new maxillary complete denture as well as an implant-supported mandibular prosthesis was recommended. Four dental implants (Straumann Dental implant system, Bone level, NC) were planned for placement in the anterior sextant of the mandible to improve the support, retention, and stability of her lower prosthesis (Figs. 13.1 and 13.2).

13.2 Implant Placement Strategy

Clinical assessment of the edentulous mandible reveals a "U-shaped" arch with severe residual ridge resorption especially in the posterior areas. The excessive amount of resorption has resulted in the left mental nerve being located on the crest of the ridge (Fig. 13.3). The floor of her mouth is very mobile; muscle and frenum attachments are located high on the ridge, her soft tissue is thin, and the buccal vestibule is shallow.

The preliminary assessment was completed, and a removable complete denture to be supported by a Dolder bar on four implants placed in the interforaminal region was planned. The two posterior implants were placed as close as possible to the mental foramen without jeopardizing the nerve. The anterior implants were placed as far anteriorly as possible without compromising distribution (in this situation, the lateral incisor positions) (Fig. 13.4). This careful planning of the implant position should maximize the anterior-

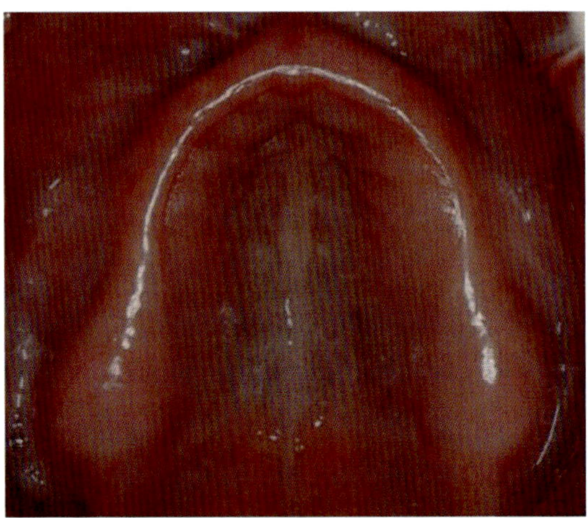

Fig. 13.1 Maxillary residual ridge

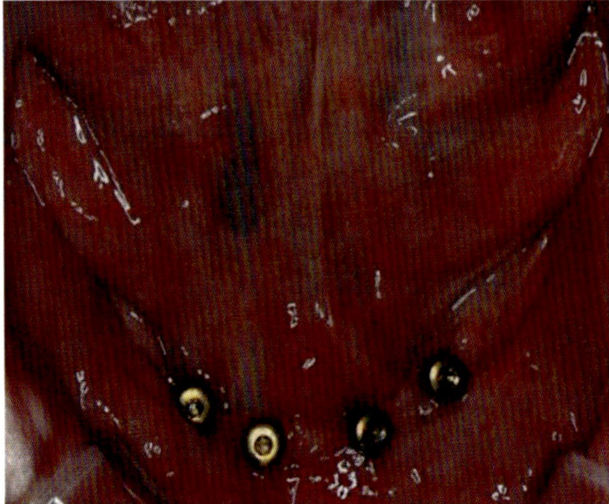

Fig. 13.2 Mandibular residual ridge following implant placement. Surgery: Dr. Veronique Benhamou, Periodontist

posterior spread and allow for the fabrication of a Dolder bar with bilateral distal extensions. Such a bar design would entirely support the mandibular overdenture and greatly increase retention, stability, and support. This will enhance the comfort of the prosthesis by minimizing any pressure on the soft tissue during function, therefore preventing any impingement of the left mental nerve.

Although the survival and success rate of different loading protocols (immediate, early, and conventional) seem to be similar, some authors have reported a tendency toward a slight increase of failure rates when implants are immediately loaded [1, 2]. A conventional delayed approach was favored in this situation due to several factors including quantity and quality of the bone as well as the surgeon's preference.

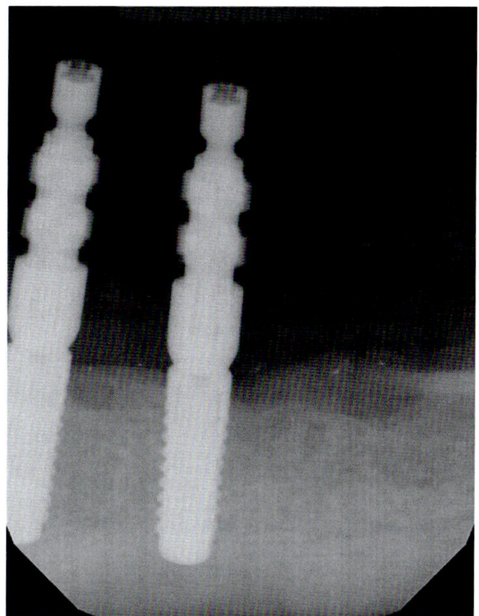

Fig. 13.3 Left mental nerve located on crest of residual ridge due to severe resorption

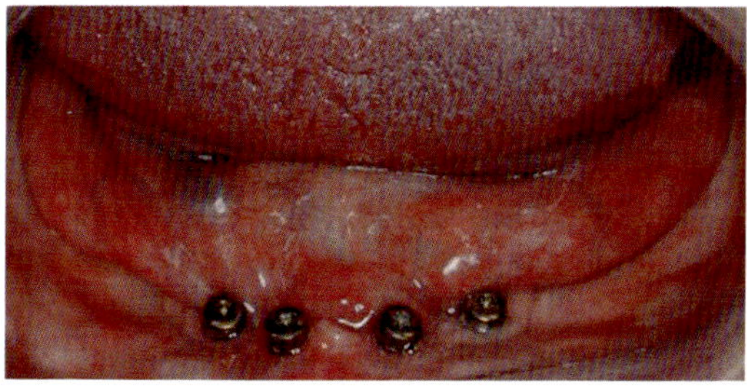

Fig. 13.4 Strategic implant placement in the interforaminal region resulting in even distribution and maximizing A-P spread

13.3 Clinical Procedures

13.3.1 Abutment Selection

Transmucosal abutments were used to move the prosthetic interface closer to the level of the soft tissue. This will facilitate the prosthetic procedures as well as allow the splinting of the four implants. The abutments are selected based on the height of the soft tissue around each implant (measured from the platform of the implant to the lowest contour of the gingiva) (Fig. 13.5a, b). The required height of the abutment to be selected corresponds exactly to the soft tissue measurement described previously or is the next lowest height available. In doing so, the margin of the prosthetic interface will be located either at the level or slightly below the gingiva (Fig. 13.6).

Four Straumann multi-base abutments are inserted and torqued using the torque wrench following the manufacturer's recommendation.

13.3.2 Preliminary Impression

After ensuring that the tissues are healthy, preliminary impressions of the maxillary and mandibular arches (Fig. 13.7a, b) are completed using irreversible hydrocolloid (*Jeltrate Alginate, Dentsply Caulk, Canada*) with the help of stock edentulous metal trays (*Patterson Dental Supply, Canada*). Impressions are then poured in Type III

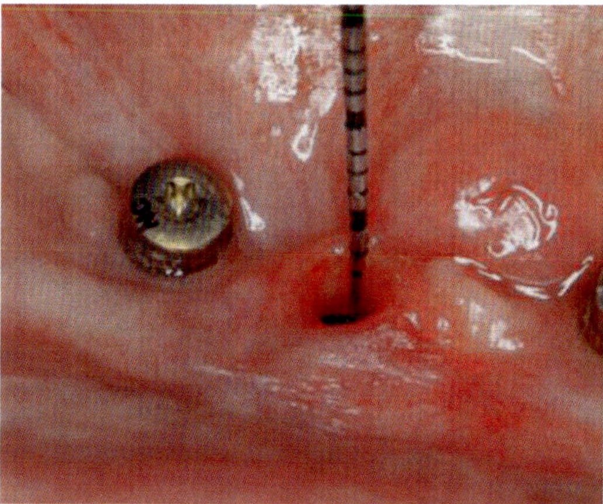

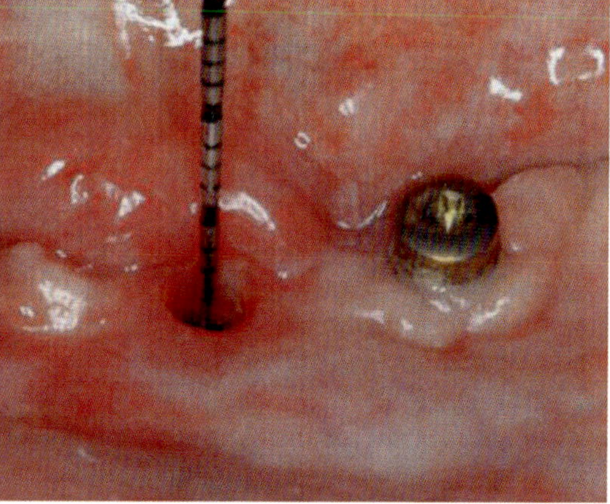

Fig. 13.5 Measurement of soft tissue height for multi-base abutment selection

gypsum (*GC America Inc., USA*) to produce the preliminary casts (Fig. 13.8a, b) for the fabrication of custom trays.

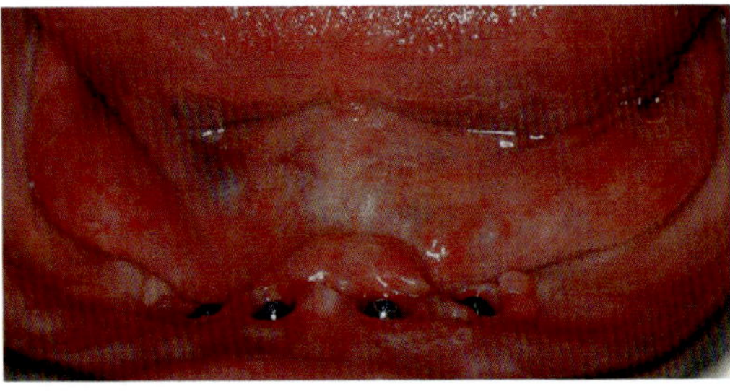

Fig. 13.6 Multi-base abutments inserted and torqued in position following manufacturer's recommendation

13.3.3 Border Molding and Final Impressions of the Upper Arch

The outline of the custom trays was designed based on anatomical landmarks, muscles, and frenal attachments, as well as to accommodate for the space requirement for the border-molding material (Fig. 13.9a, b). The maxillary custom tray was fabricated using a light polymerizing acrylic resin material (*Triad TruTray, Dentsply. Canada*). The custom tray was subsequently tried intraorally and evaluated for proper fit, and the extensions were verified and adjusted to allow space for the modeling compound material

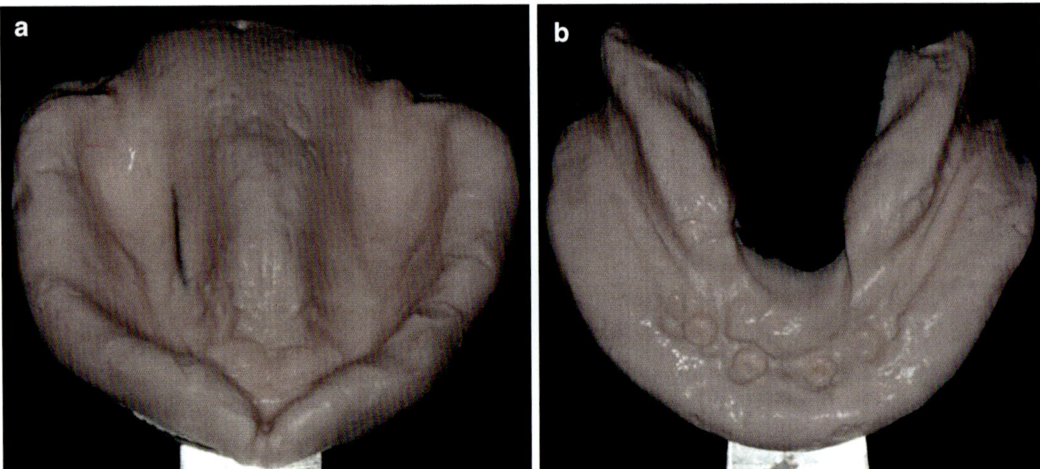

Fig. 13.7 (**a** and **b**) Alginate impression (irreversible hydrocolloid) of the maxillary and mandibular arches using edentulous stock trays

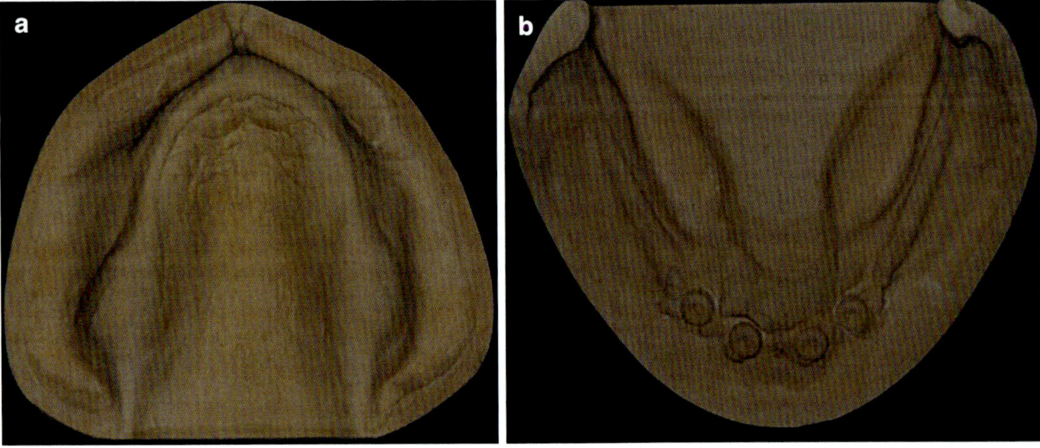

Fig. 13.8 (**a** and **b**) Preliminary models of the maxillary and mandibular arches poured in Type III dental stone

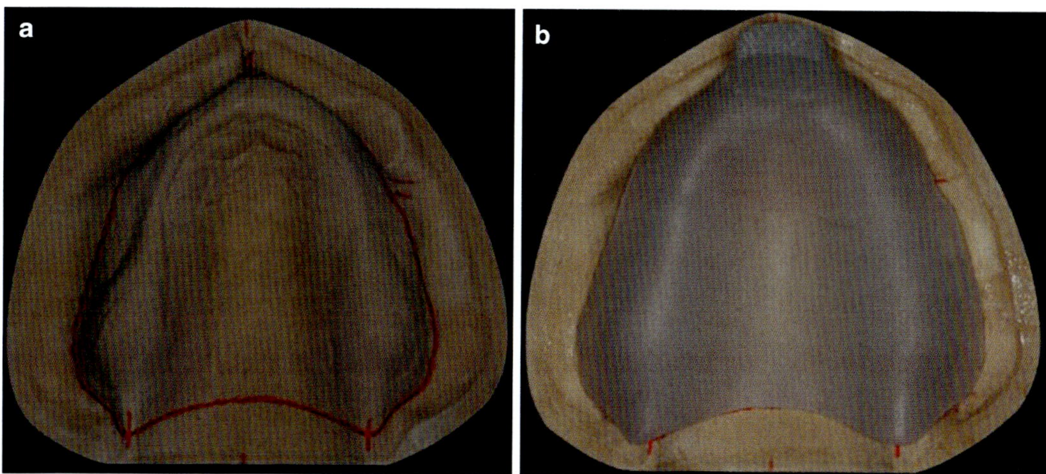

Fig. 13.9 (**a** and **b**) Design and fabrication of the maxillary custom tray for final impression

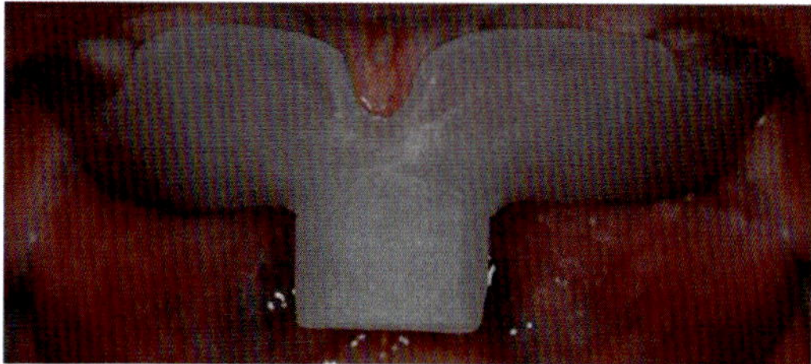

Fig. 13.10 Clinical try-in of the maxillary custom tray prior to the border-molding procedure

(Fig. 13.10). Bolder molding of the periphery was performed using dental compounds (Fig. 13.11a, b) and the manipulation of the patient's tissue to capture the muscles and soft tissue attachments. Final impression of the maxillary arch was taken using a polysulfide rubber material (*Permlastic™, Kerr Dental*).

13.3.4 Border Molding and Final Impressions of the Lower Arch

A mandibular custom tray was fabricated using a light polymerizing acrylic resin material (*Triad TruTray, Dentsply. Canada*) using the same principle as the maxillary arch (Fig. 13.12a, b). Additional space was provided in the anterior sextant to accommodate the implant pickup impression copings. The custom tray was tried intraorally, evaluated for proper adaptation, and the extensions were adjusted approximately

2 mm short of the mucobuccal fold (Fig. 13.13). The custom tray was border molded to the muscles and soft tissue attachments using dental compound (*Kerr Dental, Canada*).

The long-term success of multiunit implant-supported prostheses depends on a multitude of factors of which proper fit and passivity of the superstructure are of prime importance [3]. Multiple studies [4–6] have reported that splinting of the impression copings may improve the accuracy of the final impression and the resulting master cast.

The splinting process is generally done either directly in the mouth or indirectly using a master model. In this situation, a direct technique was preferred, as it requires fewer clinical steps, appointments, and lab work, which ultimately results in a decrease in the cost. The pickup abutment level impression copings were connected to the multi-base abutments. Radiographs were taken to confirm their proper fit (Fig. 13.3). Dental floss was used to link the impression copings together to act as a scaffold onto which a light cured acrylic material (*TRIAD Dual- line, Dentsply. Canada*) was applied to connect all the impression copings together. The splint was subsequently sectioned between each coping and reconnected using the same light cured material (Fig. 13.14). This process of sectioning and reconnecting is done to improve accuracy by reducing internal stresses caused by the

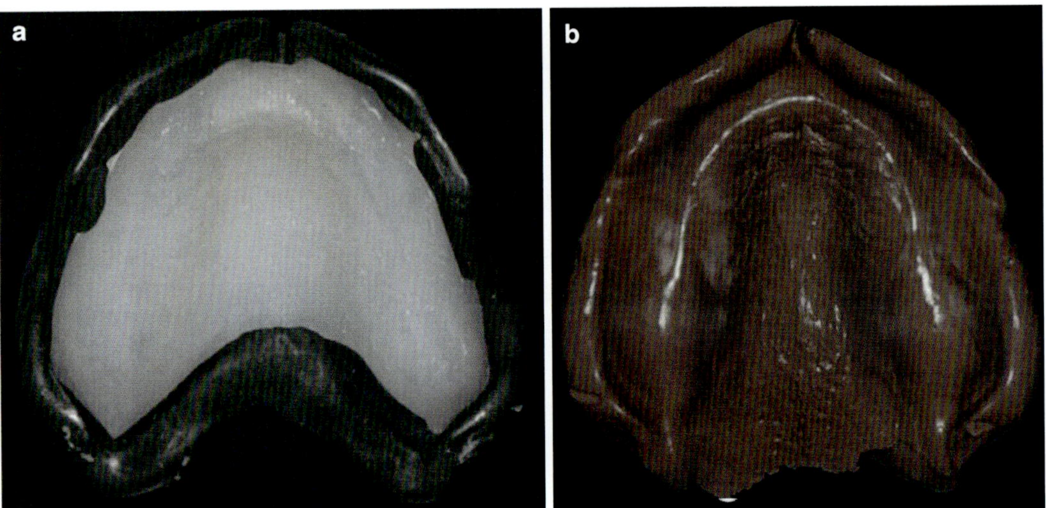

Fig. 13.11 (**a** and **b**) Border-molding procedure is performed using dental compound, and subsequently final impression is made using polysulfide impression material

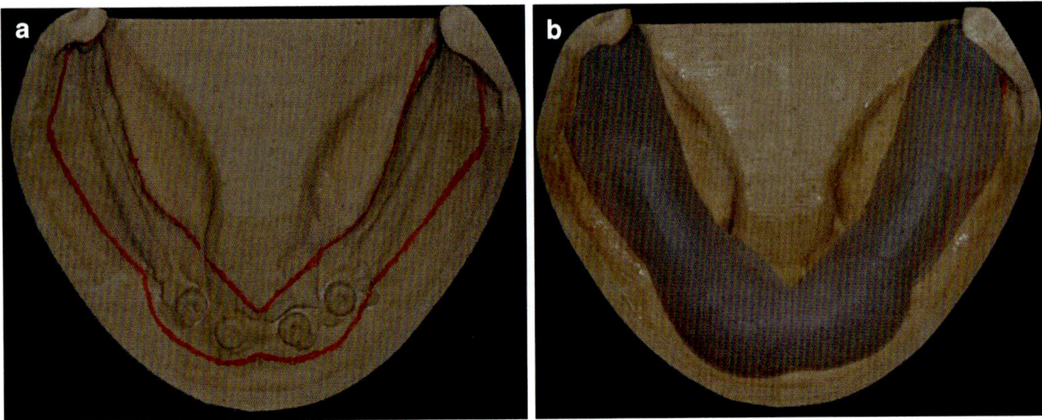

Fig. 13.12 (**a** and **b**) Design and fabrication of the mandibular custom tray for final impression

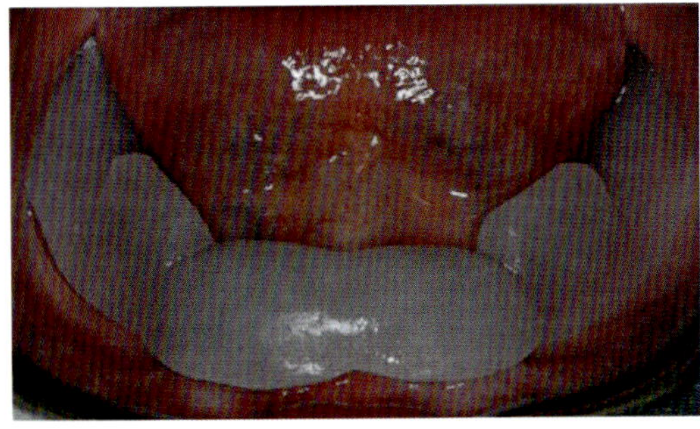

Fig. 13.13 Try-in of the custom trays prior to the border-molding procedure

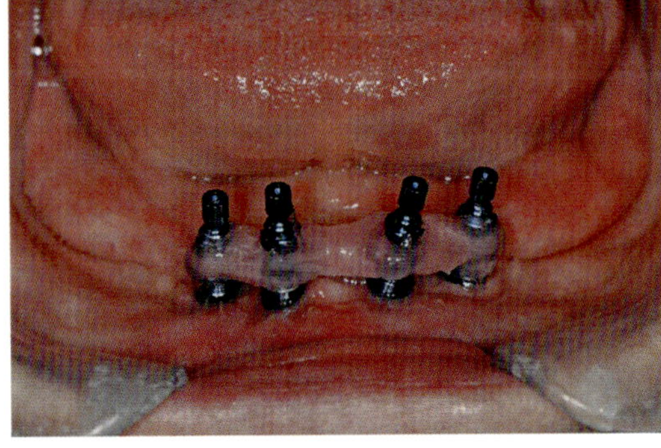

Fig. 13.14 Abutment level pickup impression copings were placed onto the multi-base abutments and splinted together using a light curing resin

polymerization process of the material [7]. An open-tray final impression was taken using the previously border-molded custom tray and a high consistency addition type polyvinyl siloxane impression material (*Affinis, Coltene Dental*) (Fig. 13.15).

The maxillary final impression is poured in Type III gypsum (*GC America Inc., USA*) to generate the master cast (Fig. 13.16a). Laboratory abutment analogs are attached to the pickup impression copings, and the mandibular final impression is poured using type IV gypsum (*Fujirock EP, GC America, USA*) with a soft tissue analog to produce the definitive mandibular cast (Fig. 13.16b).

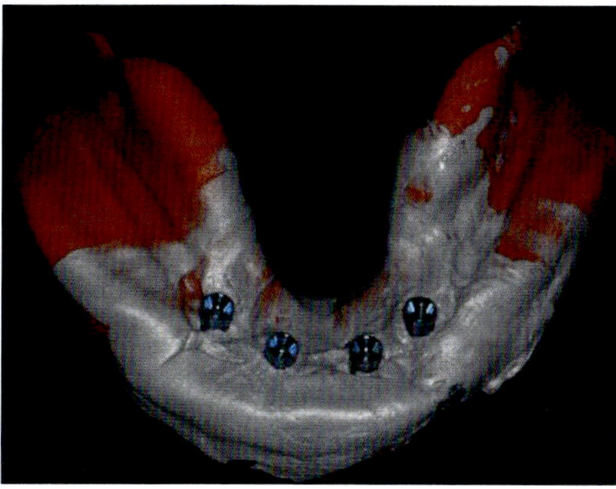

Fig. 13.15 Open-tray mandibular final impression of splinted impression copings using light and heavy bodied polyvinyl siloxane impression material

13.3.5 Wax Rim Adjustments

The maxillary occlusal wax rim was tried clinically and adjusted to establish the anterior and posterior occlusal planes based on lip support, anterior display, esthetic and phonetic parameters, and Camper's plane (Fig. 13.17a–c). The mandibular wax rim was then adjusted to the maxillary record base at the appropriate vertical dimension of occlusion. The vertical dimension was determined using phonetic [8] and facial measurements taken at the physiologic rest space [9] (Fig. 13.18a).

Maxillomandibular relationship was then recorded in centric relation using a fast set bite registration material (*Blue Bite, Polyvinylsiloxane, Henry Schein, Canada*). The recorded position was verified for reproducibility to confirm its accuracy (Fig. 13.18b). A facebow record was also taken to allow for proper positioning of the maxillary cast during mounting on a semi-adjustable articulator. Teeth shade and mold are selected and approved by the patient. All records are sent to the dental laboratory to have the casts mounted and denture teeth set in wax per the determined parameters. Bilateral balanced occlusion is recommended for complete denture therapy, although very little clinical evidence is available to support the use of this occlusal scheme for complete dentures and implant-retained/supported prostheses.

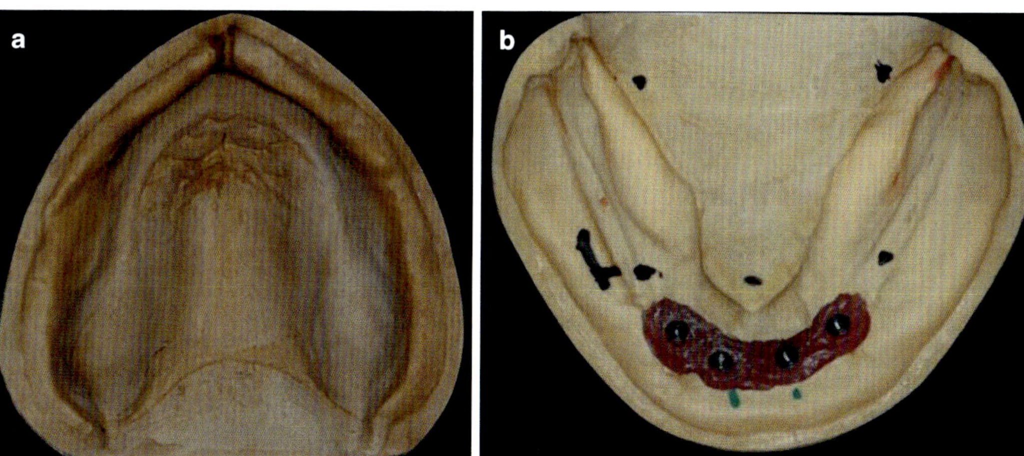

Fig. 13.16 (**a** and **b**) Master casts of the maxillary and mandibular arches

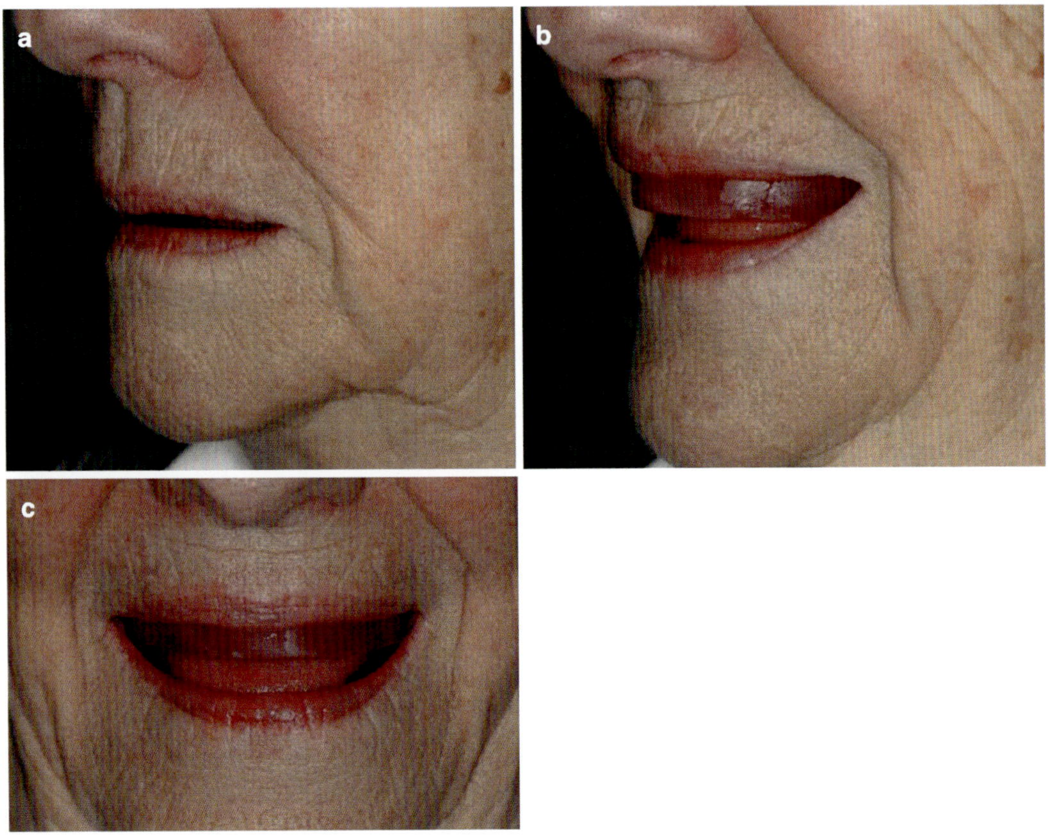

Fig. 13.17 Wax rim adjustments: (**a**) Lip support, (**b**) esthetic, and (**c**) occlusal plane alignment

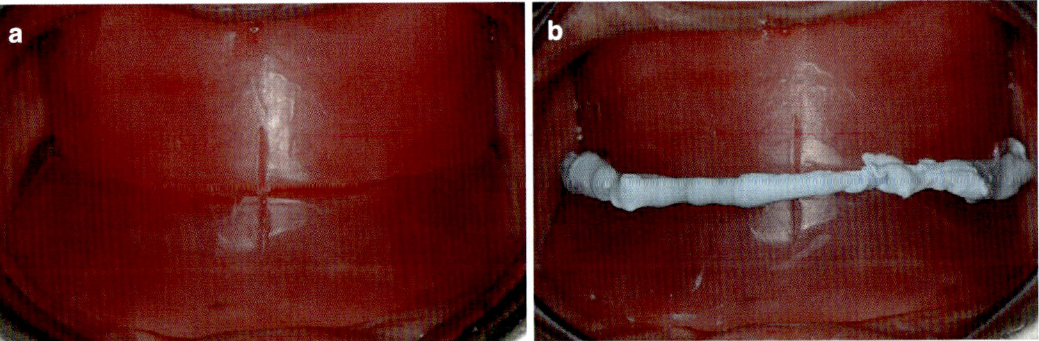

Fig. 13.18 (**a** and **b**) Wax rims are adjusted to the proper vertical dimension of occlusion and the maxillomandibular relationship recorded in centric relation using chin point guidance technique and a fast set silicone bite registration material

13.3.6 The Trial Denture

The teeth are set in wax (Fig. 13.19) and tried clinically to evaluate the esthetics, phonetics, function, stability, and occlusion (Fig. 13.20). Centric relation and vertical dimension of occlusion are confirmed. Once all parameters are verified and the patient is satisfied with esthetics and function, the case is returned to the dental laboratory for the design and fabrication of the mandibular Dolder bar.

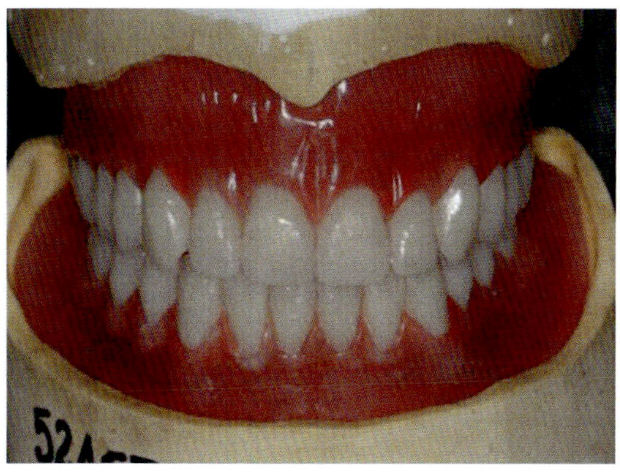

Fig. 13.19 Mounting on semi-adjustable articulator and setting of denture teeth per the determined parameters

13.3.7 Computer-Aided Design and Computer-Aided Manufacturing (CAD/CAM)

Once all the setup completed and verified clinically, the bar can be designed and manufactured. Most bar-type attachment systems consist of a metallic bar connected to the implant and a clip mechanism nested in the denture base. Most of the retentive bars are often distinguished by the morphological characteristics of their walls and their composition (Ackermann bar/spherical shape, Dolder bar/U shape or ovoid shape, Hader bar/keyhole

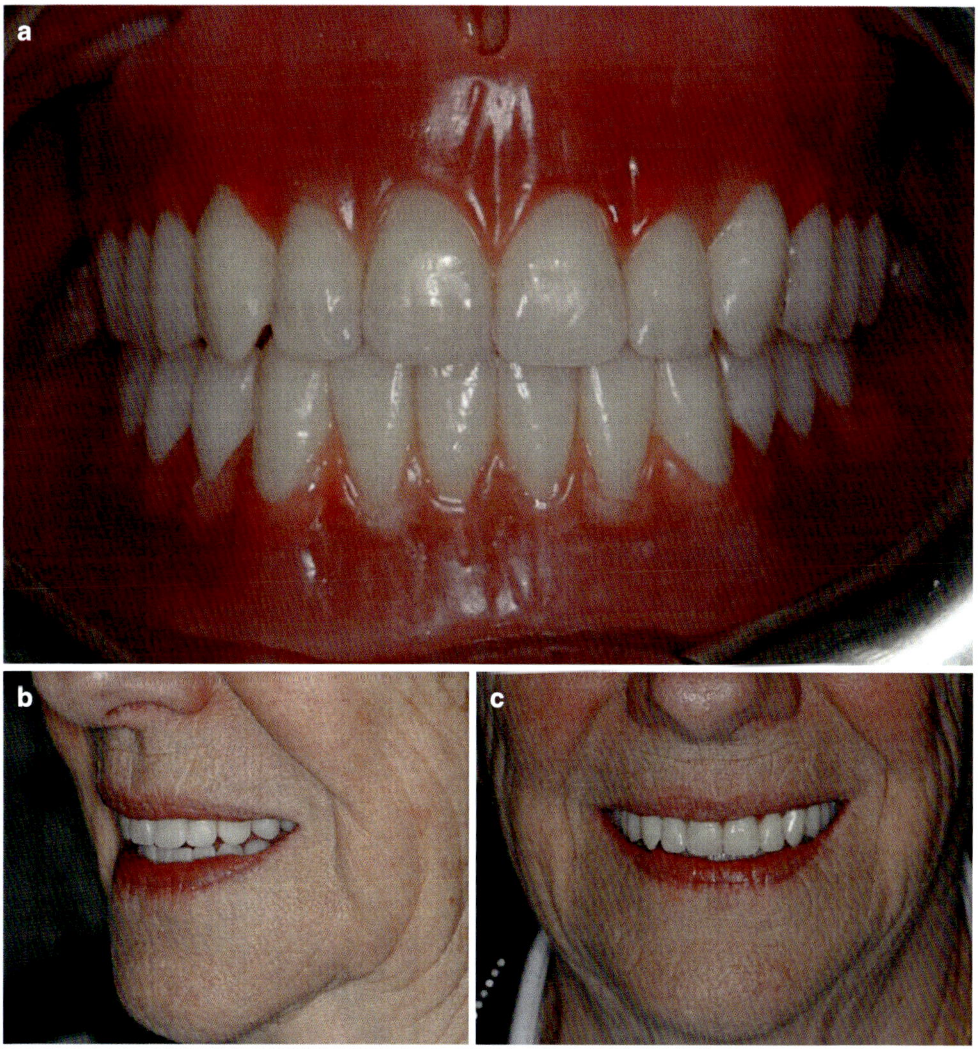

Fig. 13.20 (**a–c**) Denture teeth try-in to evaluate esthetics, phonetics, function, stability, occlusion and vertical dimension of occlusion during excursive movements

shape). Based on the later, bars can also be characterized as resilient or non-resilient. Resilient bars are designed to allow movement around their axis and are often recommended for the restoration of implants retained prostheses to accommodate the movement of the denture during mastication. The non-resilient designs are often recommended for implant-supported prostheses. They are characterized by parallel walls, which once engaged by the clip assembly, limit significantly the movement of the dentures.

A variety of methods exist for the fabrication of bars. The conventional method consisted of prefabricated bars that are adjusted (cut to desired dimension) and soldered to the abutments that are connected to the implants. Plastic patterns for various types of bars are also available and can be casted to produce the final bar. Bars can also be designed virtually by computer and fabricated by milling machines. The later method is today the most commonly used technique as it is assumed to offer advantages such as precision, accuracy, strength, and individualized design that the traditional methods do not [10]. Katsoulis et al. [11] compared the conventional soldered technique of bar fabrication to the new CAD/CAM approach and observed that milled bars resulted in less technical complications and fractures.

Bar design is dependent on several factors such as the available restorative space, the implant position, the amount of retention desired, the type of attachment systems, and the type of prosthesis desired (rigid vs. resilient).

When designing the bar, it is critical to determine the restorative space available, as the bar attachment system requires more space than a prosthesis using a stud attachment system (as described in a previous chapter). Sawdosky et al. reported that a minimum of 10–12 mm of space was required for a bar overdenture. This space is measured from the implant platform to the occlusal plane. The tooth setup is often used as a guideline in the

design process, and it is an essential component for the design phase. This information is digitally acquired by scanning the mandibular master cast as well as the tooth arrangement (Fig. 13.21a). Once the background information is captured, the virtual design process can begin (Fig. 13.21b, c). When designing the bar, certain important criteria should be respected: the bar should be positioned within the confine of the prosthesis and directly over the crest of the ridge (Fig. 13.21b), a space of about 2 mm or more between the bar and the soft tissue should be left to allow for proper hygiene (Fig. 13.22), and if a distal extension is planned, the later should not extend beyond 1.5 times the distance between the most anterior and most posterior implants [12–14]. Once the virtual design process is completed, the information is sent to a production center to have the bar milled from a titanium block.

13.3.8 Bar Try-In

The Dolder bar is tried intraorally and verified for proper fit and passivity. Alternate finger pressure, direct vision and tactile sensation, radiographs, one-screw test, and screw resistance test [15, 16] are all different methods that have been documented in the literature to evaluate the fit of a framework. Kan et al. [17] suggested using a combination of these different methods to verify and confirm the fit of a framework. The design of the bar is also evaluated visually to ensure that it is not impinging on the tissue and that adequate space is available for proper maintenance.

13.3.9 Second Trial Denture

The bar is returned to the laboratory, and the initial mandibular tooth setup is modified to fit onto the bar. Another clinical trial of the tooth arrangement is then performed. The mandibular tooth setup is tried over the bar and reevaluated to confirm that the parameters

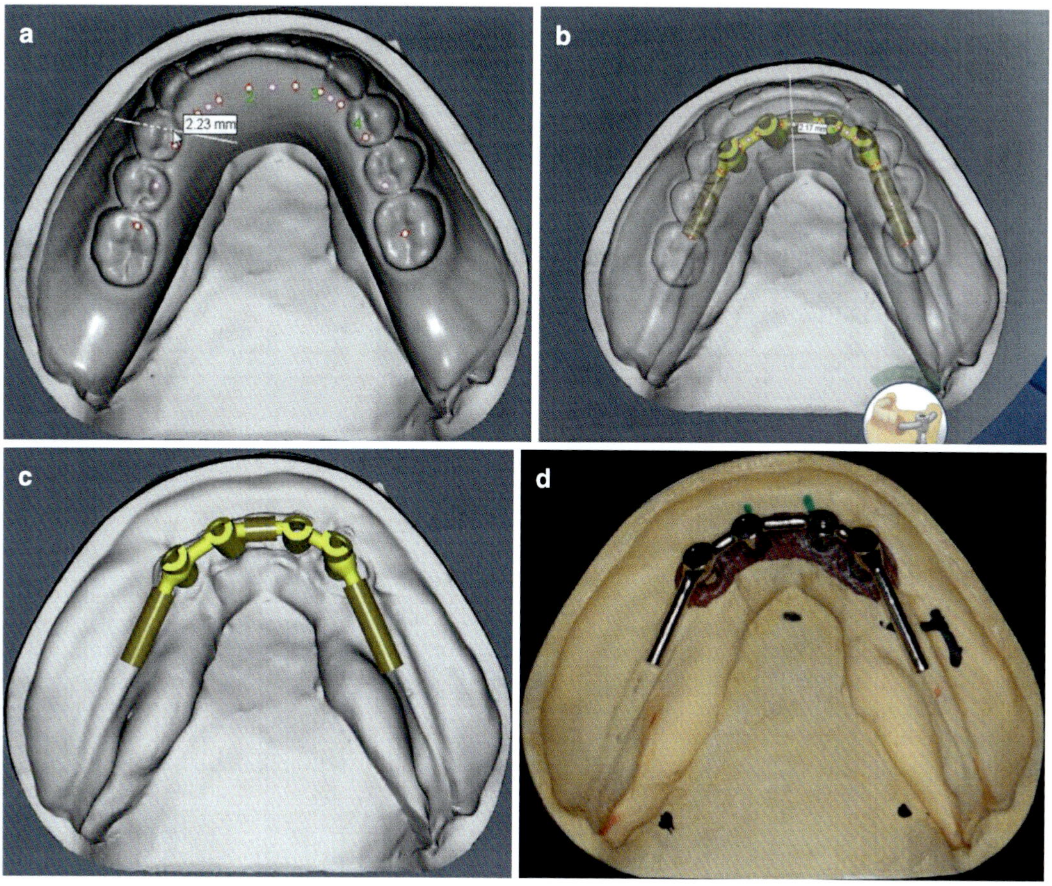

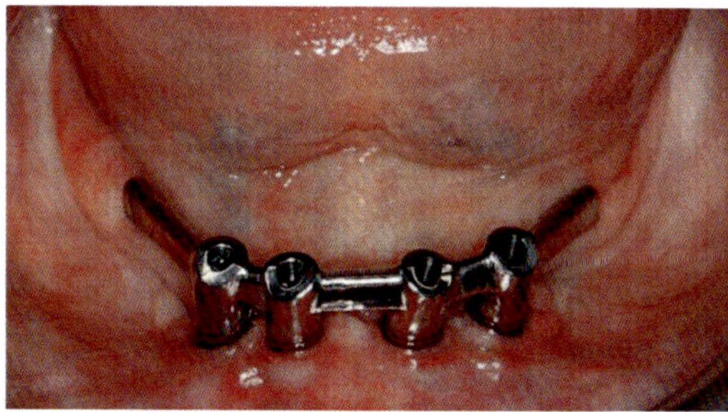

Fig. 13.21 (**a**) Digital scan of the mandibular master cast and tooth setup (**b**) 3-D virtual design of the Dolder bar beneath the planned prosthesis (**c**) Final design of Dolder bar (**d**) Manufactured Dolder bar

Fig. 13.22 Clearance of 2 mm between bar and tissue to allow for proper hygiene

established in the initial clinical trial (i.e., esthetics, phonetics, function, stability, occlusion, and vertical dimension of occlusion) were all maintained. Centric relation is reconfirmed. For implant-supported prostheses, tooth arrangement should not extend beyond the milled bar, which usually limits the occlusion to the first molars. Once all parameters are verified and the patient is satisfied with esthetics and function, the case is returned to the dental laboratory for processing and incorporation of the metal retentive clips (Fig. 13.23). Depending on the type of bars used, the retention mechanism/clips come in different materials. Metal clips are usually more resistant to wear, and their dimension can be customized to fit exactly onto the bar (especially important in small inter-implant segment), while plastic clips are easier to replace.

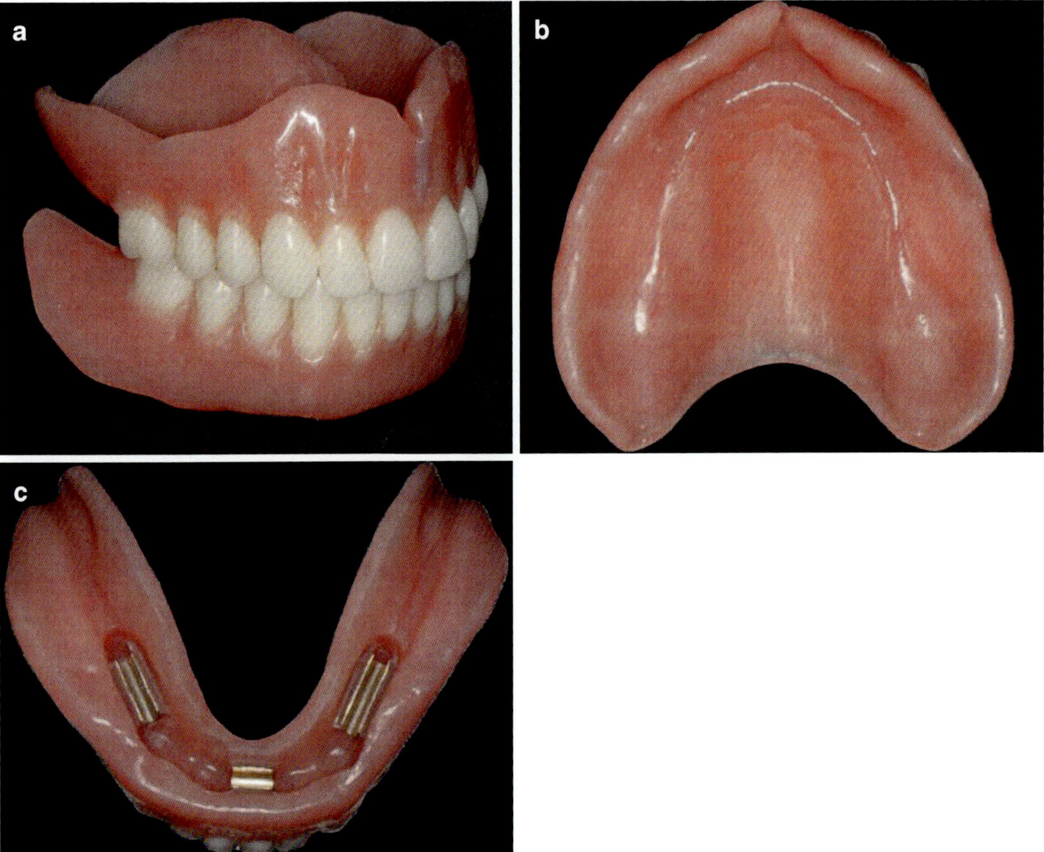

Fig. 13.23 (**a**) Acrylized removable prostheses (**b**) Maxillary complete denture (**c**) Mandibular overdenture with three retentive metal clips positioned in the anterior section and on the distal extensions

13.3.10 Delivery

The Dolder bar is seated in position, and the prosthetic screws are torqued to the manufacturer's recommendation using a torque wrench. The access holes are closed with cotton pellets and a composite material. This cotton protects the head of the prosthetic screws and allows for the removal of the bar at a latter appointment should there be a need. The mandibular implant-supported removable denture is tried onto the bar and evaluated for proper seating, fit, peripheral extension, retention, and stability. If necessary, the metal retentive clips can be adjusted to either increase or decrease the retention as needed. The occlusion is verified last and adjusted if any interference is detected in centric occlusion and eccentric movements (Fig. 13.24). The patient is shown how to insert and remove her prosthesis. Home care is explained, and the patient is shown to use an interdental brush to clean and remove plaque from the undersurface areas of the bar (Fig. 13.25). The patient is also instructed to remove her prostheses at night.

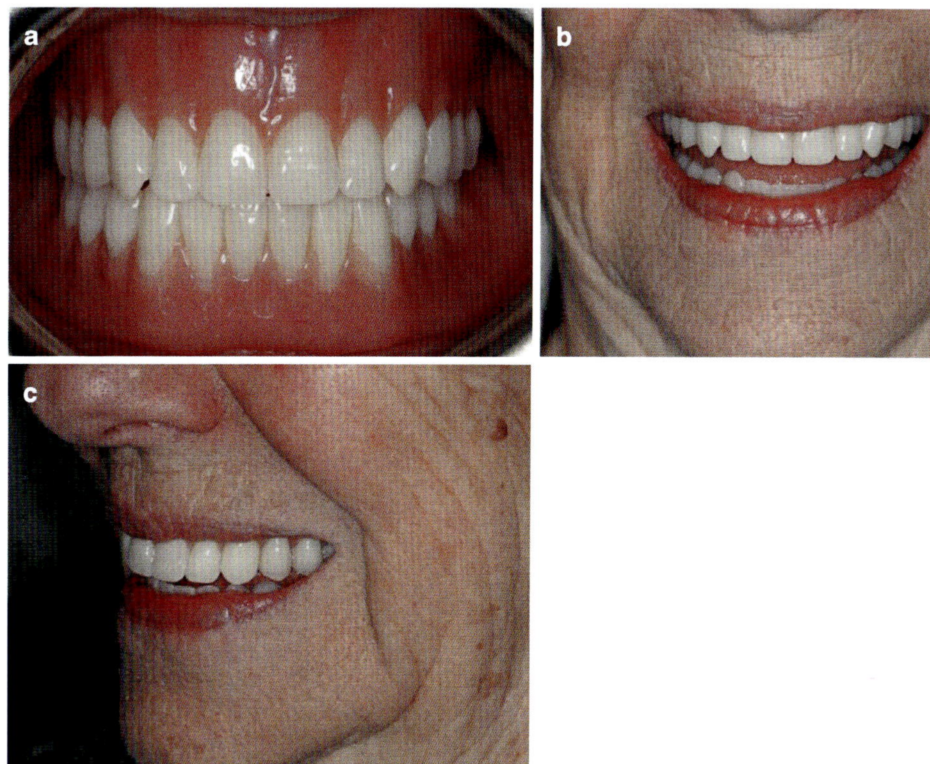

Fig. 13.24 (**a–c**) Delivery of complete upper denture and removable implant-supported mandibular overdenture

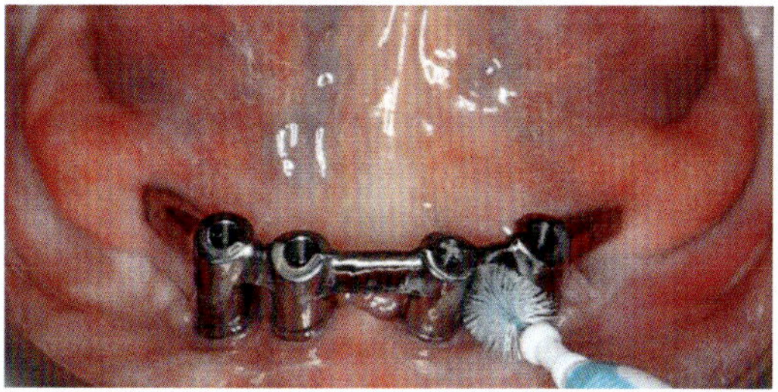

Fig. 13.25 Careful design of the bar allows for ease of maintenance

References

1. De Smet E, Duyck J, Vander Sloten J, Jacobs R, Naert I. Timing of loading – immediate, early, or delayed – in the outcome of implants in the edentulous mandible: a prospective clinical trial. Int J Oral Maxillofac Implants. 2007;22:580–94.
2. Esposito M, Grusovin MG, Achille H, Coulthard P, Worthington HV. Interventions for replacing missing teeth: different times for loading dental implants. Cochrane Database Syst Rev. 2009;21:CD003878.
3. Papaspyridakos P, Lal K, White GS, Weber HP, Gallucci GO. Effect of splinted and nonsplinted impression techniques on the accuracy of fit of fixed implant prostheses in edentulous patients: a comparative study. Int J Oral Maxillofac Implants. 2011;26(6):1267–72.
4. Assif D, Nissan J, Varsano I, et al. Accuracy of implant impression splinted techniques: effect of splinting material. Int J Oral Maxillofac Implants. 1999;14:885–8.
5. Buzayan M, Baig MR, Yunus N. Evaluation of accuracy of complete-arch multiple-unit abutment-level dental implant impressions using different impression and splinting materials. Int J Oral Maxillofac Implants. 2013;28(6):1512–20.
6. Papaspyridakos P, Chen CJ, Gallucci GO, Doukoudakis A, Weber HP, Chronopoulos V. Accuracy of implant impressions for partially and completely edentulous patients: a systematic review. Int J Oral Maxillofac Implants. 2014;29(4):836–45.
7. Wee AG. Comparison of impression materials for direct multi-implant impressions. J Prosthet Dent. 2000;83:323–31.

8. Pound E. Utilizing speech to simplify a personalized denture service. J Prosthet Dent. 1970;24(6):586–600.

9. Turrell AJ. Clinical assessment of vertical dimension. J Prosthet Dent. 1972;28(3):238–46.

10. Jemt T. Three-dimensional distortion of gold alloy castings and welded titanium frameworks. Measurements of the precision of fit between completed implant prostheses and the master casts in routine edentulous situations. J Oral Rehabil. 1995;22(8):557–64.

11. Katsoulis J, Wälchli J, Kobel S, Gholami H, Mericske-Stern R. Complications with computer-aided designed/computer-assisted manufactured titanium and soldered gold bars for mandibular implant-overdentures: short-term observations. Clin Implant Dent Relat Res. 2015;17(Suppl 1):75–85.

12. English CE. Critical A-P spread. Implant Soc. 1990;1(1):2–3.

13. Rangert B, Jemt T, Jörneus L. Forces and moments on Branemark implants. Int J Oral Maxillofac Implants. 1989;4(3):241–7.

14. Semper W, Heberer S, Nelson K. Retrospective analysis of bar-retained dentures with cantilever extension: marginal bone level changes around dental implants over time. Int J Oral Maxillofac Implants. 2010;25:385–93.

15. Jemt T. Failures and complications in 391 consecutively inserted fixed prostheses supported by Brånemark implant in the edentulous jaw: a study of treatment from the time of prostheses placement to the first annual check up. Int J Oral Maxillofac Implants 1991;6:270–6.

16. Yanase RT, Binon PP, Jemt T, Gulbransen HJ, Parel S. Current issue form. How do you test a cast framework for a full arch fixed implant supported prosthesis? Int J Oral Maxillofac Implants. 1994;9:471–4.

17. Kan JY, Rungcharassaeng K, Bohsali K, Goodacre CJ, Lang BR. Clinical methods for evaluating implant framework fit. J Prosthet Dent. 1999;81(1):7–13.

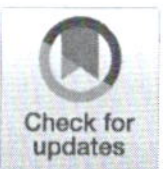

Case Presentation: Implant-Supported Fixed Mandibular Prostheses

14

Samer Abi Nader and Samer Mesmar

Abstract

This chapter will present a clinical case describing the treatment of a lower edentulous patient with an implant-supported fixed prosthesis. The surgical strategies underlining the placement and the distribution of the dental implants will be highlighted and discussed, as well as the concepts that underscore the design of the final prosthetic outcome.

The various clinical and laboratory steps starting from the planning to the completion of the prostheses will be presented. This includes the use of cone beam computer tomography in the planning process to prepare and plan for implant placement, the various impression technics, as well as the computer-aided design and manufacturing (CAD/CAM) of the titanium bar.

14.1 Patient History and Background

A 66-year-old female presented with the following chief concern: "My lower denture is very loose and I am having a hard time chewing and talk-ing, I want something fixed." The patient has been wearing her current set of tissue-supported removable dental prostheses for 4 years. She is satisfied with the overall performance of her maxillary denture. However, She is concerned with the absence of retention and stability of the mandibular prosthesis.

During the clinical examination, a moderately resorbed mandibular residual ridge was noted. In addition, high muscle attachments and shallow buccal and lingual vestibules were observed (Fig. 14.1). The overall prosthetic parameters of the current prostheses were acceptable in terms of teeth arrangement and display, maxillo-mandibular relashionship and occlusal vertical dimension (Fig. 14.2).

Patient's medical history consisted of a controlled hypertension and hyperthyroidism with medication. There is no history of smoking or known allergies.

14.2 Implant Placement Strategy

A cone beam computer tomography (CBCT) was performed in order to evaluate the bone volume in the mandibular arch as well as the location of anatomical structures. A preliminary assessment was completed, and four implants (NobelSpeedy Groovy) were planned for placement in the anterior sextant (Nobel Clinician, Nobel Biocare) (Fig. 14.3). A distal inclination was planned for the two posterior implants in order to improve the distribution and increase the anteroposterior spread. This

S. A. Nader, BSc, DMD, MSc, FRCD(C) (✉)
Department of Restorative Dentistry,
Faculty of Dentistry,
McGill University, Montreal, QC, Canada
e-mail: samer.abinader@mcgill.ca

S. Mesmar, DMD, MSc, FRCD(C)
Division of Prosthodontics, McGill University
Health Centre, Montreal, QC, Canada

© Springer International Publishing AG, part of Springer Nature 2018
E. Emami, J. Feine (eds.), *Mandibular Implant Prostheses*,
https://doi.org/10.1007/978-3-319-71181-2_14

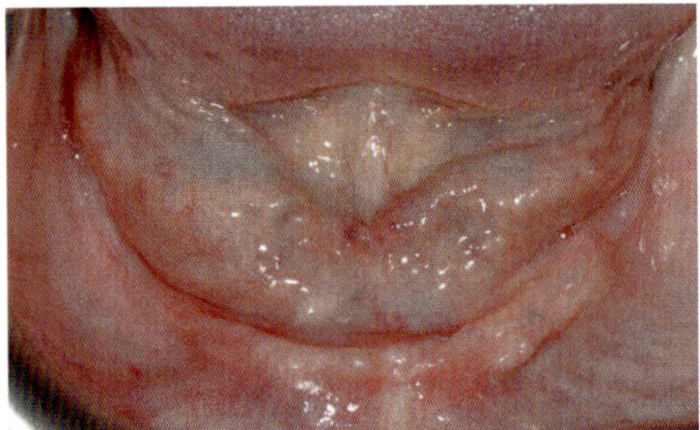

Fig. 14.1 Preoperative mandibular ridge

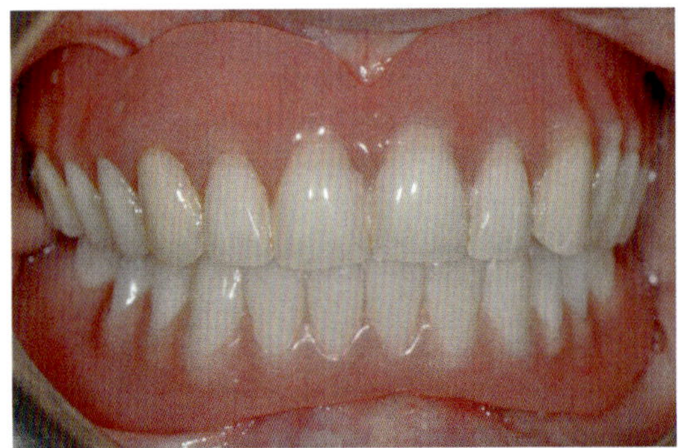

Fig. 14.2 Preoperative complete upper and lower prostheses

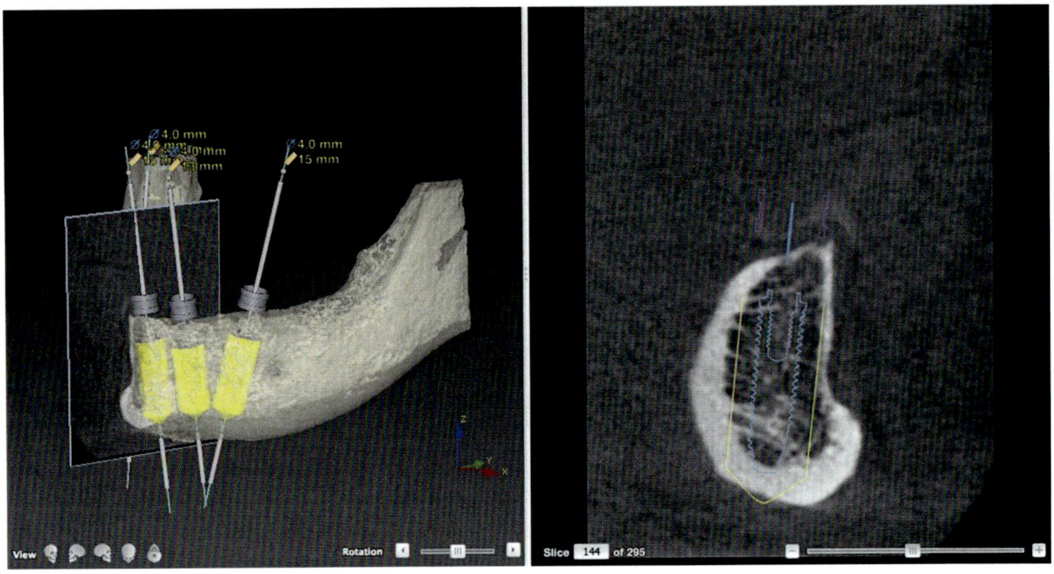

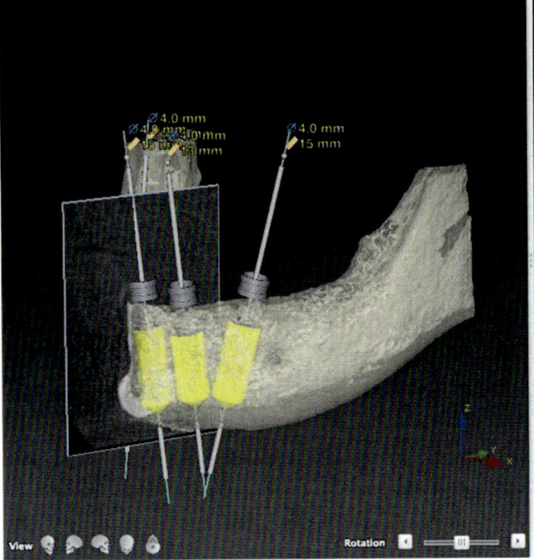

Fig. 14.3 Cone beam computer tomography illustrating the anticipated surgical placement of the four implants

surgical strategy will minimize the prosthetic cantilever as well as avoid the anterior loop of the inferior alveolar nerve [1]. This careful planning of the implant position should allow for the fabrication of a fixed implant supported prosthesis. This type of prosthetic design will significantly increase the stability of her lower prosthesis and greatly enhance her comfort during function.

With the mandibular prosthesis being adequate, a duplicate was made in acrylic in preparation for surgery (Fig. 14.4). The duplicate will be utilized during the surgical procedure to calibrate bone reduction to ensure the presence of sufficient restorative space for the prescribed treatment as well as target implant placement. The addition of beryllium sulfate in the acrylic

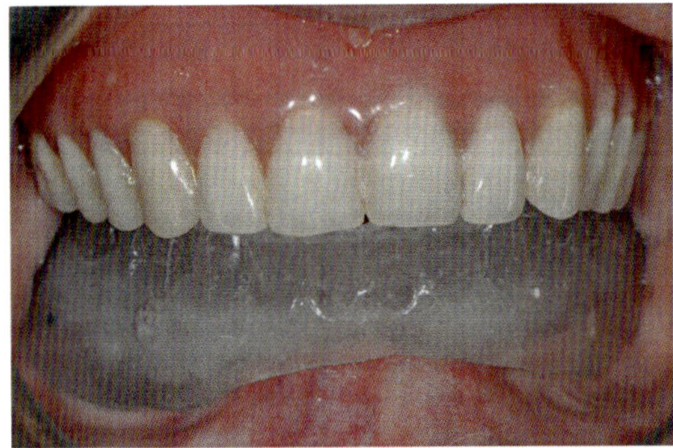

Fig. 14.4 Mandibular prosthesis duplicate in acrylic

mix would have provided a radiopaque medium. Wearing the latter during the CBCT would have provided a prosthetic guideline for further planning on the digital medium.

14.3 Clinical Procedures

14.3.1 Abutment Selection

Once the surgical procedure completed, healing abutments were placed during the healing period. After osteo-integration is confirmed and the soft tissue fully matured, the patient is ready for abutment selection (Fig. 14.5). Four multiunit abutments (Nobel Biocare) were selected and placed on the implants. The abutment selection was done to provide a prosthetic interface that is located at the level of the soft tissues as well as correct the posterior implant angulation (Fig. 14.6). The angle correction is necessary to align the access holes of all four implants within the occlusal table of the lower teeth. The surgical guide is generally used for this step; it provides a guideline to position the angulated abutments (Fig. 14.7). The abutments are then torqued to the recommended manufacturer values using a torque controller.

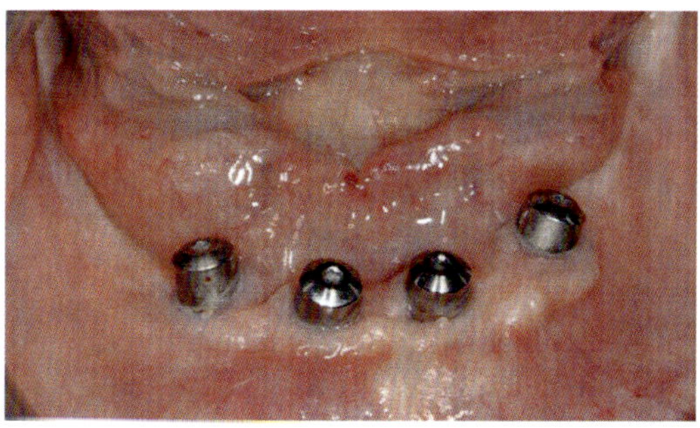

Fig. 14.5 Mandibular residual ridge following implant placement. Surgery: Dr. Veronique Benhamou, Periodontist

14.3.2 Preliminary and Final Impressions of the Upper Arch

An impression of the maxillary ridge was taken using an irreversible hydrocolloid material *(Jeltrate Alginate, Dentsply Caulk, Canada)* and a stock trays for edentulous arch *(Patterson Dental Supply, Canada)* (Fig. 14.8a). The impression was then poured with type III stone *(GC America Inc., USA)* in order to produce a preliminary cast for custom tray fabrication.

The maxillary custom tray was fabricated using a light-cured acrylic material *(Triad TruTray, Dentsply, Canada)*. The extensions were trimmed to allow space for dental compound material used to border mold the periphery. After the custom tray was verified intraorally, border molding was performed, using dental compounds *(Kerr Dental, Canada)*, by having the patient execute various movements to capture the functional periphery (Fig. 14.8b). Subsequently, the final impression of the maxillary arch was taken using a polysulfide rubber material *(Permlastic™, Kerr Dental)* (Fig. 14.8c). A working cast was then produced (Fig. 14.8d) and baseplate with wax rim fabricated.

14.3.3 Preliminary and Final Impressions of the Lower Arch

Fixed implant-supported prostheses depend solely on dental implants for their support, retention, and stability. Therefore, the registration of a functional periphery using the border-molding technique and a custom tray is not indicated for this prosthetic design. The use of a stock tray to register the anatomical details of the mandible,

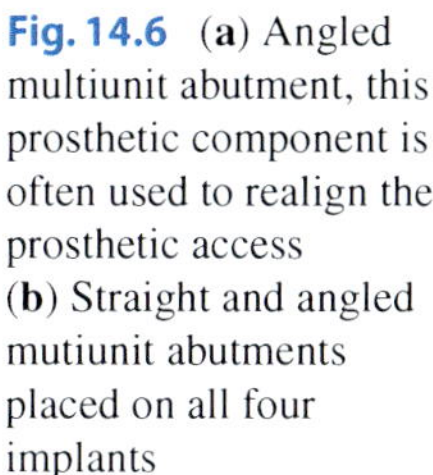
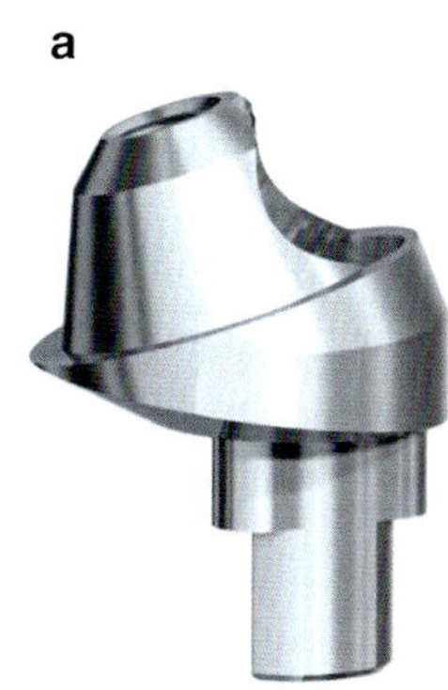
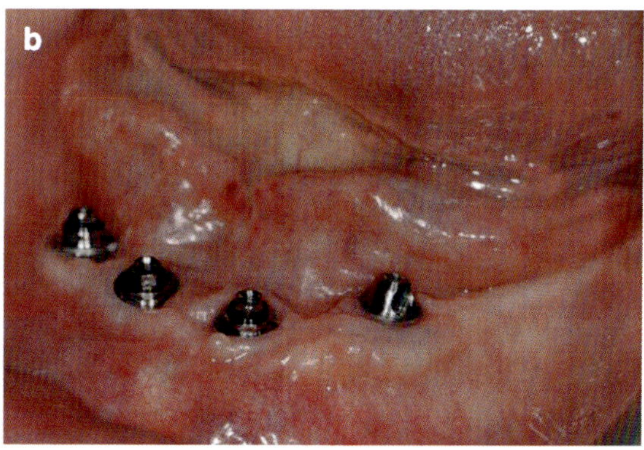

Fig. 14.6 (**a**) Angled multiunit abutment, this prosthetic component is often used to realign the prosthetic access (**b**) Straight and angled mutiunit abutments placed on all four implants

as well as register the implant position, is generally sufficient. Various techniques have been described in the literature to take the mandibular impression [2]. The main differences are related to the concept of splinting vs. non-splinting the impression copings during the process.

When assessing the success rate of fixed implant-supported dental prostheses, multiple factors are important to consider [3]. One of the major considerations is the passive fit of the superstructure attached to the implants. Passivity of fit is important to the success of any prosthesis due to the nature of

the implant-bone interface [3]. Several clinical and technical variables can affect this parameter, namely, the impression material, impression and pouring techniques, the die stone properties, machining tolerance of prosthetic components, in addition to implant angulation, and depth [4]. Several articles have been published to assess the effect of splinting the impression copings when taking an impression of multiple implants [5]. It has been reported that splinting may reduce the variance in the implant analog position within the cast, therefore producing a more accurate working model [6]. Moreover, ensuring that the components are joined intraorally using an auto-polymerizing acrylic material seems to improve the accuracy of the final impression [7].

The fabrication of the splint is generally done intraorally. However, the use of a model greatly facilitates the procedure and reduces chair time during the final impression appointment. Pickup impression copings were connected to the multiunit abutments on the mandibular arch (Fig. 14.9); a non-splinted preliminary impression using polyvinyl siloxane *(Affinis, Coltene Dental)* was taken using a stock tray *(COE, GC America, USA)* (Fig. 14.10) and poured using ISO type IV dental stone *(Snap-Stone, Whip Mix, USA)*. This preliminary cast will be utilized for splint fabrication (Fig. 14.11a).

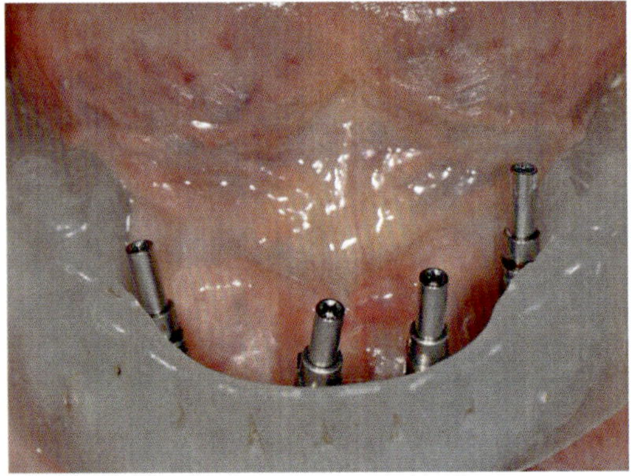

Fig. 14.7 Abutment selection and alignment

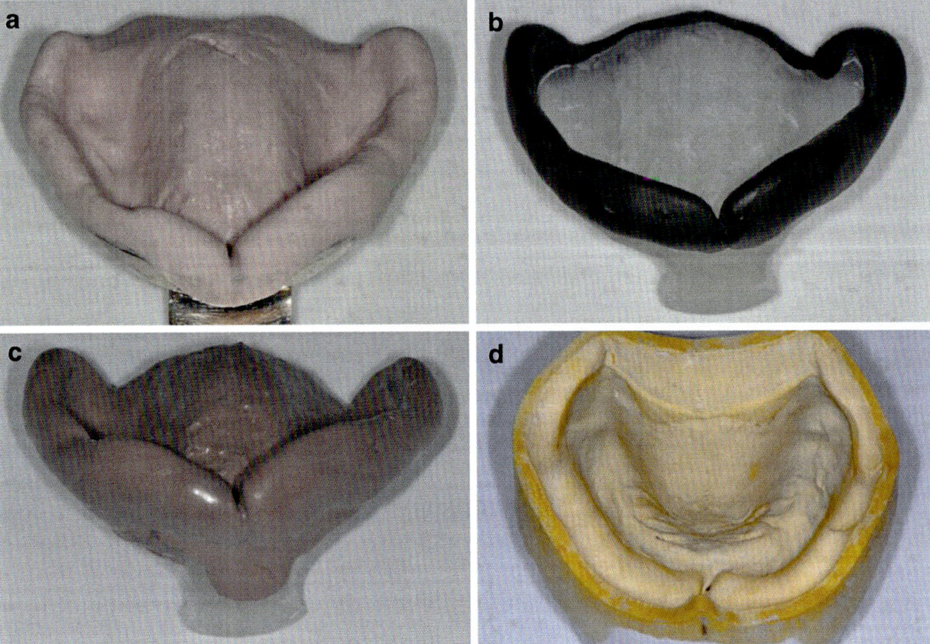

Fig. 14.8 (**a**) Preliminary maxillary impression (**b**) Custom tray and border molding (**c**) Final maxillary impression (**d**) Final maxillary cast

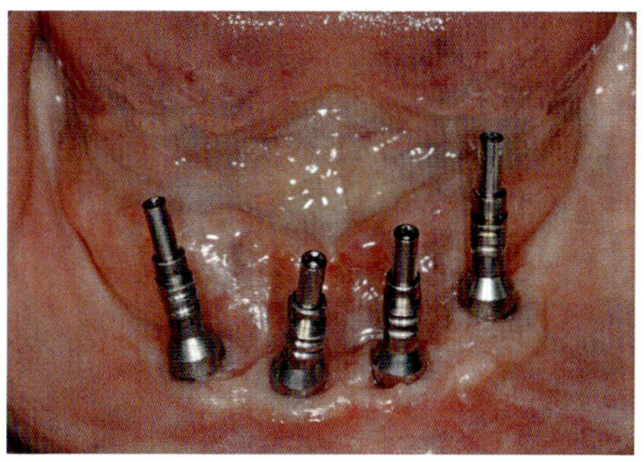

Fig. 14.9 Abutment level impression copings placed onto multiunit abutments

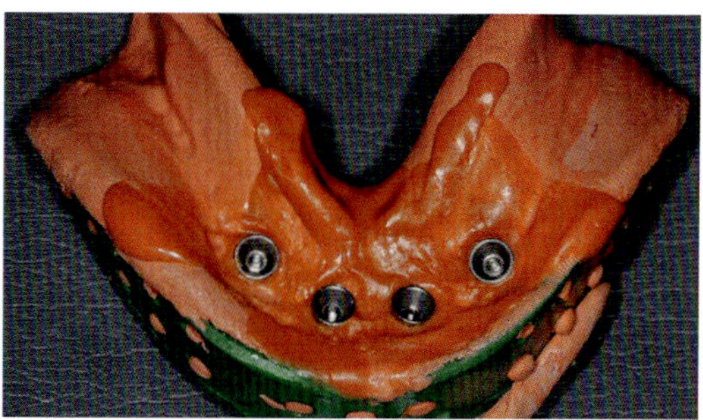

Fig. 14.10 Non-splinted preliminary impression using polyvinyl siloxane

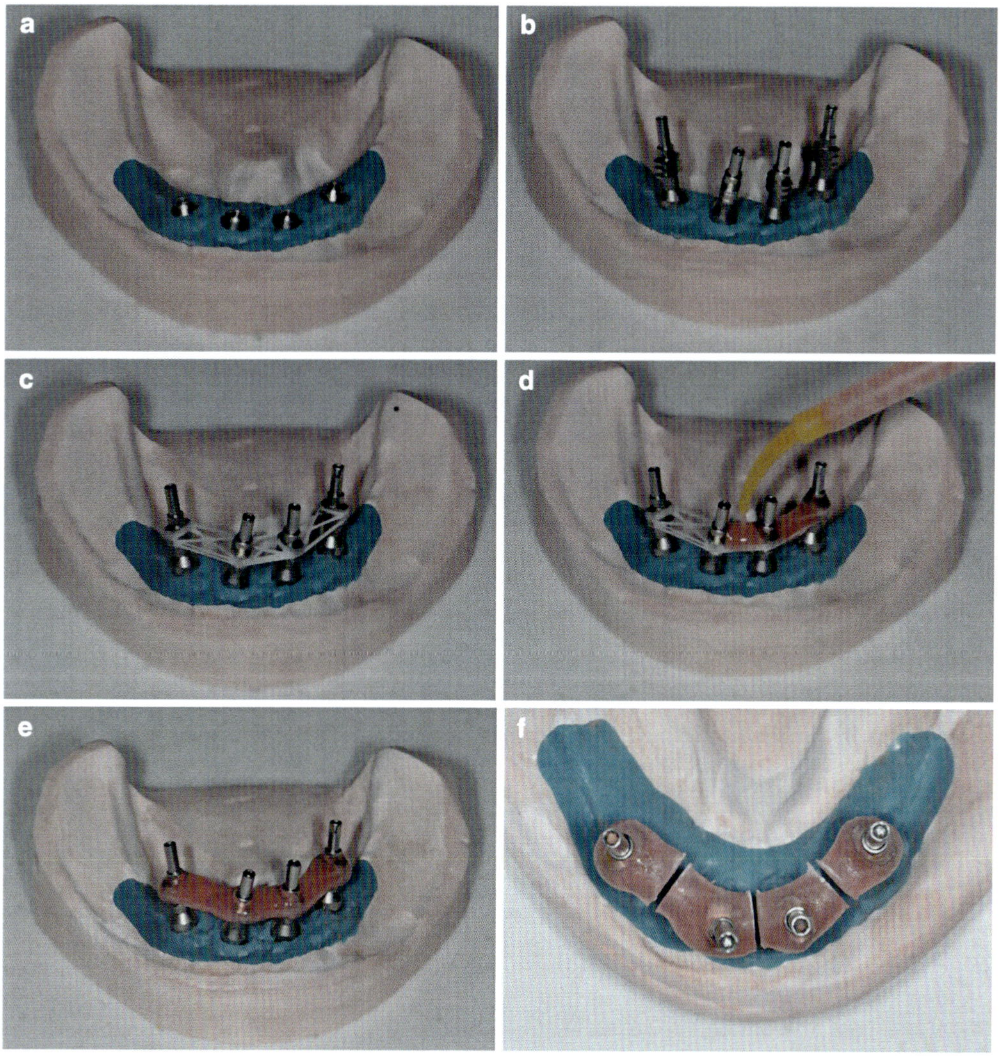

Fig. 14.11 (**a**) Preliminary cast used for splint fabrication (**b**) Abutment level impression copings placed onto multiunit abutment analogs (**c**) Dental floss tied around impression copings to support splinting material (**d**) Syringing with light curing composite material (**e**) Impression copings splinted. (**f**) Sectioning of the splint in between impression copings

The splint fabrication starts by connecting the abutment level impression copings on the multiunit abutment analogs (Fig. 14.11b). A dental floss is then tied around the impression copings to support the splinting material (Fig. 14.11c). A light-curing composite material is syringed *(TRIAD Dual-line, Dentsply. Canada)* onto the meshwork created by the floss in order to splint the impression copings (Fig. 14.11d). Once the splint is completed (Fig. 14.11e), it is sectioned in between the corresponding impression copings (Fig. 14.11d). A stock tray (COE, GC America, USA) is then adjusted by creating a window allowing for an open-tray impression technique (Fig. 14.12). As discussed earlier, the use of a custom tray to capture the functional border of the mandible is not indicated for an implant-supported fixed mandibular denture. The next steps consist of placing the sectioned splint intraorally and confirm seating clinically and/or radiographically (Fig. 14.13a). A self-cured acrylic *(Pattern resin LS, GC America, USA)* is then used to splint all sections (Fig. 14.13b). Once the material has fully set, the impression is made using a polyvinyl siloxane material *(Affinis, Coltene Dental)* (Fig. 14.14a). The impression is poured using ISO type IV stone *(Fujirock EP, GC America, USA)* with a soft tissue analog to produce the definitive cast (Fig. 14.14b).

A verification jig can be fabricated using the same steps described earlier. The jig is splinted on the final model using a pattern resin and transferred to the oral cavity in order to verify the seat and confirm the precision of the final model prior to the fabrication of the titanium bar. Once both the final upper and lower impressions are completed and definitive casts produced, the occlusion wax rims are fabricated for intraoral adjustments.

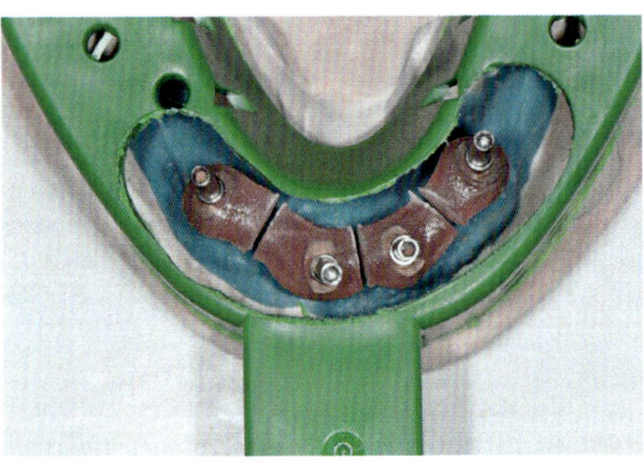

Fig. 14.12 Adjustment of stock tray for an open impression technique

14.3.4 Wax Rim Adjustments

The adjustments of maxillary and mandibular occlusion rims are then completed as described in detail in the previous chapters. The lip support, incisal display, midline, and occlusal plane are all adjusted and recorded on the upper rim following the conventional complete denture protocols (Fig. 14.15a, b). The physiological rest position and the vertical dimension of occlusion are determined using the lower wax rim.

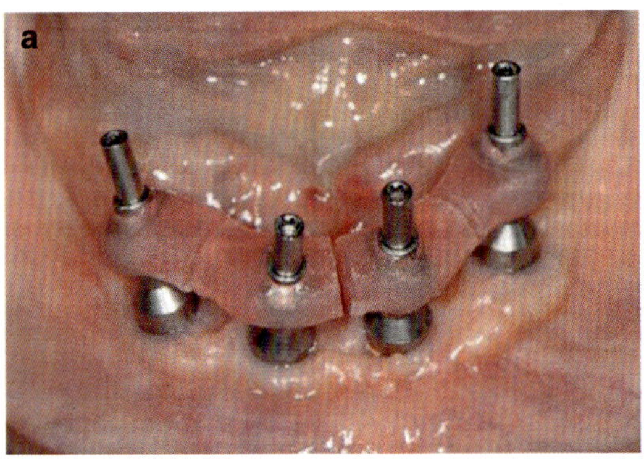
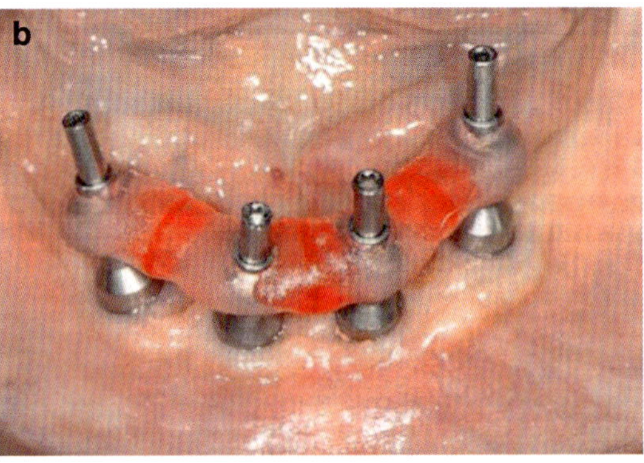

Fig. 14.13 (a) Placement of sectioned splint intraorally (b) Splinting intraorally of each section using auto-polymerizing acrylic

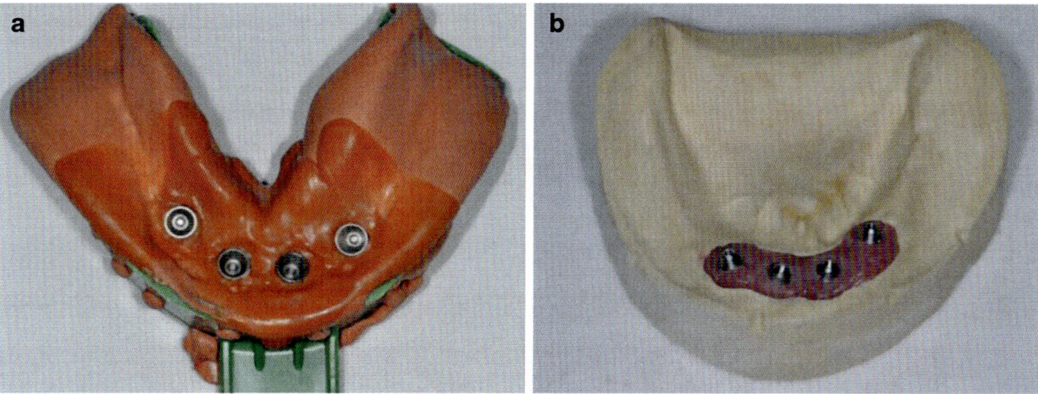

Fig. 14.14 (**a**) Final impression with the splinted impression copings (**b**) Definitive cast with soft tissue analogue around the implant replicas

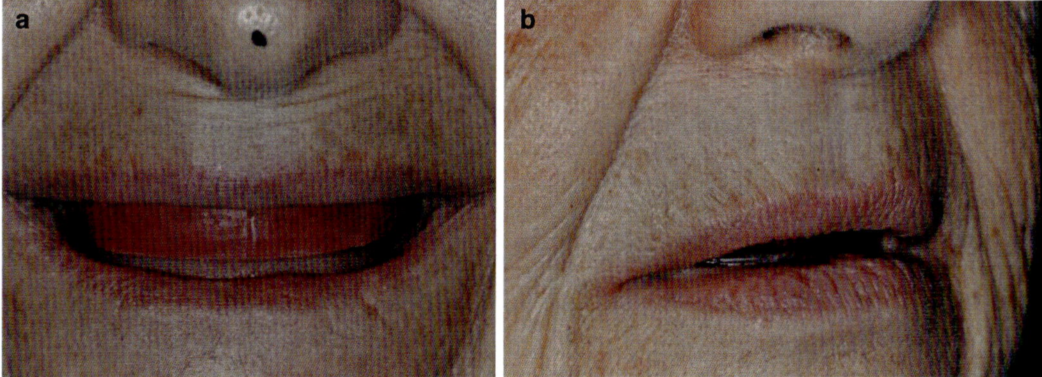

Fig. 14.15 Wax rim adjustments: (**a**) esthetic, occlusal plane alignment and (**b**) lip support

Maxillo-mandibular relationship is then recorded in centric relation using a fast set bite registration material (*Jet Blue Bite registration material, Coltene Whaledent*) (Fig. 14.16). The recorded position is then verified for reproducibility. All records are sent to the dental laboratory to have the casts mounted and denture teeth set according to the determined parameters. Balanced occlusion is recommended for complete denture therapy, although very little clinical evidence is available to support the use of this occlusal scheme for complete dentures and implant-retained/implant-supported prosthesis.

14.3.5 The Trial Denture

The tooth setup is tried clinically to evaluate the esthetics, phonetics, function, stability, and occlusal contacts during mandibular move-ments (Fig. 14.17). Once all parameters are verified and the patient is content with esthetics and function (Fig. 14.18a, b), the case is sent back to the dental laboratory to request the design and fabrication of the mandibular bar.

14.3.6 Computer-Aided Design and Computer-Aided Manufacturing (CAD/CAM)

The design process is started by scanning the mandibular working model as well as the tooth setup into the selected software. Various bar designs are available from different manufacturer that can adapt to different implant or abutment platforms. Most of the design features are dependent on the available restorative space and the restorative material selected.

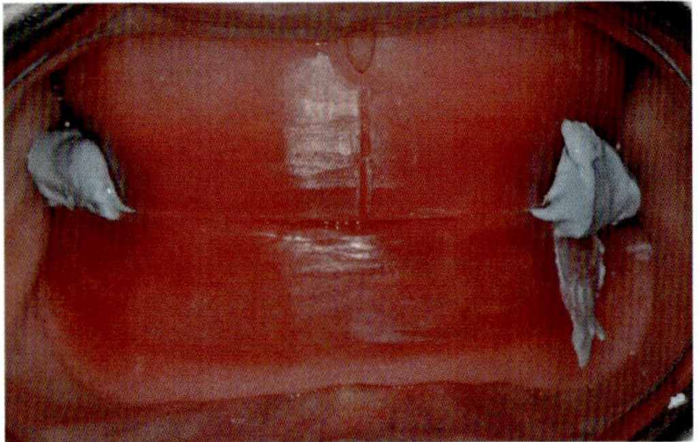

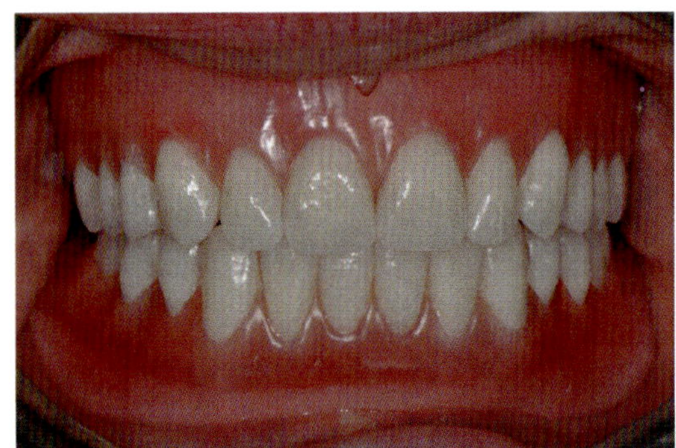

Fig. 14.16 Intermaxillary relationship recorded in centric relation

Fig. 14.17 Denture teeth try-in

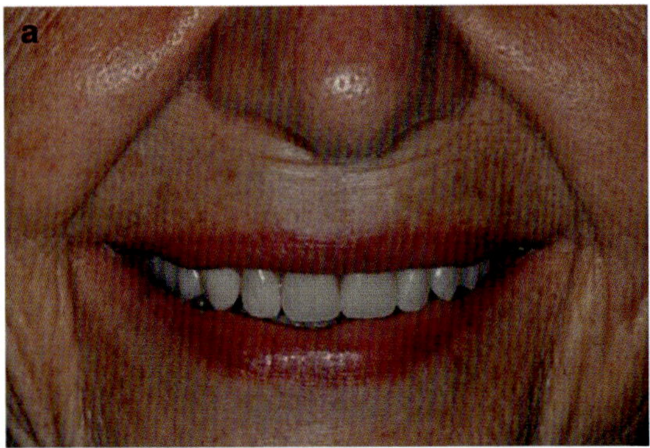

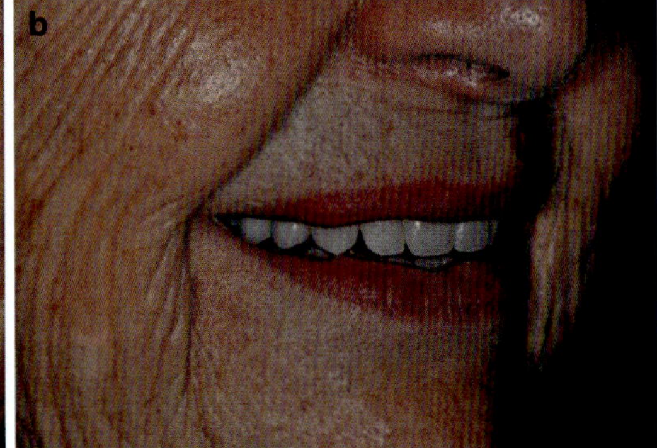

Fig. 14.18 (**a**, **b**) Denture teeth try-in to evaluate esthetics, phonetics, function, stability, and occlusal contacts during mandibular movements

Fixed implant-supported prostheses have different space requirements depending on the selected design and restorative material. It is very important to assess the available restorative space prior to communicating the options of prostheses to the patient. These options can be divided into three distinct categories: porcelain fused to metal-, zirconia-, or metal-acrylic-based prostheses. Restorative space is usually measured from the implant platform to the opposing dentition or plane of occlusion. For a fixed porcelain fused to metal or zirconia prosthesis, a minimum of 7–8 mm is required depending if it is a screw-retained or cemented restoration [8]. A metal-acrylic prosthesis, a minimum of 12–14 mm, is required to allow space for the metal bar and enough thickness for the acrylic supporting the denture teeth [9]. Other factors such as phonetics, esthetics, patient expectation, hygiene, and maintenance also need to be assessed carefully prior to deciding on the type of prosthesis recommended [10].

For implant-supported metal-acrylic fixed prosthesis, metal bars provide the support and strength required. Conventionally, metal bars were fabricated using a casting method, which is labor-intensive and technique sensitive [8]. CAD/CAM technology introduced a milling process to fabricate the metal bars.

Today, titanium milled bars have become the "standard of care" for the treatment of the lower edentulous arch with a fixed implant-supported prosthesis. Several articles have demonstrated their superior fit and passivity when compared to conventional casted bars [11, 12].

The titanium bar is usually fabricated out of a solid block medical grade titanium and milled using a *5-axis milling machine*. Titanium is well suited for this purpose because of its resistance to corrosion, biocompatibility, low cost and favorable mechanical properties. The final product is a one-piece titanium bar that is not susceptible to any deformation or errors which may result with the casting and soldering procedures [13]. The bar generally incorporates retentive features for improved mechanical retention of the acrylic. The framework has to support the denture teeth with a suggested minimum height of 4 mm [14].

The design features of the bar are heavily influenced by the final position of the prosthetic teeth. Support and retentive characteristics are strategically planned in order to optimize the final result. The two most common designs for the mandibular arch are the "wrap-around" and the "Montreal" bars. The "wrap-around" bar allows for the placement of acrylic on the intaglio surface and will permit for easier modifications of the fitting area (Fig. 14.19a, b). The "Montreal" bar is a more complex design featuring a full titanium surface in contact with the soft tissues (Fig. 14.20a, b). Highly polished titanium is generally more hygienic because it is less retentive to plaque. This feature may be of interest in cases were oral hygiene is a challenge.

14.3.7 Bar Try-In

The bar is returned to the laboratory after milling, finishing, and polishing. The mandibular denture teeth are then remounted on the bar using a remount jig (Fig. 14.21) in order to preserve all the prosthetic parameters that were previously established and verified clinically (Fig. 14.22). The case is then sent back to the clinician for a final try-in with the teeth in wax to confirm the passive fit of the bar intraorally, as well as verify all the necessary clinical parameters (Fig. 14.23). Several methods have been described in the literature for evaluating framework fit: alternate finger pressure, direct vision and tactile sensation, radiographs, one-screw test, and screw resistance test [15, 16]. A combination of these different methods should be used to verify the fit [17]. This step will also provide the clinician and the patient with the anticipated final contours of

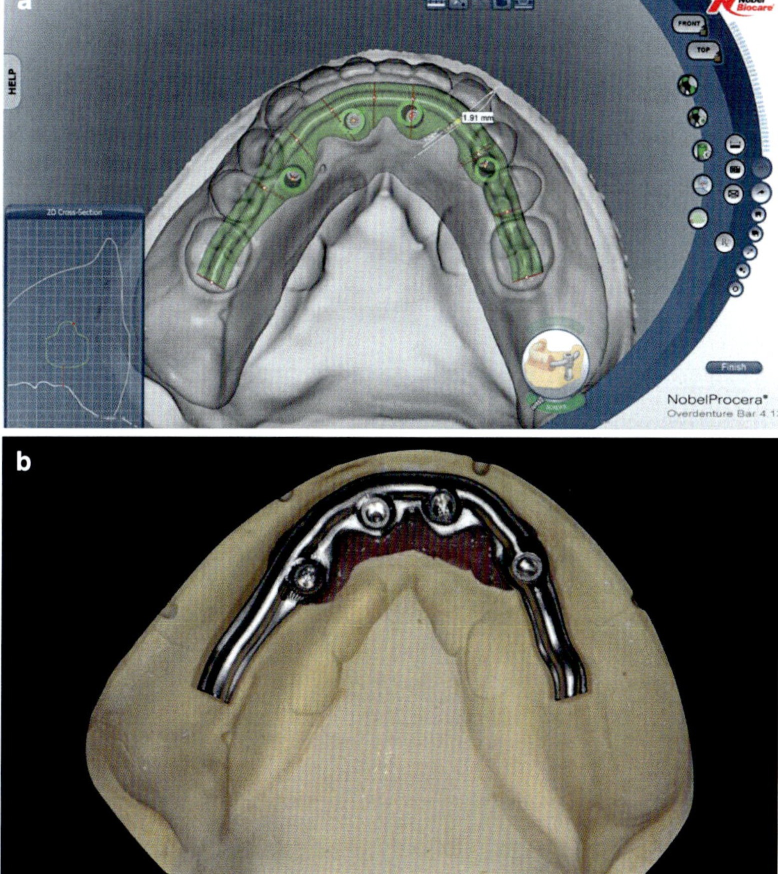

Fig. 14.19 (**a**) Occlusal and sectional views of the CAD software "NobelProcera™" demonstrating denture teeth position over the designed wrap-around bar (**b**) Completed bar in titanium

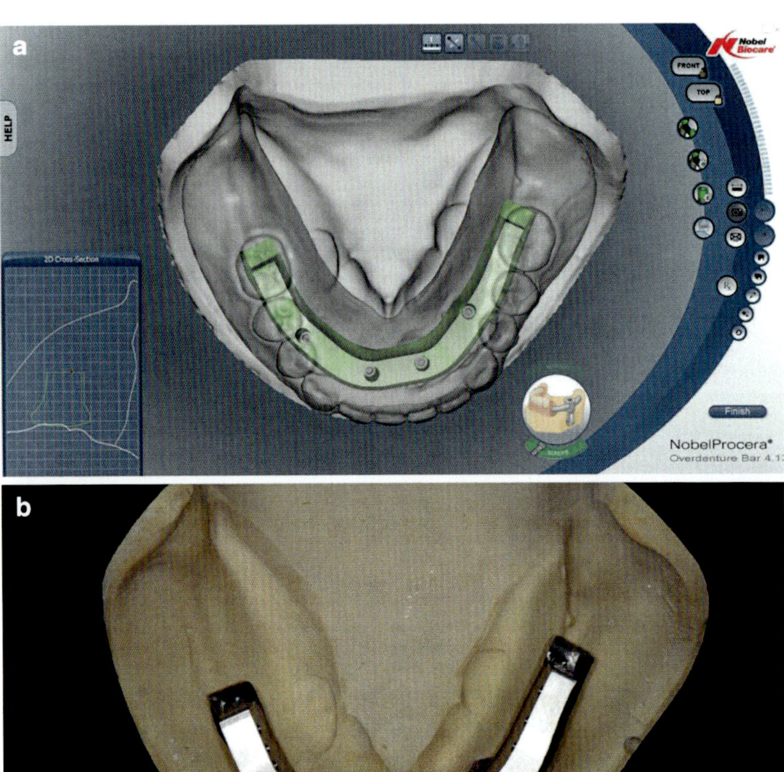

Fig. 14.20 (**a**) Occlusal and sectional views of the CAD software "NobelProcera™" demonstrating denture teeth position over the designed bar "Montreal" (**b**) Completed bar in titanium with added lingual and buccal channels to enhance the retention of the resin

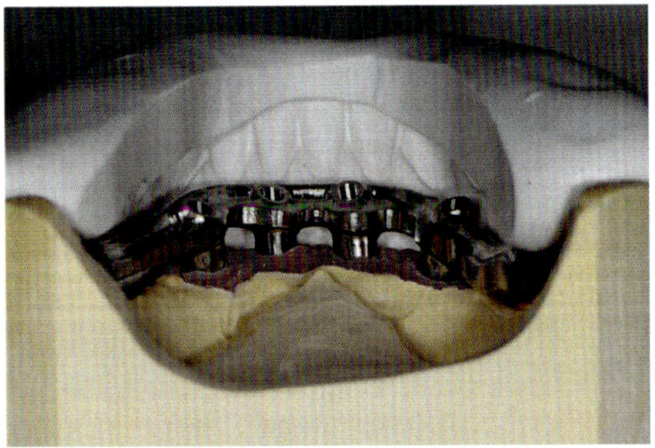

Fig. 14.21 Teeth being transferred onto the bar using a silicone positioning index

the prosthesis and would allow for some minor modifications prior to final processing. This is generally more critical for the maxillary prosthesis as the gingival and buccal contours have an influence on the phonetic and the esthetic outcomes. Once all parameters are reverified and the patient is satisfied with esthetics and function, the prostheses are sent back to the dental laboratory for final processing.

14.3.7.1 Design Principle of Prosthetic Contours

The design principles of the prosthetic contours for the fixed implant-supported prosthesis are centered on creating a prosthesis that is cleanable by the patient. This is an essential component of the treatment to allow patients to properly care for their restoration. Fixed prosthesis should not possess any flanges extending beyond the position of the implants (Fig. 14.24) which is critical in providing access for maintenance. The presence of flanges will hinder the removal of any food particles that accumulate between the denture and the soft tissues possibly causing biological complications in the long run. Essentially, the intaglio surface of the prosthesis that is in contact

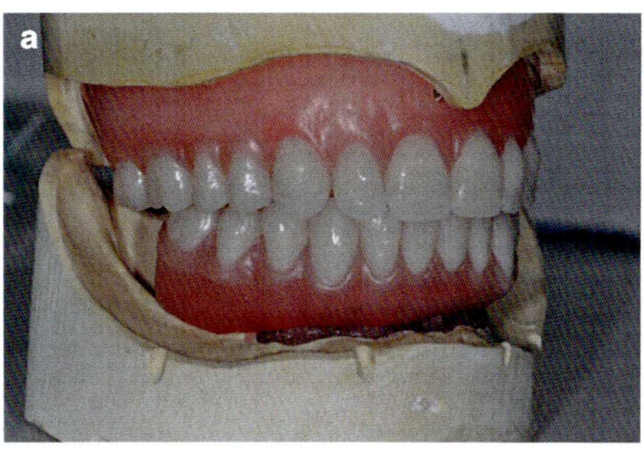 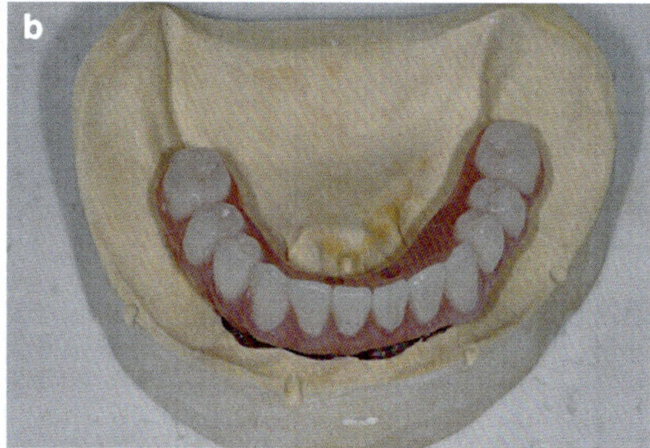

Fig. 14.22 Remounting the mandibular denture teeth on the titanium framework according to the predetermined parameters

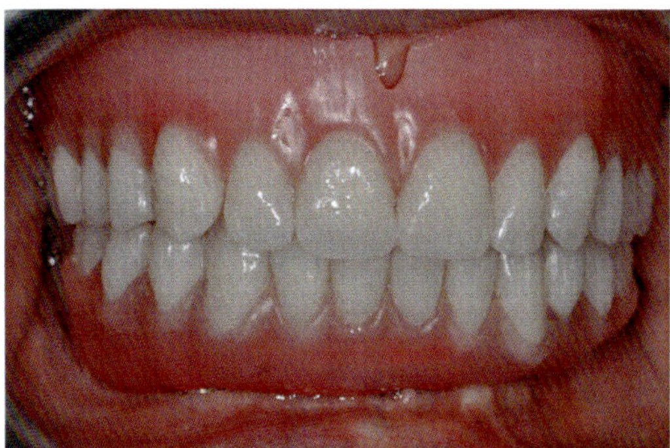

Fig. 14.23 Bar and denture try-in to evaluate passivity and prosthetic parameters

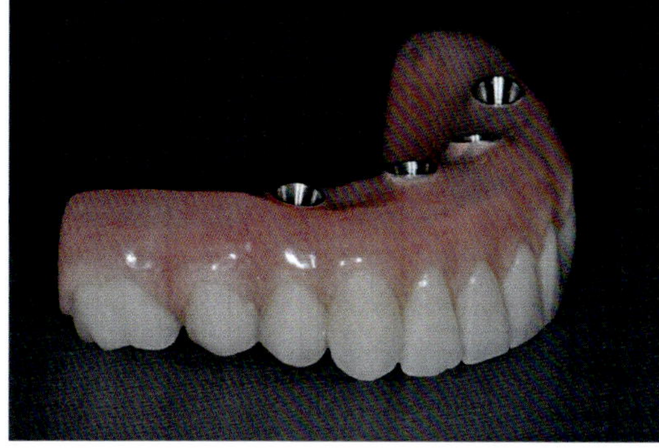

Fig. 14.24 Prosthetic contours of implant-supported fixed mandibular prosthesis

with soft tissues should be convex to discourage the accumulation of debris and allow for easier plaque removal on a daily basis. Lastly, the prosthesis should be in contact with the soft tissues without creating any hindrance for hygienic care. This is in contrast with the original design where a space was intentionally created to allow for maintenance. This intimate contact will minimize the accumulation of large food debris as well as limit the airflow bellow the prosthesis during speech.

14.3.7.2 Delivery of the Final Prosthesis

The final upper and lower prosthesis are acrylized and prepared for delivery to the patient (Fig. 14.25). The lower prosthesis is placed in position and evaluated for proper seating and fit as described earlier. The prosthetic screws are torqued to the manufacturers' recommendation using a torque wrench (15 N/CM). The access holes are sealed with cotton pellets and a composite material; this will ensure the possibility to reaccess the prosthetic screws if needed without any difficulties. The upper prosthesis is also seated and the presence of pressure spots assessed. The clinical parameters are verified, and all the esthetic and functional parameters are reconfirmed. The desired occlusal scheme is reassessed, and minor adjustments are done accordingly (Fig. 14.26).

Hygiene instructions are given to the patient in order to ensure proper care for the lower and the upper prosthesis. The maintenance of this type of prosthesis is considered more challenging. Abi Nader et al. in 2015 [18] determined that plaque often accumulates on the fitting surface of the denture in proximity to the soft tissues. This accumulation was more significant on the lingual areas of the prosthesis; this is possibly due to a more

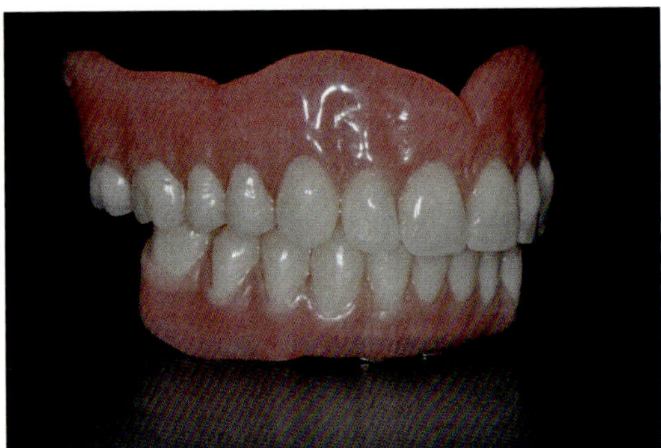

Fig. 14.25 Completed upper and lower prosthesis

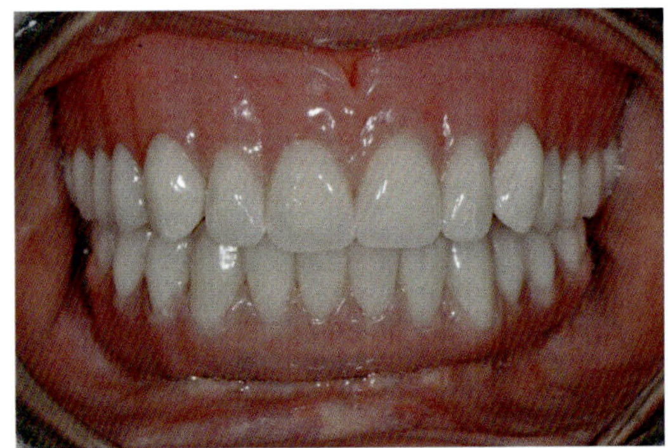

Fig. 14.26 Delivery of complete upper denture and fixed implant-supported mandibular prosthesis

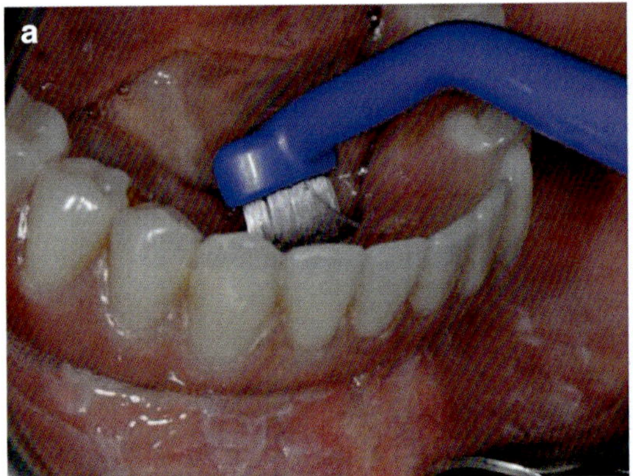

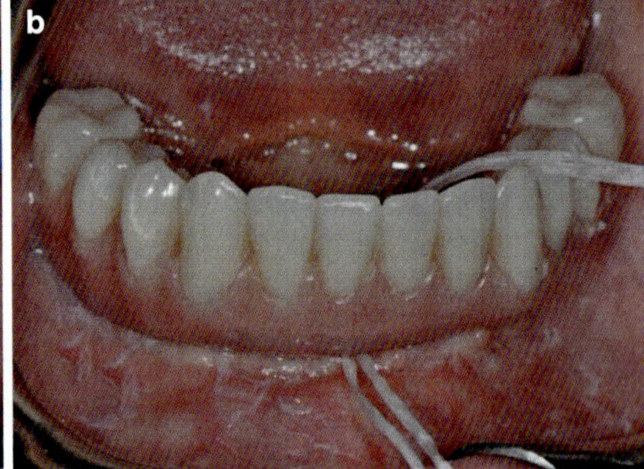

Fig. 14.27 (**a**) Implant care toothbrush to clean the lingual of the fixed mandibular prosthesis (TePe). (**b**) Dental floss to access and maintain the fitting surfaces of the fixed denture

restricted access. A rigorous daily maintenance routine is recommended in order to ensure plaque control. Home care is explained, and the patient is provided with all the necessary tools in order to optimize plaque removal (Fig. 14.27 a, b).

References

1. Malo P, Nobre M d A, Lopes A, Moss SM, Molina GJ. A longitudinal study of the survival of All-on-4 implants in the mandible with up to 10 years of follow-up. J Am Dent Assoc. 2011;142(3):310–32.
2. Assif D, Nissan J, Varsano I, Singer A. Accuracy of implant impression splinted techniques: effect of splinting material. Int J Oral Maxillofac Implants. 1999;14(6):885–8.
3. Papaspyridakos P, Lal K, White GS, Weber HP, Gallucci GO. Effect of splinted and nonsplinted impression techniques on the accuracy of fit of fixed implant prostheses in edentulous patients: a comparative study. Int J Oral Maxillofac Implants. 2011;26(6):1267–72.
4. Papaspyridakos P, Chen CJ, Gallucci GO, Doukoudakis A, Weber HP, Chronopoulos V. Accuracy of implant impressions for partially and completely edentulous patients: a systematic review. Int J Oral Maxillofac Implants. 2014;29(4):836–45.
5. Buzayan M, Baig MR, Yunus N. Evaluation of accuracy of complete-arch multiple-unit abutment-level dental implant impressions using different impression and splinting materials. Int J Oral Maxillofac Implants. 2013;28(6):1512–20.
6. Papaspyridakos P, Benic GI, Hogsett VL, White GS, Lal K, Gallucci GO. Accuracy of implant casts generated with splinted and non-splinted impression techniques for edentulous patients: an optical scanning study. Clin Oral Implants Res. 2012;23(6):676–81.
7. Papaspyridakos P, Hirayama H, Weber H-P, Papaspyridakos P, Chronopoulos V, Chen C-J, Ho C-H, et al. Full-arch implant fixed prostheses: a comparative study on the effect of connection type and impression technique on accuracy of fit. Clin Oral Implants Res. 2015a;27(9):1099–105.

8. Thalji G, Bryington M, De Kok IJ, Cooper LF. Prosthodontic management of implant therapy. Dent Clin N Am. 2014;58:207–25.

9. Sawdosky SJ, et al. Evidence-based criteria for differential treatment planning of implant restorations for the maxillary edentulous patient. J Prosthodont. 2015;24(6):433–46.

10. Phillips K, Wong KM. Vertical space requirement for the fixed-detachable, implant-supported prosthesis. Compend Contin Educ Dent. 2002;23:750–6.

11. Al-Fadda SA, Zarb GA, Finer Y. A comparison of the accuracy of fit of 2 methods for fabricating implant-prosthodontic frameworks. Int J Prosthodont. 2007;20(2):125–31.

12. Sierraalta M, Vivas JL, Razzoog ME, Wang RF. Precision of fit of titanium and cast implant frameworks using a new matching formula. Int J Dentistry. 2012;2012 Article ID 374315, 9 pages.

13. Jemt T. Three-dimensional distortion of gold alloy castings and welded titanium frameworks. Measurements of the precision of fit between completed implant prostheses and the master casts in routine edentulous situations. J Oral Rehabil. 1995;22(8):557–64.

14. Drago C, Howell K. Concepts for designing and fabricating metal implant frameworks for hybrid implant prostheses. J Prosthodont. 2012;21(5):413–24.

15. Jemt T. Failures and complications in 391 consecutively inserted fixed prostheses supported by Brånemark implant in the edentulous jaw: a study of treatment from the time of prostheses placement to the first annual check up. Int J Oral Maxillofac Implants. 1991;6:270–6.

16. Yanase RT, Binon PP, Jemt T, Gulbransen HJ, Parel S. Current issue form. How do you test a cast framework for a full arch fixed implant supported prosthesis? Int J Oral Maxillofac Implants. 1994;9:471–4.

17. Kan JY, Rungcharassaeng K, Bohsali K, Goodacre CJ, Lang BR. Clinical methods for evaluating implant framework fit. J Prosthet Dent. 1999;81(1):7–13.

18. Abi Nader S, Eimar H, Momani M, Shang K, Daniel NG, Tamimi F. Plaque accumulation beneath maxillary All-on-4™ implant-supported prostheses. Clin Implant Dent Relat Res. 2015;17(5):932–7.

Occlusal Consideration for Mandibular Implant Overdentures

15

Igor J. Pesun

Abstract

Guidelines for the occlusion of mandibular implant-supported overdentures are presented based on best available evidence. Often the cause for late implant failure is due to occlusal overload. Various occlusal schemes have been described in the literature, but none have been determined as being superior over another. More research is required to evaluate the prognosis of various occlusal schemes following treatment. Moreover, the lack of devices for monitoring objectively the degree of force placed on implants makes the topic a clinical challenge where proper tooth selection is important. In this chapter, the records required to set denture teeth and their relation to one another are described. Based on the setting of the articulator and patient situation, the occlusal scheme can be linked to specific treatment protocols. Particularly, the various occlusal schemes that the posterior denture teeth can be arranged are described and are related to several specific patient scenarios.

I. J. Pesun, DMD, MSc, FACP, FRCDC
Division of Prosthodontics, Department of
Restorative Dentistry, College of Dentistry,
University of Manitoba, Winnipeg, MB, Canada
e-mail: Igor.Pesun@umanitoba.ca

Occlusion as it related to the implant-assisted mandibular complete dentures can vary significantly depending on the type of implant prosthesis and patient factors. The goal is to develop an aesthetic and functional occlusal scheme. Functionally the occlusion should distribute forces to prevent damage to the existing soft tissue and implants. Occlusion is a known factor that can affect the long-term prognosis of a dental implant. Occlusal forces on the osseointegrated implants have demonstrated that occlusal overloading appears to be the main cause of bone loss around mandibular implants [1]. Full-arch prostheses that are implant-retained and soft tissue-supported should have an occlusal scheme that relates to that of complete dentures for patients that have ideal ridge configurations. The occlusal scheme depends not only on the support of the implant but also that of the opposing dentition. If the opposing dentition is a removable soft tissue-supported dentition, it should be closer to that expected for a complete denture. If the opposing dentition is fixed, then the occlusal scheme should incorporate the concepts of a mutually protected occlusion we want to create for a fully dentate occlusion. Although there is significant literature that relates to the surgical techniques and the implant bone and soft tissue interface, the literature on occlusion is lacking.

This chapter will review the collection of jaw relation records, their application to the laboratory situation by mounting and setting of the

© Springer International Publishing AG, part of Springer Nature 2018

E. Emami, J. Feine (eds.), *Mandibular Implant Prostheses*,
https://doi.org/10.1007/978-3-319-71181-2_15

articulator and how the manipulation of the articulator settings will affect the overall occlusion of the final prosthesis. The chapter will conclude with a review of the different occlusal scheme that can be developed and the current indications for each occlusal scheme based on the type of restoration that is being fabricated.

15.1 Jaw Relation Records

To develop an appropriate occlusal scheme for edentulous patients, it is important to collect appropriate jaw relation records. Jaw relation records include three types of records: intra-arch, inter-arch and gleno-maxillary.

15.1.1 Intra-arch Records

Intra-arch records reflect the relationship between the teeth, implants and soft tissue in the same arch. This record is most commonly known as an impression. There is a wide range of intra-arch recording medium, and the use of the appropriate material is dependent of the situations that one is addressing.

Thermoplastic materials include waxes and modelling plastic impression compound. These are used to border moulding final impressions. The goal of border moulding is to capture the dynamic borders for complete dentures. Proper denture extension captured during the final impression procedure will ensure adequate retention, support and stabilization of complete dentures.

Rigid materials include plaster and metallic oxides. These are most commonly used as wash impression materials for complete denture impressions or for inter-arch records.

Elastic materials include alginates, polysulfides, polyethers and polyvinyl siloxanes (PVS). Alginates are generally used for diagnostic impressions or removable partial denture final impressions. Polysulfide, polyether and polyvinyl siloxane materials are used for final impressions for fixed and removable restorations.

Polyvinyl siloxanes (PVS) are the most popular material used in practice. They are very stable over time. Polyvinyl siloxane's various viscosities allow it to be used in many applications. PVS was initially developed for final impressioning for fixed restorations and is now used for all types of intra-arch and inter-arch records. Various formulations are used for diagnostic and final impressions. For complete denture impressions, the heavy body materials can be used for border moulding similar to the thermoplastic materials, whereas the light body materials can be used as wash material similar to the rigid materials. The accuracy of PVS materials makes it the ideal material in implant dentistry where the tolerances of fit of multiple abutment implant prosthesis relate to the long-term success of these prostheses.

The introduction of digital technologies has resulted in multiple systems available to make final impressions. Intraoral scanners are very accurate when used to make hard tissue impressions of teeth and scan bodies. Intraoral scanners are not able to accurately record the movable soft tissues intra-orally. To accurately digitize the edentulous soft tissue, laboratory scanners are used to scan casts or the impressions made with the aforementioned materials.

15.1.2 Inter-arch Record

Inter-arch records aim to reflect the relationship between the arches in various positions, to allow for the patient's casts to be mounted allowing for the fabrication of a dental prosthesis. These records capture the anterior-posterior, lateral and vertical relationships between the maxillary and mandibular arches. Inter-arch record positions that are collected are dependent on what information the dentist feels is necessary to mount the casts and set the articulator. The records include centric relation (CR), centric occlusion (CO), maxillary intercuspation (MIP), protrusive and lateral. The dentist can physically guide the patient into these positions or let the patients go into the position under the direction of the dentist. There has been significant debate over the years as what is the correct position of the condyles in the glenoid fossa. Irrespective of ones position on how the record is made, the one thing that is consistent is that these recorded positions need to be repeatably reproduced.

When making a CR, CO or MIP record, the vertical dimension of occlusion VDO must also be properly recorded. The VDO affects the function, occlusion and stability of the restorations and the overall aesthetics of the final restorations. A modification of the inter-arch space requires close attention to the occlusal scheme developed. The greater the VDO, the longer the length of the lever arm that results in greater lateral forces acting on the implants.

The vertical dimension of occlusion can be determined by various techniques. When determining the VDO, it is helpful to use several of the techniques to confirm the chosen VDO. The difference between the VDO and the vertical dimension of rest (VDR) is known as the inter-occlusal distance (IOD) using the following formula: VDR − VDO = IOD. IOD is different for patients whether they were Angle Class 1, 2 or 3. For patients that are Class 1, the IOD is in the range of 2–4 mm and Class 2 in the range of 4–5 mm and Class 3 in the range of 1–2 mm (Fig. 15.1).

There are multiple techniques that have been described and evaluated to determine VDO. Most involve simply evaluating the patient clinically. VDO can be evaluated by looking at the patient's facial aesthetics from the facial and lateral view. Facial aesthetics [1] is considered balanced when each one third of the face is considered to be equal. The thirds are measured from the crown of the head to the nasion, the nasion to the base of the nose and the base of the nose to the base of the chin. This last measurement is the one that is the most variable and requires several additional measurements to confirm the ideal VDO. The closest speaking space [2] is dynamically determined by having the patient talk, and the dentist observes the anterior teeth and evaluates how close the teeth come together. Let "S" be your guide [3] is similar in that you have the patient count from sixty (60) to seventy (70) and make the similar evaluation as above. A measurement of the VDO can also be done after the patient swallows [4] as the mandible drops back with swallowing bringing it to the ideal VDO at which point the VDR is measured.

Making measurements using technology has also been evaluated but has not been shown to be any more accurate than those listed above. Orthodontists have used cephalometric [5] evaluation of patients to evaluate facial aesthetics based on anatomical averages. Bite force [6] should be the greatest at the VDO and can be determined using the Boos Bimeter. The VDR is when the muscles of the face are at rest, and this can be evaluated using biofeedback [7]. Studies have shown that this technique results in the

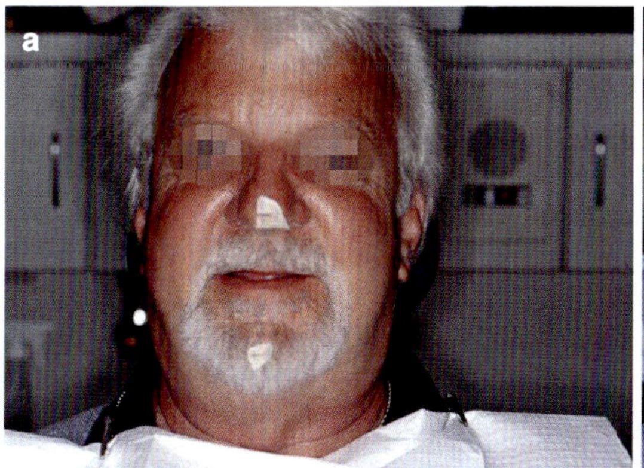
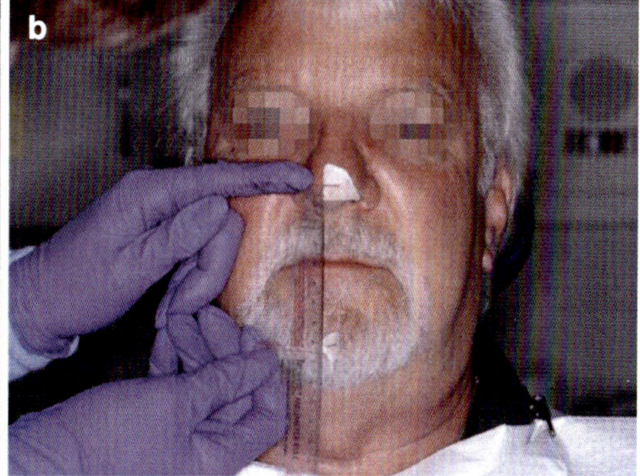

Fig. 15.1 (**a**) Determining the vertical dimension of rest: patient sitting up straight and nothing in the patient's mouth. (**b**) Recording the vertical dimension of occlusion: patient sitting straight up with the occlusal rims in the patient mouth

Table 15.1 Techniques for determining vertical dimension of occlusion

1. Facial aesthetics
2. Closest speaking space
3. Let "S" be your guide
4. Swallowing
5. Cephalometric evaluation
6. Bite force – Boos Bimeter
7. Biofeedback
8. Pre-extraction records
9. Ensuring the maxillary and mandibular ridges are parallel to each other

patients being restored to a significantly open VDO resulting in patients having myofascial pain. Pre-extraction records [7] can record the facial form with lateral photographs or a Willis gauge. A Willis gauge records the distance from the base of the nose to the gonion before the teeth are extracted and relates that to the post-extraction situation. Once the casts are mounted, the maxillary and mandibular ridges should be parallel to each other [7] (Table 15.1).

Recording medium for inter-arch records is similar to those described early in the section on intra-arch records. Irrespective of which material is used, it is important that the bite registration materials have the following features: short working/set time, viscosity that is mousse like when being placed but is very rigid once set so that it has the ability to be trimmed.

Once the VDO has been determined, the mandible also needs to be set in the correct position that the dentist wants to capture. To capture these positions, there are several bite registration techniques. Basically these are categorized as either a closed-bite registration or open-bite registration technique. Closed-bite registration techniques have the patient placed in the desired position, and the registration material is injected into the patient's mouth. For dentate patients or those with implants, the facial contour is captured. This is also how most digital technologies capture the inter-arch relationship. For the edentulous patient, record bases are stabilized in the patient's mouth before the material is injected between the bases. The record bases can be wax rims or utilize a central bearing point. Using a central bearing point is useful for those patients who have difficulty in being guided into position to be recorded (Fig. 15.2a–c).

Open-bite registration technique involves placing bite registration material on a stabilized base and occlusion rim and then guiding the patient into position. For this technique to be successful, the patient will need to be easily guided into a repeatable position (Fig. 15.3a, b).

15.1.3 Gleno-Maxillary Record

Gleno-maxillary records reflect the relationship between the glenoid fossa and the maxillary dentition (Fig. 15.4). Bonwill described an average equilateral triangle of 110 mm (4 in.) with the apices at the centre of the condyles and the mesial-incisal point angle of the mandibular central incisors [2]. The importance of this record is most important in cases where VDO might need to be changed and where the loss of all of the posterior teeth requires the development of an appropriate occlusal scheme.

The maxillary dentition orientation is recorded on a bite fork. The third point of reference attempts to relate the occlusal plane to be parallel to the Frankfort horizontal plane. How this is determined is dependent of the type of face bow that is used. Examples include the nasion (Whipmix), infraorbital notch (Hanau) or 43 mm superior to the distal incisal line angle of the maxillary right central incisor (Denar).

The location of the glenoid fossa can be determined using various techniques. The most accurate technique involves finding the transverse horizontal axis. The need for the accuracy to this level can be questioned when evaluating the geometry of the mandibular movement. Weinberg calculated that the error at the second molar would be 0.2 mm if the average condylar axis is within 5 mm of the transverse horizontal axis [3]. This minimal error usually results in flatter cusps which is desirable in that it reduces the lateral forces on the prostheses. With this minimal error in occlusion, the most common average used value for the condylar axis involves using external auditory meatus as a simple repeatable

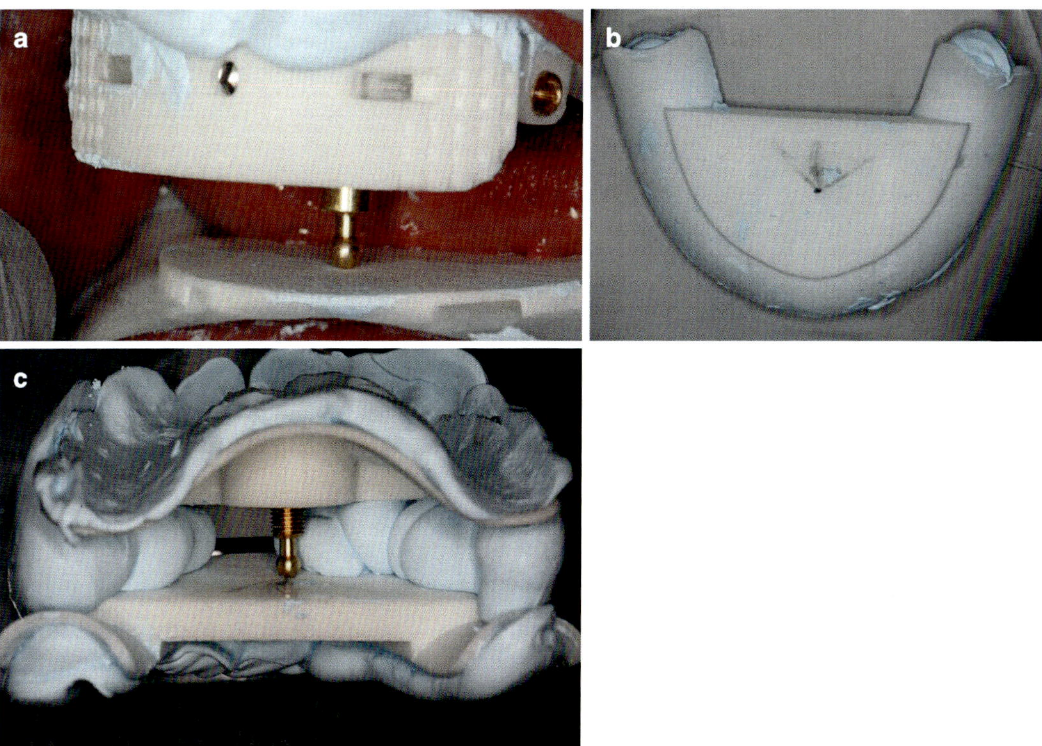

Fig. 15.2 (**a**) Central bearing point set at correct vertical dimension of occlusion. (**b**) Gothic arch tracing with the centric relation position at the apex of the tracing. (**c**) Central bearing point closed-mouth jaw relation record

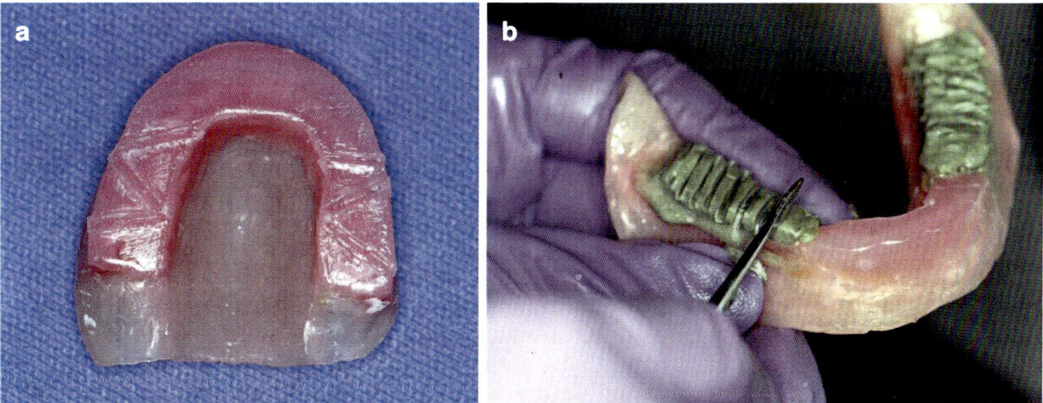

Fig. 15.3 Preparation of the stabilized base and wax occlusion rims for a open-mouth centric relation record. (**a**) Place grooves in maxillary rim and place stabilized base and rim in the patient's mouth. (**b**) Build up the posterior mandibular rim with wax, soften and place in the patient's mouth and have patient close into centric position

location to record a repeatable relationship to glenoid fossa. Ear bows sits within the external auditory meatus and takes into account that the transverse horizontal axis within the glenoid fossa is an average distance of 8–14 mm anterior to the external auditory meatus.

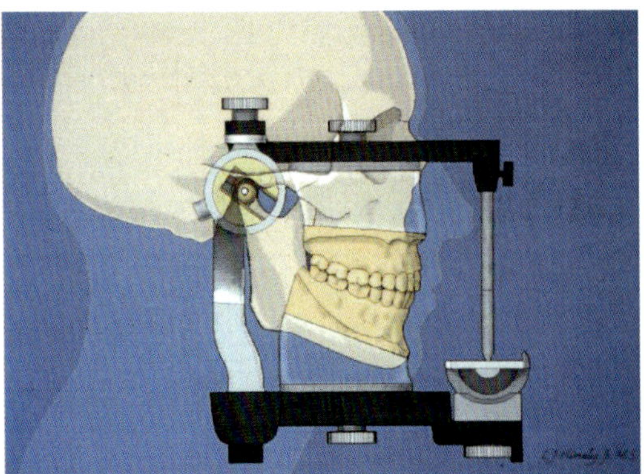

Fig. 15.4 Relationship between the patient's dental arches and an articulator

15.2 Articulators and Their Relation to Occlusion

Articulators are an analog of masticatory geometry not of masticatory function. Based on how close to the actual movement the articulator can mimic that of the patient is how articulators are classified. Some simply relate the casts to each other in a static position that is nonadjustable. The relationship allows for a vertical or hinge opening to be evaluated. An average value articulator allows for the mounting of the casts with a gleno-maxillary record, but the remaining values of the intra-condylar distance, the Bennet angle, condylar curvature and condylar angle are preset at anatomical averages. The casts can be moved in protrusive and lateral movements, but they are based on these anatomical averages and will not exactly reproduce the patient's mandibular movements. This articulator is adequate for cases where the anterior guidance is very steep and the occlusal scheme is canine guidance. Semi-adjustable articulators have adjustable features that each manufacture selects as being the most important for their line of articulators. For most removable and simple fixed prosthodontic treatment, semi-adjustable articulators are adequate. Highly or fully adjustable articulators are used in restoring complex fixed prosthodontic cases (Table 15.2).

The choice of articulator should be made based on articulator cost and the benefits the

Table 15.2 Articulator classification

1. Nonadjustable
(a) Vertical alignment
(b) Hinge
2. Average value
3. Semi-adjustable
4. Highly or fully adjustable

articulator will bring to the treatment being undertaken. Articulator costs relate to the clinic time required to set up the articulator, the cost of articulator itself and the time it takes to communicate the required information to the laboratory. The benefits of an articulator relate to its ability to provide a higher quality of service. Although the setup time for articulators is greater on the front end of treatment, it can significantly reduce the clinic time required to deliver restorations. This is achieved by reducing the inaccuracies in occlusion by accurately recording mandibular movement and transferring it to the articulator. When choosing an articulator, it should be the simplest instrument that meets the requirements of the dental treatment and has features in common with the restoration being fabricated.

15.3 Factors Affecting Occlusion

Hanau described five factors (Hanau's Quint) that affected a balanced occlusion [4] (Table 15.3). The posterior factor that cannot be modified by the dentist is the condylar inclination, which is determined by the patient's anatomy. The restoring dentist can control all the remaining four factors as they all relate to the teeth and their arrangement. The arrangement of the anterior teeth influences the horizontal and vertical overlap known as the incisal guidance. The posterior teeth have a cuspal inclination that can be changed by selecting teeth of varying cuspal angles. The occlusal plane inclination and the compensating curve refer to the arrangement of all of the teeth. The occlusal plane can be raised or lowered, and the compensating curve of the occlusal plane can be increased or decreased.

When setting denture teeth or completing a full-mouth reconstruction, the dentist can change

Table 15.3 Hanau's Quint

1. Condylar inclination/guidance (CG)
2. Incisal guidance (IG)
3. Cuspal inclination/height (CH)
4. Occlusal plane inclination (OP)
5. Compensating curve (CC)

all of these factors with the exception of the condylar inclination. Using appropriate jaw relation records will help in setting the articulator. Theilman elaborated on the Hanau's Quint and described the interrelationship of these five factors with the formula: $\mathbf{CG \times IG = CH \times CC \times OP}$. By changing the interrelationship, the dentist can develop the type of occlusal scheme that they seek to create for their patient. This can range from canine disocclusion to a fully bilateral balanced occlusion. When all five factors with in Hanau's Quint are in "balance", all teeth contact in excursive positions.

Condylar inclination is the one factor that the dentist has no control over since it is based on the anatomy of the patient. The condylar inclination recorded for setting the articulator is made by making functionally generated path, protrusive and/or lateral jaw registrations from the patient.

The incisal guidance, which is controlled by the clinician, plays a key role in the proper placement of the anterior teeth. In general it is suggested that the incisal guidance for the complete denture patient be minimized (within the confines of aesthetics and phonetics) to reduce horizontal forces of occlusion. Cusp height, cusp angulations and compensating curves are affected by these determinants and affect the final aesthetic result.

Geometry dictates that three points define a plane. To define the occlusal plane, the anterior point is the mesial-incisal point angle of the mandibular central incisors. The posterior determinates of the occlusal plane are located one half to two thirds the way up the retromolar pad. Although the occlusal plane can be located where needed for the edentulous patient, it cannot be substantially changed since functional requirements dictate its position.

The degree of cuspal inclination is dependent on multiple factors (residual ridges, neuromuscular control, aesthetics, etc.). However in general it is best to reduce cuspal inclination to help reduce horizontal forces of occlusion. The compensating curve is very helpful in obtaining balanced occlusion, and depending on the posterior tooth forms, it can easily be modified to facilitate posterior tooth contacts in eccentric positions.

15.4 Posterior Tooth Selection

Anterior teeth selection is aesthetically oriented. The maxillary anterior teeth are designed for the aesthetics and phonetics, whereas the lingual of the maxillary anterior teeth and the facial of the mandibular anterior teeth are designed to provide the incisal guidance for the patient. The degree of horizontal overlap and vertical overlap is how incisal guidance can affect the occlusion.

The patient's anatomy determines the condylar guidance and is recorded with the appropriate jaw relation record to set it on the articulator. The incisal guidance is determined by the arrangement of the anterior teeth. The remaining determinates of occlusion are all related to the posterior teeth. This makes the selection of posterior teeth functionally oriented. The design and selection of posterior teeth have been discussed in the earliest prosthodontic literature as a factor in denture success.

There are four factors to consider when selecting posterior denture teeth. These include the mesiodistal length of posterior teeth, occlusogingival height, degree of cusp height and least importantly the shade (Table 15.4).

The posterior tooth shade is selected to match the shade of anterior teeth. Even so these teeth have a shade that is slightly lower in value to take into account the increased thickness of the dentin posterior teeth have.

There are several methods to determine the mesiodistal length of posterior denture teeth. Denture teeth have anterior/posterior tooth mould conversion charts. The posterior teeth length is based on an anatomical average. The posterior teeth should be based on measuring the distance

Table 15.4 Posterior teeth selection

1. Shade
2. Mesiodistal length of posterior teeth
3. Occluso-gingival height
4. Degree of cusp height

Table 15.5 Classification of denture teeth cusp heights

0° teeth (monoplane, rational)
10° teeth (functional, anatoline)
20° teeth
30° teeth (Pilkington-turner)
33° teeth
40° teeth (Euroline, Biostabil)

from the distal of canine to the anterior of maxillary tuberosity or anterior to the ascending ramus of mandible. There is a need for a compromise often and can be achieved by leaving a space distal to the canine or the elimination of the premolar.

The occluso-gingival height of posterior teeth is dependent of the inter-ridge space available. Ideally the longest tooth that will fill this space should be chosen. If there is insufficient inter-ridge space, choose a shorter tooth and be prepared to thin the trial base to the point of even setting the denture teeth on the ridge. The cervical portion of the tooth is trimmed.

Denture teeth are manufactured with a wide range of degrees of cusp heights. These are dependent on the type of occlusal scheme that the dentist wants to develop for their patient. The cusp height angles range from 0 to 40 degrees (Table 15.5).

15.5 Occlusal Schemes for Complete Dentures

Occlusal schemes are greatly influenced by the degree of cusp height of the posterior teeth that are selected. Denture occlusal schemes can be broken down into three types: bilateral balanced, monoplane or lingualized. Patient surveys have indicated that overall not one occlusal scheme is superior to another based on function. Even with these studies, there are indications for the choice

of one denture occlusal scheme over another. The remainder of this chapter will review each of these occlusal schemes, describing how the teeth are arranged and the indications of when each of these schemes should be used. These schemes are only important when the teeth are in contact. It is important to remember that once a bolus is placed between the teeth, what occlusal scheme is used is irrelevant as occlusal schemes only relate to when the teeth are in contact. Teeth are only in contact during parafunctional habits or during swallowing. As these are active positions, it is important to make sure that the centric relation position of the dentures is a stable position. For patients with parafunctional habits, it is important that as the denture occlusion is such that when the patient moves into positions away from the centric relation position, the occlusal scheme should be designed to stabilize the denture into place and distribute the forces over a greater area. This becomes even more important for implant prosthesis where occlusal forces overtime can result in bone loss around the implant.

15.5.1 Bilaterally Balanced Occlusion

Bilaterally balance occlusion is one of the most complex occlusal schemes to set teeth in. The goal of bilateral balanced occlusion is where all of the posterior teeth should be in simultaneous contact when the patient contacts their teeth in the centric relation/occlusion position. As the patient moves into lateral excursion, the teeth have continuous smooth bilateral gliding to any eccentric position within the normal range of mandibular function. The contact is required on both on the working and the balancing side dentition, namely, there is cross-arch contact or "balanced occlusion". Maxillary teeth should travel across the inter-cusp spaces and grooves of the mandibular teeth. These contacts are smooth without inter-arch interferences. Bilateral balanced occlusion requires a minimum of three contacts for establishing a plane of equilibrium. To achieve balanced occlusion, the factors described in Hanau's Quint must be utilized. This would require mounting the case with a face bow,

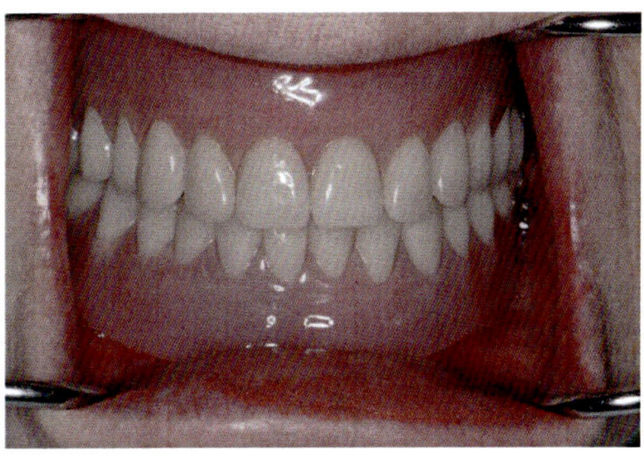

Fig. 15.5 Bilateral balanced denture setup

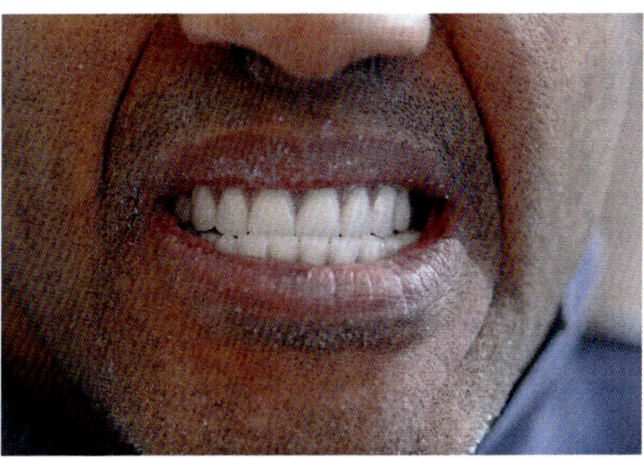

Fig. 15.6 A patient with minimal mandibular coordination with dentures with monoplane occlusion

centric jaw record and protrusive records to set up a semi-adjustable articulator. The setup of teeth in bilateral balanced occlusion requires the most time and complexity of records to be completed. The teeth used to achieve this type of occlusion will have adequate cusp heights that will result in proper balance of the occlusion. There is a restriction of posterior tooth positions that is allowed by cuspal anatomy. This also limits the position of the anterior teeth. Patients with good ridge height and anatomy or implants to stabilize the dentures are indications for this type of occlusion. The benefits of this occlusal scheme are that aesthetically the posteriors appear more natural. Chewing is also more efficient than with any other tooth setup (Fig. 15.5).

The realeff: resiliency and like effect that presents with the resilient mucosa that tissue-supported dentures experience, results in a decrease in the tolerances that dentures need to be made to, simplifying the balancing of the teeth in any type of occlusal scheme. Hanau stated the less realeff, the more the instrument would simulate mandibular movements [4]. Even so with dentures, once a bolus enters between teeth, balance exits, and the denture occlusal scheme would have very little to do with denture stability.

15.5.2 Monoplane Occlusion

Monoplane occlusion is the polar opposite of that of bilaterally balanced occlusion. It is a simple occlusal scheme where the posterior tooth anatomy is flat and the cusp angles are at 0 degrees. There are no curves or cusps on the occlusal of the teeth. The flat occlusal surfaces sit against the flat occlusal surface of the opposing teeth. This makes the setup of the teeth very simple. And there can be a wide range of posterior teeth positions. To mount the casts to complete this setup, a centric relation jaw record is needed and can be setup on a simple articulator. The anterior teeth can be setup with a horizontal overlap but not any vertical overlap. The lower posterior teeth are set up after the anterior teeth and are set in a flat plane to the middle of the retromolar pad. The upper teeth are set to contact the lower teeth with no attempt to have contact on excursive movements. All teeth just pass over one another during excursive movements usually with nothing to provide guidance.

This setup results in reduced lateral stresses on the mucosa. It is indicated for patients with uncoordinated closures where it is difficult to capture a repeatable jaw centric relation record. Patients with parafunctional habits also find this type of occlusal scheme more comfortable as it reduces lateral forces on the residual ridge. This lack of lateral interferences helps the denture be more stable for those patients with poor ridge anatomy (Fig. 15.6).

There are compromises with this setup. The flat premolars may appear less aesthetic when compared to the posterior teeth. The lack of cusps results in a less efficient chewing ability. The anterior aesthetics is affected by the need of more horizontal overlap and no vertical overlap.

Monoplane teeth can also be arranged to a balanced articulation. To achieve a balanced articulation, a centric relation jaw record is required with a face bow to mount the cast, and records are required to set the condylar inclinations on a semi-adjustable articulator. The anterior teeth are set with horizontal overlap and slight vertical overlap. To achieved a balance occlusion, a compensating curve is incorporated that goes from the anterior to the posterior (Curve of Spee) and a medio-lateral curve (Curve of Wilson) with the buccal cusps higher than the lingual cusps. The posteriors teeth are set to contact on at least 1 point on nonworking and balancing movement. Overall this is a simple tooth arrangement to set up although it does take slightly more laboratory setup time. It also allows for more aesthetic overlap of anterior teeth than that found in an unbalanced monoplane occlusion, but the premolars still appear flat if visible. The posterior point contact maintains denture base stability on excursions or parafunction.

15.5.3 Lingualized Occlusion

Lingualized occlusion has been around for over 80 years but the last scheme to be introduced to the profession and may use a variety of tooth moulds. Some manufacturers produce specific moulds for this occlusal concept. This is a very versatile type of occlusal scheme. These teeth can be arranged in a balanced or non-balancing scheme.

All that is required is a centric jaw record if a non-balanced occlusal scheme is desired. For those patients who have poor ridges, a monoplane or flat occlusal plane that is not balanced can be established. The maxillary teeth are chosen based on aesthetics resulting in the upper premolars appearing natural. The mandibular teeth are chosen to have none to minimal cusp height. The monoplane lower posterior teeth are set to retromolar pad. The anatomical upper posterior teeth are set with only lingual cusps contacting the central groove of the mandibular teeth. The buccal cusps are raised off the occlusal plane. When setting the teeth, some range of posterior

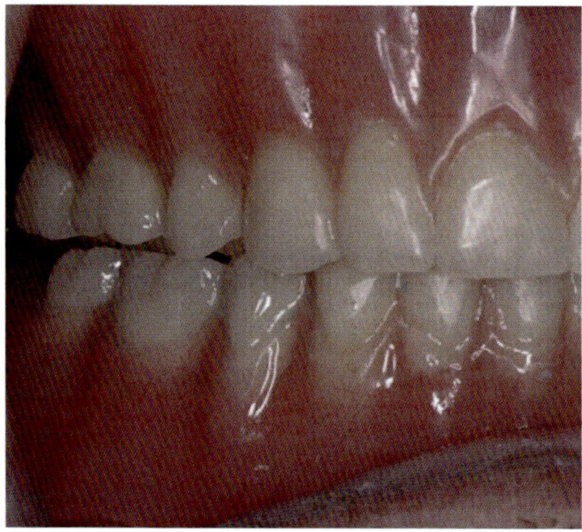

Fig. 15.7 Dentures with lingualized occlusion (Note the buccal cusps are above the level of the occlusal plane)

tooth position is allowed. With the introduction of the cusped maxillary teeth into the occlusal scheme, there is a reported slightly better chewing ability than with monoplane teeth but not as efficient as fully cusped teeth.

This occlusal scheme can also be set up as a balanced lingualized occlusion. Additional records such as the face bow and eccentric records to set the condylar inclination on the articulator are then also needed. To achieve a balanced lingualized occlusion, some grinding may be needed to create upper cusp tip/lower fossa contacts. By altering the mandibular teeth cusp angulations, the occlusal scheme can be fully balanced for those patients with good ridges or implants. Lingualized occlusion helps to eliminate or reduce lateral stress [5]. This eliminates contacting of the maxillary buccal cusp on the working side, thus lingualizing or centralizing the forces on the prosthesis. It might be argued that this reduction of the horizontal lever arm is insignificant, but any reduction in the lateral stresses generated should be considered advantagous (Fig. 15.7).

15.5.4 Buccalized Occlusion

Buccalized occlusion is a variant on lingualized occlusion where the buccal cusps of the mandibular teeth contact the central groove of the maxillary teeth. To achieve buccalized occlusion, the mandibular teeth have significantly greater cusp heights than the maxillary teeth. Buccalized occlusal scheme has similar advantages and disadvantages to that of lingualized occlusal schemes with the exception of the aesthetics of the maxillary premolars. The maxillary premolars appear flatter that one would expect to be natural.

15.5.5 Anatomical Variations

The description above of the occlusal schemes is for patients who are considered to have an orthognathic mandible (Angle Class 1). Patients with a prominent maxilla and/or a retrognathic mandible (Angle Class 2) may need a modified denture tooth setup. The horizontal and vertical overlap relationship to restore their facial form, dental aesthetics and speech will need to be revised to take this into account. The upper teeth may need to be set to the lingual with their labial inclination very vertical or even retruded. The mandibular teeth are set to the facial to correct for the skeletal mismatch. When setting the maxillary posterior teeth, often the first premolars are deleted similar to what takes place during the orthodontic therapy using serial extraction.

Patients with a combination of a prominent long mandible with small retruded maxillae are prognathic (Angle Class 3). Upper anterior teeth are set to the facial with no horizontal or vertical overlap and only light "end-to-end" incisal contact. The mandibular teeth are inclined lingually and distally back from the larger mandible to meet upper teeth. There is a limit to how far anterior the maxillary incisors can be put facially as too much tension can be placed on the denture by the upper lip musculature. This would result in dislodgement of the denture. The posteriors are often set in a "crossbite" relationship with the maxillary buccal cusps positioned lingual to the mandibular teeth and an enhanced lateral occlusal curvature (Curve of Wilson) to best accommodate the small maxillary/large mandibular arches [6].

15.6 Selection of Occlusal Scheme for Implant-Supported Restorations

The goal of patient restorations is to be able to achieve adequate retention, stability and support for the restoration while preventing damage to the underlying soft and hard tissues and dental implant. Overall this relates to the residual anatomy that remains after the extraction of the teeth. Support is determined by the extension of the denture bases and the introduction of dental implants. Implants can add to provide additional support for tissue-supported dentures.

The selection of an occlusal scheme for implant-supported complete denture restorations is dependent on the occlusal philosophy that one subscribes to and what one is trying to achieve. This is even though there are no clinical experimental data to substantiate these assumptions. Occlusal scheme choice is based on the literature pertaining to the development of occlusion for natural tooth-borne restorations and transposes these principles to develop the occlusion for implant-borne prostheses. The goals that are set out for all occlusal schemes agree on a stable non-traumatic posterior occlusion with simultaneous contacts in the centric cusp to fossa relation occlusion position. Interfering occlusal contacts need to be reduced, and as a result there are reduced lateral stresses. The emphasis is that the forces should be as vertical as possible.

15.6.1 Considerations

When examining a patient, one has to evaluate multiple factors to determine the appropriate occlusal scheme for full-mouth restorations. The denture stability is dependent on the anatomy of the residual ridge. Adequate ridges that have parallel sides to them allow for greater stability and retention. The height of the muscle attachments will also affect the retention and stability. Closer to the crest of the residual ridge, the muscle attachments attach; the dentures will be increasingly unstable.

The maxillary denture retention is based on achieving suction. The extension of the dentures must be correctly recorded to create the suction cup effect. The posterior border of dentures must not extend beyond the vibrating line. Dependent on the House classification of palatal mobility, the palatal seal location becomes important to identify.

Overall complete upper dentures are more stable than complete lower dentures. This has resulted in the McGill consensus statement that treatment of the edentulous mandible should include the use of minimally two implants to provide adequate retention, support and stability of the lower denture. The use of implants will make the mandibular denture more stable than the maxillary denture. Keep in mind that the arch in which implants are placed becomes the dominant arch. The maxillary edentulous arch now becomes the weaker arch and the subject of patient complaints as to the inadequacy of stability, retention and support of the prosthesis.

To achieve a stable set of dentures, the peripheries need to be captured properly, and an occlusal scheme needs to be correctly chosen.

15.6.2 Guidelines

The needs of each patient are not always obvious and may require a great deal of analysis before a final occlusal scheme is selected. When selecting an occlusal scheme, the greater the stability of the bases on the patient's residual ridges, the less the type of occlusal scheme is relevant. It should be carefully noted that regardless of the scheme of occlusion used when implants are placed in one arch, there is always the possibility of rendering an opposing complete denture unstable. Therefore the occlusion must be carefully developed to provide support, stability and retention to the soft tissue-supported opposing prosthesis. It is recommended that in the edentulous patient, the type of occlusion used should follow the precepts of a bilateral balanced or a lingualized balanced occlusion.

References

1. Lindqvist LW, et al. Bone resorption around fixtures in edentulous patients treated with mandibular fixed integrated prostheses. J Prosthet Dent. 1988;59:59–63.
2. Bonwill WGA. The scientific articulation of the human teeth as founded on geometrical, mathematical, and mechanical laws. Dental Items of Interest, pp. 617–43, October 1899. In Vol. I, Classic Prosthodontic Articles. A.C.O.P., pp. 1–28.
3. Weinberg LA. An evaluation of basic articulators and their concepts. Part II. Arbitrary, positional, semiadjustable articulators. J Prosthet Dent. 1963;13:644–63.
4. Hanau RL. Articulation defined, analyzed, and formulated. J Am Dent Assoc. 1926;13:1694.
5. Lang BR, Razzoog ME. Lingualized integration: tooth molds and an occlusal scheme for edentulous implant patients. Implant Dent. 1992;1:204–11.
6. Zarb G. Prosthodontic treatment for edentulous patients. 13th ed. St Louis: Mosby; 2013. p. 225–6.
7. Zarb G. Prosthodontic treatment for edentulous patients. 13th ed. Mosby; 2013. p. 275–7.

Part IV

Treatment Assessment: Clinician and Patient Perspectives

Clinical Outcomes

16

Raphael F. de Souza

Abstract

The clinical outcomes of implant-retained over-dentures can be depicted in several ways. Perhaps the most intuitive manner is to classify each implant and prosthesis as successful or not. Treating edentulous patients with implants will also place them at risk of certain problems, including prosthetic complications and unfavorable soft and hard tissue responses. These adverse events add to those already expected following conventional denture treatment. In this chapter, the main success criteria for implants are described. Success rates are provided for the main treatment methods based on mandibular overdentures retained by different attachments and implant numbers. Some eventual complications and maintenance events are also described, including changes in the peri-implant complex and supporting tissues. The chapter also reviews the maintenance of overdentures per se, including attachments and other prosthetic parts.

R. F. de Souza, D.D.S., M.Sc., Ph.D.
Division of Oral Health and Society, Faculty of Dentistry, McGill University, Montreal, QC, Canada

Department of Dental Materials and Prosthetics, School of Dentistry of Ribeirao Preto, University of Sao Paulo, Ribeirao Preto, SP, Brazil

16.1 Introduction

Treatment of edentulism in all its modalities elicits a wide range of responses from patients. Both conventional removable dentures and implant-retained prostheses aim to improve oral function but have some maintenance requirements. The provision of overdentures follows the same operative principles used for conventional dentures; both modalities demand short-term post-insertion adjustments and preservation of fitting on supporting tissues. However, fixtures and superjacent components render maintenance more demanding than with complete dentures. Oral rehabilitation with implants demands specific care to maintain long-term survival and good performance of implants, their attachments, as well as to prevent specific complications.

The performance of mandibular-retained overdentures has led to their recommendation as a standard of care for edentulism [1, 2]. This improved performance can be described both from a clinician-based viewpoint and from patient perspectives.

This chapter deals with clinical outcomes of mandibular overdenture treatment, including the survival and success rates, clinical complications, and maintenance.

© Springer International Publishing AG, part of Springer Nature 2018
E. Emami, J. Feine (eds.), *Mandibular Implant Prostheses*,
https://doi.org/10.1007/978-3-319-71181-2_16

16.2 Survival and Success Rates

Up until relatively recently, success and survival rates were the main criteria considered in most studies on dental implants [3]. Despite their use as synonyms in several instances, success and survival refer to different concepts. Success criteria were first introduced by Albrektsson et al. [4], which were based mainly on the osseointegration success. According to these criteria, a successful individual implant must:

1. Present no mobility when tested clinically.
2. Demonstrate no evidence of peri-implant radiolucency.
3. Have less than 0.2 mm of vertical bone loss annually after the first year in function.
4. Show no persistent and/or irreversible signs and symptoms, including pain, infections, violation of the mandibular canal, paresthesia, or neuropathy.

In order to consider an implant system as successful, the same criteria recommend 5- and 10-year success rates of at least 85% and 80%, respectively.

Buser et al. [5] also proposed a widely used guideline for classifying implant success. This involved the following five criteria:

1. No persistent patient-reported complaint, such as pain, foreign body sensation, or dysesthesia.
2. No recurrent peri-implant infection with suppuration.
3. No clinically detectable mobility.
4. No continuous radiolucency around the implant.
5. Possibility of restoration.

In 2007, a consensus conference (held by the ICOI—International Congress of Oral Implantologists) revised the definitions of implant success with four precise criteria to be considered over a period of at least 12 months following functional restoration [6]:

1. Absence of pain or tenderness during function, palpation, and percussion.
2. No visible mobility following vertical and horizontal percussion with loads limited to 500 gf.
3. Crestal bone resorption lower than 2 mm vertically at any postsurgical time, checked by periapical radiographs.
4. No history of exudate.

According to this classification system, early success refers to a span of 1–3 years, intermediate success to 3–7 years, and long-term success to more than 7 years.

Table 16.1 provides a summary of these three guidelines for implant success criteria. It is important to highlight that prosthetic restorability is a common requirement.

Lately, the definition of success has evolved to consider other aspects, including prosthetic success and patient-reported outcomes. A systematic review by Papaspyridakos et al. [7] examined the most frequent success criteria used by randomized trials and prospective cohort studies. Most frequent success criteria at the implant level were mobility, pain, peri-implant bone loss, and radiolucency, whereas soft tissue-level criteria included probing pocket depth, bleeding, and suppuration. The review also observed the use of prosthetic-related criteria—technical complications and maintenance needs, adequate function, and esthetics—and patient-reported aspects, discomfort, satisfaction with appearance, and perceived function/masticatory ability. All included studies on overdentures quantified implant success rate based on Albrektsson et al. [4] and/or Buser et al. [5], however.

Survival refers to those cases in which the implants are still in the oral cavity but cannot fulfill all success criteria. For instance, implants may be successfully osseointegrated but placed in a position that precludes adequate restoration. A surviving implant is unsuccessful if peri-implant bone resorption exceeds acceptability criteria. For instance, an implant with 3 mm of vertical bone loss 12 months after the insertion of a mandibular overdenture could not be considered a clinical success.

In summary, implant success refers to "ideal" clinical conditions, whereas survival is one of the criteria for success [6].

Relatively high success rates are one of the reasons for recommending implant overdentures as a treatment for mandibular edentulous arches. Early reports of two-implant-retained

Table 16.1 Comparative summary of the major success criteria used in dental implantology

	Success criteria		
	Albrektsson et al. [4]	Buser et al. [5]	Misch et al. [6]
Absence of clinical mobility	✓	✓	✓ (vertical/horizontal percussion: 500 gf)
No peri-implant radiolucency	✓	✓	–
Acceptable vertical bone loss	✓ (<0.2 mm/year, after 1st year)	–	✓ (<2 mm, any time)
Absence of signs and symptoms	✓ (persistent and/or irreversible events, e.g., pain/paresthesia/ neuropathy, infection, violation of the mandibular canal)	✓ (persistent patient-reported complaint; recurrent infection with suppuration)	✓ (pain/tenderness on function, palpation, or percussion; exudate)

prostheses have reported a cumulative implant failure rate of 1.2% over 30 months, with the use of straight bar attachments [8]. Reports from a few years later provide evidence that different attachment types would not lead to more frequent implant failures, at least with the use of standard-sized implants. In other words, implant success rates using ball attachments or magnets were reported to be similar to Dolder bars [9]. A systematic review compared implant overdentures retained by bars to unsplinted attachment systems and found no difference in success or survival rates of implants after 3 years or more [10].

Treatment with mandibular overdentures generally shows high implant success and survival rates, as confirmed by subsequent reports. Ferrigno et al. [11] found nearly identical implant success rates using ball attachments on two implants compared to four fixtures united by a milled bar. After 5 years, the former option was successful for nearly 95% of 76 implants, whereas the latter resulted in 96% successful fixtures (total $n = 72$ implants). At least for standard-sized implants, these variations in numbers do not exert considerable influence on success and survival rates [12]. A study from our group confirms the good predictability of two-implant overdentures in terms of these outcomes, as a single fixture failed in 40 patients treated with ball attachments [13]. Interestingly, this failure had no correlation with osseointegration.

Other modalities of implant-retained mandibular overdentures merit consideration. Some recent studies have purported the use of a single implant placed in the symphysis area. In terms of success and survival rates, this approach seems similar to two implants in the anterior area, as disclosed by a systematic review [14]. The use of four or two mini-implants has also been reported recently. These are very narrow (<3 mm) one-piece implants presenting a threaded shaft and an attachment patrix, normally a ball-shaped extremity. Our study observed success rates between 80 and 90% after 12 months of loading, depending on the number of mini-implants [13]. As long as that study used 2 mm-wide fixtures, it could be concluded that a middle term between standard implants and that diameter may present more favorable long-term results. However, this should be further investigated.

Dentures themselves can also be evaluated to determine success and survival. A surviving prosthesis can be in use regardless of its condition, whereas success implies achieving treatment goals, including appropriate retention and stability provided by attachments. However, numbers can vary widely due to different methods used by each study [12]. Survival rates tend to be approximately similar to those found for separate fixtures. These rates just represent the number of cases of continuous denture wearing and can be at least 92% following 2 or more years. Such numbers can be much lower for success if patients do not undergo a strict maintenance program following treatment with mandibular overdentures. In our experience, this treatment method demands periodic return to replace attachment components, reline, and make minor adjustments. A success rate of 94% was observed for 120 patients treated with mandibular overdentures on either standard fixtures or mini-implants, given that adequate maintenance was provided [13]. Although a scheduled recall regimen of a single appointment each year may work well for conventional denture wearers [15], we prefer to reappoint overdenture wearers after 6 months, at least during the initial 2 years.

Table 16.2 summarizes results from recent systematic reviews comparing implant success and/or survival rates for different types of treatment methods based on mandibular overdentures. It presents some key findings, considering the major relevance of this kind of study as a source of evidence for clinical decision-making.

16.3 Clinical Complications and Maintenance

16.3.1 Changes in Denture-Supporting Tissues

A major concern when providing dental care is to preserve existing structures. However, mandibular overdentures will interact directly with the underlying edentate ridge and oral mucosa and may adversely affect those structures. This relationship must be harmonious and avoid overdependence on implant retention and stability, mainly when more conservative approaches, e.g., two-implant-retained hybrid prostheses, are used. In this way, one can avoid the overload of attachment systems, prostheses, or fixtures, while the odds of developing soft tissue lesions or accelerated residual ridge resorption will be reasonably low.

Table 16.2 Summary of results for success and survival rates of implants and overdentures, as reported by systematic reviews

Systematic review	Comparison	Type of studies	Main results
Andreiotelli et al. [16]	Different attachment types and implant numbers, both arches	– RCT ($n = 4$), prospective cohort studies ($n = 14$) – Follow-up >5 years	– Different treatment does not seem to influence implant or overdenture survival/success rates (bar-clip, ball attachments, magnets, or telescopic crowns)
Stoumpis and Kohal [10]	Splinted versus unsplinted implants, both arches	– RCT ($n = 2$), prospective ($n = 3$) and retrospective ($n = 1$) cohort studies – Follow-up >3 years	– Implant survival rate, mandible, 95.3–100%; maxilla, 90–95.5% – No difference between bar-clip and ball attachments (five studies separately); magnets (one study)
Kim et al. [17]	Different attachment types and implant numbers, mandible	– 14 clinical studies, excluding case/technical reports – Follow-up >1 year	– Mean implant survival rate was over 98% (range 91.7–100%) – No evidence of effect from attachment systems (bar clip, ball, or magnets)
Dantas et al. [12]	Two versus four implants, mandible	– RCT ($n = 1$) and non-randomized controlled trials ($n = 4$), prospective ($n = 5$) and retrospective ($n = 1$) cohort studies	– A single prospective cohort study reported both conditions of interest (10-year overdenture survival, two ball attachments, 98.8%; four-implant-retained bar, 97.7% (ns)) – Other studies reported one of the two treatment modalities, without evident difference
Srinivasan et al. [14]	Single versus two implants, mandible	– RCT ($n = 2$), prospective cohort studies ($n = 28$) – Follow-up >1 year	– *Meta-analysis* for two RCT, risk difference for implant survival—One versus two implants, 0.05; 95% confidence interval, −0.07 to 0.18 (ns)

RCT randomized controlled trial; *ns* nonsignificant

16.3.1.1 Residual Ridge Resorption

Tooth loss will invariably lead to progressive reduction of residual ridges, with considerable variation among patients. Although residual ridge resorption is associated with a series of factors that include metabolism and anatomy, there are a few interventions a clinician can perform to prevent or minimize it. One of them is the insertion of dental implants. Both mandibular overdentures and fixed dentures have been associated with lower residual ridge loss. In truth, the non-dependence of the edentulous ridge to receive loads directly from fixed dentures can result even in some posterior bone apposition over the years [18]. Mandibular overdentures will lead to a modest ridge resorption pattern over time, even with only two implants in the anterior area. Following this treatment, Raedel et al. [19] observed an average rate of 1.5 mm resorption in the posterior ridge after 10 years. Interindividual variation is considerably wide, however. It is important to highlight that overdenture rotation around attachments may lead to varied loading on the posterior ridge, which must be minimized by adequate treatment provision and maintenance.

Good standard practices for conventional complete denture treatment also deserve mention, including optimal dentures and adequate wearing habits [20]. Such practices will minimize compressive load on edentulous ridges, a known factor associated with bone resorption. As long as most implant-assisted mandibular overdenture designs rely on tissue support, one should expect these approaches to be important following these treatment modalities. Overdenture fabrication should follow the same good standard procedures expected for conventional prostheses, including satisfactory base extension and fit, in order to dissipate load evenly and to the maximum area of the ridge possible. The same could be expected from occlusion, although the evidence supporting different occlusal schemes is scarce and controversial. Overnight denture wearing should also be avoided in order to prevent further unnecessary compressive strength over edentulous ridges.

16.3.1.2 Soft Tissue Lesions

Despite the clinical success of dental implants, some mucosal lesions may be associated with implanted materials and components. The most common type is mucosal hyperplasia, which is relatively more frequent with bar-retained overdentures [21]. Stud attachments may also be associated with hyperplastic tissue if abutments do not have a minimum height, e.g., their transmucosal portion should be 1 mm above the peri-implant mucosa. Mild cases may be managed by changing prosthetic design or repairs on denture bases, but surgical removal is usually the treatment of choice for well-defined lesions. Removal of the causative factor following surgery is mandatory for avoiding recurrence.

Other lesions are rare, fortunately, but may include reactive lesions such as peripheral giant cell lesions, pyogenic granuloma, and traumatic ulcerative granuloma [22–24]. Differential diagnosis may be a bit more challenging in some of these cases but feasible by careful clinical observation associated with biopsies. As for typical hyperplastic lesions, removal or reduction of a chronic irritation associated with implant components is mandatory for their management.

There have also been reports in the literature of malignant lesions in implant sites [25]. Although they are not caused by implants, the remote possibility of such atypical lesions associated with the peri-implant mucosa merits careful diagnostic appraisal.

16.3.2 Peri-implant Complications

Perhaps the most concerning complication related to peri-implant tissues is the bone loss that occurs following implant insertion. Bone resorption is classically described as occurring more intensely during the first post-insertion year, with slightly lower rates during subsequent periods. Bone loss is not so pronounced for mandibular overdentures, even when two unsplinted fixtures are used. Contemporary implant systems can achieve mean vertical bone loss of approximately 0.3 mm during the first year followed by 0.1 mm in the subsequent year [26]. The use of bar-clip attachments, even with higher numbers of implants, does not reduce such values [27]. An advantage of splinting implants would be a better distribution of forces on fixtures; however, this does not seem to be significant when standard fixtures are used for mandibular overdentures.

The mechanism linked to peri-implant bone resorption merits some consideration, in order to understand its clinical implications. Albrektsson et al. [28] report that the placement of a dental implant leads to an inflammatory process following the osteotomy. At first, this is an acute process that may lead to primary clinical failure, which is rare when present-day implants are installed by well-trained professionals. However, successful implants will invariably undergo a mild chronic inflammatory process termed foreign body equilibrium. In this steady state, the bone encapsulates the implant with increasingly thicker mineralized tissue. Resorption tends to be more intense during the first days due to adaption to healing and loading, which may not be determinant for subsequent bone level changes. Bone loss may increase over time in the presence of some factors that can lead to imbalance in this foreign body equilibrium. These factors include poor implants or clinical handling, poor patient-related conditions (e.g., anatomical conditions, systemic diseases), or changes in the distribution of loads.

Within the context of bone loss, infection may be also a factor with potential to disrupt the inflammatory equilibrium. Bacteria may lead to mucositis when bone levels are clinically adequate, which is a reversible inflammatory disease of soft tissues around implants. This is characterized by erythema, swelling, and bleeding on probing. This alteration is treatable solely by removing peri-implant biofilm, both by professional cleaning and adequate oral hygiene [29]. The latter approach may be critical in the case of elderly patients, who may have reduced dexterity and therefore difficulties with oral hygiene. Therefore, the use of overdentures retained by a reduced number of unsplinted implants enables easier cleaning and therefore may minimize the risk of mucositis for such patients.

Peri-implantitis seems to be an aggravated response to already imbalanced implants following bone loss rather than a disease analogous to periodontitis [28, 30]. Severe bone resorption due to imbalanced foreign body equilibrium may lead to harboring of submucosal biofilm, thus leading to a more severe clinical condition. In other words, the presence of microorganisms and suppuration may not necessarily be the primary cause of bone resorption but an aggravation of the process. Although the therapeutic approach to peri-implantitis is very similar to the one used for periodontitis [29], their different etiologies should be taken into consideration when managing diseased peri-implant sites. Consequently, the abovementioned factors that may imbalance osseointegration should be approached also.

16.3.3 Prosthetic Complications

16.3.3.1 Attachment System

Any attachment system will invariably suffer some wear with ongoing use. Although there are several in vitro studies describing certain changes occurring on attachment components after cyclic loading, their findings tend to be optimistic compared to what happens to actual patients [31]. The presence of a bolus, saliva, and plaque is associated with varied types and degrees of forces in the oral cavity. Average maintenance needs may also vary among different patients considerably. For instance, some patients may severely deform the attachment parts after receiving an overdenture. This happens due to incorrect insertion using oblique paths and even seating dentures by biting; from a clinical perspective, this problem seems more pronounced in the elderly with lower dexterity and extremely resorbed ridges. Furthermore, an atrophic ridge will make the denture insertion path less intuitive and transfer a higher percentage of load directly onto attachment components.

Occurrence of attachment maintenance may vary considerably for different systems. A nylon capsule-based O-Ring system could require substitution of retentive matrices for more than 50% of patients after 6 months [13]. However, a more reasonable scenario for most mechanical stud attachments is to expect some reactivation or substitution of matrices for half of overdenture wearers during a single year [32].

The use of magnetic attachments may lead to lower maintenance needs, due to their long-lasting retentive force [33]. Contemporary magnets have overcome corrosion-related problems of older systems, while detaching from denture bases is their major complication. Compared to O-Ring attachments, bar-clip systems were preliminarily shown as less prone to wear due to insertion-removal cycles or functional forces. However, a systematic review shows some controversial data in clinical studies comparing the number of maintenance events for these systems. Longer time needed for changing bars or clips should be considered as well [17].

16.3.3.2 Other Denture Components

Overdenture bases may also break after some period of use, requiring either repairs or remaking. Fractures may occur with complete dentures regardless of the implants, often when patients drop them while cleaning. In addition, the presence of matrix housings or clips increases the incidence of this problem, as they would represent sites in the denture base bulk where cracks can develop. It is reasonable to allow a minimum thickness of 1 mm of acrylic resin at the point where attachment housings would be the closest to perforate denture flanges and more resin in other areas. A study reported that approximately 15% of patients would have fractured mandibular overdentures after little more than 3 years [34]. Denture bases can be reinforced by incorporating fibers or metallic frames in order to prevent fractures. Although some in vitro studies and clinical experience may support this approach, a clinical trial could not find a statistically significant effect of reinforced mandibular dentures as a prevention method for fractured bases [35].

Many mandibular overdenture wearers have conventional complete dentures in their antagonist arch. From our experience, a few of them complain about maxillary denture stability after attachments are in use. Although a likely cause for these complaints is based on changes in patient perspectives (i.e., the maxillary dentures do not feel much better than their opposing prosthesis anymore), they may also be associated with an augmented occlusal load in the anterior area [36].

In general, a systematic review mentions no difference in prosthetic maintenance for different attachment systems, except for bars with distal extensions, which are prone to fracture [16]. The same review highlights an unclear difference between rigid and resilient bar attachments, although the latter seems associated with more maintenance events. However, a paucity of randomized trials in removable prosthodontics hinders a precise comparison between different types of attachments. This renders clinician expertise and preferences to be major determinants for the choice of attachment systems.

16.4 Final Remarks

From a clinical perspective, mandibular implant-retained overdentures are an important treatment option for edentulism due to their high success rate. Favorable outcomes do not exclude the possibility of complications of a biological or prosthetic nature, as with any oral rehabilitative procedure. The delivery of a mandibular overdenture will require continuous maintenance to prevent or minimize the impact of eventual complications. An understanding of ongoing phenomena following initial insertion will lead to more predictable clinical care and to better-informed patients.

References

1. Feine JS, Carlsson GE, Awad MA, Chehade A, Duncan WJ, Gizani S, Head T, Heydecke G, Lund JP, MacEntee M, Mericske-Stern R, Mojon P, Morais JA, Naert I, Payne AG, Penrod J, Stoker GT, Tawse-Smith A, Taylor TD, Thomason JM, Thomson WM, Wismeijer D. The McGill consensus statement on overdentures. Mandibular two-implant overdentures as first choice standard of care for edentulous patients. Gerodontology. 2002;19(1):3–4.

2. Thomason JM, Feine J, Exley C, Moynihan P, Müller F, Naert I, Ellis JS, Barclay C, Butterworth C, Scott B, Lynch C, Stewardson D, Smith P, Welfare R, Hyde P, McAndrew R, Fenlon M, Barclay S, Barker D. Mandibular two implant-supported overdentures as the first choice standard of care for edentulous patients--the York consensus statement. Br Dent J. 2009;207(4):185–6.

3. van der Wijk P, Bouma J, van Waas MA, van Oort RP, Rutten FF. The cost of dental implants as compared to that of conventional strategies. Int J Oral Maxillofac Implants. 1998;13(4):546–53.

4. Albrektsson T, Zarb G, Worthington P, Eriksson AR. The long-term efficacy of currently used dental implants: a review and proposed criteria of success. Int J Oral Maxillofac Implants. 1986;1(1):11–25.

5. Buser D, Weber HP, Lang NP. Tissue integration of non-submerged implants. 1-year results of a prospective study with 100 ITI hollow-cylinder and hollow-screw implants. Clin Oral Implants Res. 1990;1(1):33–40.

6. Misch CE, Perel ML, Wang HL, Sammartino G, Galindo-Moreno P, Trisi P, Steigmann M, Rebaudi A, Palti A, Pikos MA, Schwartz-Arad D, Choukroun J, Gutierrez-Perez JL, Marenzi G, Valavanis DK. Implant success, survival, and failure: the international congress of oral Implantologists (ICOI) Pisa Consensus conference. Implant Dent. 2008;17(1):5–15.

7. Papaspyridakos P, Chen CJ, Singh M, Weber HP, Gallucci GO. Success criteria in implant dentistry: a systematic review. J Dent Res. 2012;91(3):242–8.

8. Quirynen M, Naert I, van Steenberghe D, Teerlinck J, Dekeyser C, Theuniers G. Periodontal aspects of osseointegrated fixtures supporting an overdenture. A 4-year retrospective study. J Clin Periodontol. 1991;18(10):719–28.

9. Naert I, Quirynen M, Hooghe M, van Steenberghe DA. Comparative prospective study of splinted and unsplinted Brånemark implants in mandibular overdenture therapy: a preliminary report. J Prosthet Dent. 1994;71(5):486–92.

10. Stoumpis C, Kohal RJ. To splint or not to splint oral implants in the implant-supported overdenture therapy? A systematic literature review. J Oral Rehabil. 2011;38(11):857–69.

11. Ferrigno N, Laureti M, Fanali S, Grippaudo G. A long-term follow-up study of non-submerged ITI implants in the treatment of totally edentulous jaws. Part I: ten-year life table analysis of a prospective multicenter study with 1286 implants. Clin Oral Implants Res. 2002;13(3):260–73.

12. Dantas IS, Souza MB, Morais MH, Carreiro AF, Barbosa GA. Success and survival rates of mandibular overdentures supported by two or four implants: a systematic review. Braz Oral Res. 2014;28:74–80.

13. de Souza RF, Ribeiro AB, Della Vecchia MP, Costa L, Cunha TR, Reis AC, Albuquerque RF Jr. Mini vs. standard implants for mandibular overdentures: a randomized trial. J Dent Res. 2015;94(10):1376–84.

14. Srinivasan M, Makarov NA, Herrmann FR, Müller F. Implant survival in 1- versus 2-implant mandibular overdentures: a systematic review and meta-analysis. Clin Oral Implants Res. 2016;27(1):63–72.

15. Öwall B, Käyser AF, Carlsson GE. Prosthodontics: principles and management strategies. London: Mosby-Wolfe; 1996.

16. Andreiotelli M, Att W, Strub JR. Prosthodontic complications with implant overdentures: a systematic literature review. Int J Prosthodont. 2010;23(3):195–203.

17. Kim HY, Lee JY, Shin SW, Bryant SR. Attachment systems for mandibular implant overdentures: a systematic review. J Adv Prosthodont. 2012;4(4):197–203.

18. Wright PS, Glantz PO, Randow K, Watson RM. The effects of fixed and removable implant-stabilised prostheses on posterior mandibular residual ridge resorption. Clin Oral Implants Res. 2002;13(2):169–74.

19. Raedel M, Lazarek-Scholz K, Marré B, Boening KW, Walter MH. Posterior alveolar ridge resorption in bar-retained mandibular overdentures: 10-year results of a prospective clinical trial. Clin Oral Implants Res. 2015;26(12):1397–401.

20. Carlsson GE. Implant and root supported overdentures - a literature review and some data on bone loss in edentulous jaws. J Adv Prosthodont. 2014;6(4):245–52.

21. Gotfredsen K, Holm B. Implant-supported mandibular overdentures retained with ball or bar attachments: a randomized prospective 5-year study. Int J Prosthodont. 2000;13(2):125–30.

22. Cloutier M, Charles M, Carmichael RP, Sándor GK. An analysis of peripheral giant cell granuloma associated with dental implant treatment. Oral Surg Oral Med Oral Pathol Oral Radiol Endod. 2007;103(5):618–22.

23. Dojcinovic I, Richter M, Lombardi T. Occurrence of a pyogenic granuloma in relation to a dental implant. J Oral Maxillofac Surg. 2010;68(8):1874–6.

24. dos Reis AC, León JE, Ribeiro AB, Della Vecchia MP, Cunha TR, de Souza RF. Traumatic ulcerative granuloma with stromal eosinophilia around mini dental implants without the protection of a denture base. J Prosthodont. 2015;24(1):83–6.

25. Agostini T, Sacco R, Bertolai R, Acocella A, Colafranceschi M, Lazzeri D. Peri-implant squamous odontogenic tumor. J Craniofac Surg. 2011;22(3):1151–7.

26. Payne AG, Tawse-Smith A, Duncan WD, Kumara R. Conventional and early loading of unsplinted ITI implants supporting mandibular overdentures. Clin Oral Implants Res. 2002;13(6):603–9.

27. Romeo E, Chiapasco M, Lazza A, Casentini P, Ghisolfi M, Iorio M, Vogel G. Implant-retained mandibular overdentures with ITI implants. Clin Oral Implants Res. 2002;13(5):495–501.

28. Albrektsson T, Dahlin C, Jemt T, Sennerby L, Turri A, Wennerberg A. Is marginal bone loss around oral implants the result of a provoked foreign body reaction? Clin Implant Dent Relat Res. 2014;16(2):155–65.

29. Smeets R, Henningsen A, Jung O, Heiland M, Hammächer C, Stein JM. Definition, etiology, prevention and treatment of peri-implantitis – a review. Head Face Med. 2014;10(34)

30. Koka S, Zarb G. On osseointegration: the healing adaptation principle in the context of osseosufficiency, osseoseparation, and dental implant failure. Int J Prosthodont. 2012;25(1):48–52.

31. Chaves CAL, de Souza RF, Cunha TR, Della Vecchia MP, Ribeiro AB, Bruniera JF, Silva-Sousa YT. Preliminary in vitro study on O-ring wear in mini-implant retained overdentures. Int J Prosthodont. 2016;29(4):357–9.

32. Bryant SR, Walton JN, MacEntee MI. A 5-year randomized trial to compare 1 or 2 implants for implant overdentures. J Dent Res. 2015;94(1):36–43.

33. Cristache CM, Muntianu LA, Burlibasa M, Didilescu AC. Five-year clinical trial using three attachment systems for implant overdentures. Clin Oral Implants Res. 2014;25(2):e171–8.

34. Gonda T, Maeda Y, Walton JN, MacEntee MI. Fracture incidence in mandibular overdentures retained by one or two implants. J Prosthet Dent. 2010;103(3):178–81.

35. MacEntee MI, Walton JN, Glick N. A clinical trial of patient satisfaction and prosthodontic needs with ball and bar attachments for implant-retained complete overdentures: three-year results. J Prosthet Dent. 2005;93(1):28–37.

36. Fontijn-Tekamp FA, Slagter AP, van't Hof MA, Geertman ME, Kalk W. Bite forces with mandibular implant-retained overdentures. J Dent Res. 1998;77(10):1832–9.

Patient-Based Outcomes

17

Janice S. Ellis, Wafa A. A. Kashbour, and J. Mark Thomason

Abstract

Patient-oriented outcomes focus on the patients' 'lived experience' of medical or dental conditions rather than metrics such as prosthesis survival, operator perceived acceptability or physiological outcomes. Patient-oriented outcomes can provide important insight into how it is to live with a condition and also the management of a condition. This is perhaps most important when considering chronic conditions where treatment does not aim to cure the condition but has the intention of allowing the patient to live with it more easily [1]. Treatment of patients with tooth loss is an example of such a chronic condition where 'palliative care' rather than 'cure' is the intended outcome. This may be valuable in informing treatment planning decisions, refocusing towards aspects of treatment which are most important to the patient, their families and carers. In the research setting, it is a process that may be used to assess and assure the quality of care delivered and ensure that the objectives which patients value most are prioritised over those a clinician may have otherwise considered best [2].

This chapter examines both qualitative and quantitative examples of patient-oriented outcomes and considers these alongside patient expectations. In doing this it becomes clear that having an understanding of the patients' lived experience of implant-assisted overdentures is crucial to understanding their value and essential when providing prospective patients with accurate information to enable them to give truly informed consent. Whilst it is important for patients to know that their implant may have a 98% chance of surviving for 5 years after placement, it is probably more important for patients to understand the likely effects of implant-assisted overdentures on their quality of life *as reported by patients'* and are possibly the best means of countering unrealistic patient expectations.

17.1 Introduction

17.1.1 What Do We Mean by Patient-Oriented Outcomes?

The concept of patient-oriented (also referred to as patient-centred or patient-reported) outcomes is relatively new.

J. S. Ellis • W. A. A. Kashbour • J. M. Thomason (✉)
School of Dental Sciences, and the Centre for Oral Health Research, Newcastle University, Newcastle upon Tyne, UK
e-mail: Janice.Ellis@newcastle.ac.uk;
j.m.thomason@newcastle.ac.uk

© Springer International Publishing AG, part of Springer Nature 2018
E. Emami, J. Feine (eds.), *Mandibular Implant Prostheses*,
https://doi.org/10.1007/978-3-319-71181-2_17

Prior to the use of patient-oriented outcomes, the success or otherwise of treatment tended to focus on metrics such as prosthesis survival, operator perceived acceptability or physiological outcomes. By contrast, patient-oriented outcomes focus on the patients' 'lived experience' of medical or dental conditions, the management of those conditions and subsequent aftercare. In order to do this fully, patient-oriented outcome measures may also take into consideration patients' initial expectations of treatment, their subsequent levels of satisfaction and the impact of their medical or dental condition and its management on their quality of life. For some patients and some conditions, the outcome measure may be primarily orientated towards a patient's family, friends and/or other support network.

Patient-oriented outcomes can provide important insight into how it is to live with a condition and/or the management of a condition. This is particularly important when considering chronic conditions where treatment does not aim to cure the condition but has the intention of allowing the patient to live with it more easily. As an obvious example of this, there is no cure for tooth loss, and so treatment aims at living with tooth loss but improving the condition for the patient. In this respect patient-centred outcomes may be seen as being of greatest value when faced with a chronic medical or dental condition where 'palliative care' rather than 'cure' is the intended outcome. This in turn may be valuable in informing treatment planning decisions, by refocusing the patient-doctor shared decision-making towards aspects of treatment which are most important to the patient, their families and carers.

From a research point of view too, such measures are also increasingly being used to assess and assure the quality of care delivered, and further, to inform clinical guidelines and policy, such that the objectives which patients value most are prioritised over those a clinician may consider best.

17.1.2 Specificity of Outcomes

The phrase 'quality of life' is used by the general population as well as the scientific community and can be thought of as a general measure of wellbeing. Patients living with chronic conditions, and their subsequent management, are likely to experience some degree of impact on their quality of life. An instrument for capturing the extent to which an individual's (or a society's) quality of life is affected is an attractive concept. Its assessment or determination may include consideration of multiple aspects of an individual's life, such as their employment, financial situation, educational opportunities and attainment, living environment, feelings of safeness/security as well as physical health.

Such broad outcome measures whilst having value in some circumstances clearly lack the sensitivity to observe changes in outcomes which are condition specific. This lack of sensitivity means that if wanting to use such broadly based instruments to detect meaningful differences between treatment options, the group sizes required for each of the study groups would need to be very large in order to provide sufficient power to demonstrate significant effect.

It is useful to reflect on Marlow's hierarchy of need when considering some of the difficulties of using a generic measure such as quality of life [3]. Thus an edentulous adult struggling with poorly fitting mandibular dentures whilst living in comfortable secure housing in a peaceful environment may well report a significant impact on their quality of life due to their dental status. The same individual living in war-torn city, with intermittent water supplies and no access to medical service, may report a similar degree of impairment in quality of life but due to a completely different set of considerations. Their dentures would be just as ill fitting, move the same amount and cause a similar amount of discomfort. The former individual may not be able to go and dine out with friends and family due to fear of social embarrassment on dislodgement of their dentures. The latter may likewise be unable to socialise in this way—but due to fear for their lives on leaving their home. Therefore, whilst highly transferable, generalised assessment tools may be less useful in comparing and contrasting treatment strategies.

'Health-related quality of life' has a more specific focus on physical health, yet this measure still remains highly generic. The lived experience, of any one condition, is likely to present a quite unique model specific only to that condition. Thus a patient-oriented outcome measure that assesses the quality of life of renal dialysis patients would be hugely different to that of a patient living with an edentulous mandible. Interventions in one of these areas may bring about significant changes in this condition, but its effect on an overall quality of life measure may be masked by the impact the other condition has on the patient's quality of life. Generic patient-oriented outcome tools such as health-related quality of life may be used to assess a range of medical conditions but lack the specificity required to compare treatment modalities for the same condition and are thus less useful in informing treatment planning and policy [4].

Ideally, patient-centred outcome measures should be specific to the particular condition being considered and as such require to be individually modelled, designed and constructed. Arguably this cannot be achieved unless there is an understanding of the lived experience [5]. One approach to establishing this understanding is the utilisation of qualitative research methods which allow us to listen to and interrogate patient's accounts and stories and subsequently identify the relevant themes. Having done so, quantitative measures which allow systematic and empirical investigation of the observed phenomena can then be developed. Such instruments allow testing of a predetermined hypothesis/theory and subsequently comparison through measurement, collection of numerical data, mathematical modelling and statistical analysis.

17.1.3 Qualitative Patient-Centred Outcome Measures

Qualitative research methods have a strong basis in sociology and may use multiple approaches including semi-structured interviews and focus groups, to examine the 'why' and the 'how'. A grounded theory approach is commonly used whereby the researcher starts with no previous understanding and builds this through an iterative exploration of the phenomena [6]. The published results of qualitative research usually include illustrative quotations from patients.

There have been very few qualitative research studies applied to the area of dental implants, which is perhaps indicative not only of the challenges in developing such studies but also the potential reticence of the dental research community, who, whilst trained in quantitative research methods, are perhaps unsurprisingly reluctant to engage with research methodologies based in sociology. Most of the studies in the literature which are entirely qualitative in their methodology are relatively recent, the oldest dating from only 2002, confirming the novelty of this approach and also the relatively recent development of implant technologies.

Qualitative research of this nature allows us to explore why patients may make decisions in a particular way and are especially useful when their decision-making may seem counterintuitive. As an example, as clinicians we may be surprised when patients decline implant treatments after experiencing multiple poor outcomes with conventional treatment modalities and when the scientific literature gives us confidence in the likelihood of a positive outcomes. For a group of such patients, the reasons for refusal were explored using focus groups of patients who had declined implants even though the 'cost barrier' had been removed [7]. There are several core themes which emerge.

The first and perhaps least unexpected is patient fear of the pain of surgical placement.

I don't want it… they could give them to me; I'd still refuse. I'm too afraid of suffering.

Of particular relevance is that this appears even more acute in the older patient who may question their own vulnerability and suitability for the surgical stage and post-operative recovery period:

Your bones are already brittle, because you are older, and you have a hole. It's like planting a nail in a dry board; it can split in two it can break.

I'm afraid of the consequences. At our age too... what if there was a little problem, an infection for some reason? At 40, the body is good (at fighting it) but at 60, 65 or 70, or older still, it's not as quick to recover, eh?

This was compounded by a healthy dose of cynicism and mistrust of the dental profession and their reasons for recommendation of a new technique.

I distrust professionals a bit...because they tell lies. So as not to scare you, maybe he looks at you and says....'it would be good for him.' – so they tone it down. The guy's selling his product.

Anxieties about early and late complications, possibly as a result of conversations with friends and family, were also at the forefront of patient's refusal to go ahead with implant procedures:

Am I going to regret them? Am I going to suffer side-effects for the rest of my life?

Another interesting theme which became apparent was the reluctance of patients to be without their current prosthesis during the healing stage:

The fact that I would have no teeth in and I couldn't, if they had given me a million pounds I couldn't walk around for three weeks, I was told, with no teeth. No way would I, even in the house, in a room I wouldn't walk around.

Only one study exists which specifically considered implant-assisted mandibular complete dentures using entirely qualitative patient-centred outcomes [8] and even so the population studied was not limited to the geriatric (age range of 48–84).

This study used semi-structured interviews and thematic content analysis to explore the effects of being edentulous and subsequent prosthetic rehabilitation with implant-assisted mandibular complete dentures. The interviews explored the social, functional and emotional aspects of eating with a view to understanding the significance of any limitations upon eating behaviour [8]. The main themes that were identified included the patients' experience of being edentulous, the 'public constraint' of wearing conventional dentures and the impact of conventional dentures and implant-assisted mandibular complete dentures on eating and the enjoyment of food. The findings suggest that whilst the functional limitations of conventional dentures impose food choice and social restrictions on edentulous patients, implant-assisted mandibular complete dentures provide improved function and subsequently increased social confidence that reduces the impact of the edentulous condition on the patients' quality of life. The following direct quote from one of the study participants (64-year-old female) illustrates the key findings.

I really have got my life back ... .because I wouldn't go out anywhere to dinners ....it was so embarrassing so I just didn't. It was really bad. But after this I go out, you know I've got so much confidence.

Even in studies not specifically considering implant-assisted mandibular complete dentures, it is possible to identify themes that are relevant to this group of patients.

A study that included within its study population patients in the age range 46–80 identified an increase in confidence as a key outcome following rehabilitation with implant-assisted mandibular and maxillary complete dentures [9]. Other aspects of the patients' experience that were identified through the semi-structured interviews included improved speech clarity and the reduction in intra-oral ulceration induced by denture movement. Patients in this study were also able to identify some challenges with using implant-assisted dentures which may be of particular relevance to the geriatric patient, namely, difficulty in 'manipulating' the denture and cleaning the implants.

A recent study within the UK utilised semi-structured interviews with patients at various stages of implant treatment to explore the patient journey from the point of referral to a specialist provider up to several years post-treatment [10]. Whilst the study had a mixed population in terms of both age and type of implant restoration, a number of interesting themes emerged which are directly relevant to a geriatric patient group being rehabilitated with an implant-assisted mandibular complete denture.

The first of these relates to the patients' expectations of implant treatment. Patients often referred to the implant rehabilitation in terms of its permanency, with little understanding of the need for maintenance.

I assume they're pretty much for life. Like I don't think they'll need much maintenance but I will have sorts of regular visits to my dentist I assume like my other teeth also implant won't get decay like teeth or infection.

Patients frequently expressed their anxiety and uncertainty about their physical suitability for implant placement and also their eligibility for free implant treatment within the UK's National Health Service.

My actual dentist couldn't really set expectations because he didn't know what the wait time was with the dental hospital; didn't have an idea of how long it would all take.

I'm scared in case I'm not allowed them, or I don't qualify.

At the stage of implant placement surgery, the main theme to emerge was patients' overestimation of problems at the time of the surgery itself, which subsequently contributed to a relatively favourable reflection on the actual experience and perceived outcome.

Oh, I think I overestimated the surgery. Definitely a lot easier than what you would think it was, plus, I mean, I was knocked out. Well, I wasn't knocked out, but, you know, you're not all there. The sedation, yes, and it was really good.

However, one particular negative aspect of the patient experience was the use of surgical drapes during the implant placement procedure:

First they tried to cover my face I did not like it. I, personally, have 'claustrophobia' and in fact um I do have it quite badly. I just didn't like the feeling of feeling like I was trapped, I think that was probably my feeling at that time, when they and my eyes were covered, so but other than that it was absolutely fine.

Whilst the majority of patients reported favourable experiences of surgery, in contrast, patients experienced difficulty in the immediate postsurgical healing period, and whilst partially dentate patients could immediately perceive the advantages of fixed retained temporary restoration, patients with overdentures perceived little/no immediate advantage.

I couldn't believe the pain about an hour later. I, it was very, very extreme in the jaw bone, you know. I called into [pharmacist] for some painkillers and they didn't work anyway. But eventually it, it settled down and, and my implants have been very successful.

I think for one week I could not wear my dentures after the surgery and I told my friends and family don't come to see me I could not face people without my teeth may be that my just pride, also I can't eat I was eating only soft and soup.

Patients strongly believed in the long-term success and permanency of their implant-retained restoration; however, this belief was often associated with uncertain knowledge of the long-term care and hygiene regime. Whilst short-term enhancement of patients' quality of life was recounted, after a significant period of use, these improvements seemed to be adversely affected by longer term complications and the ongoing maintenance needs of the implant restoration.

There was never enough room to clean up there, because you couldn't get the floss up there. So I had infection after infection, inflammation after inflammation, and realised that I'd lost a lot of bone, a lot of tissue, and that the threads were exposed on one of the implants, It was something I accepted.

The connection, connection to them, they're like a press stud, um, it doesn't, it does- they don't, oh, it seems to soon wear off after maybe about, I don't know how long you see, maybe about, is it a year or it could be even a year and a half. I don't know.

No studies have been found which investigate patients' quality of life after long periods of using implant restoration involving maintenance or failure experiences. This area should be the focus of future research.

17.1.4 Quantitative Measures

Quantitative instruments or measures provide largely numerical data that can subsequently be analysed using statistical and mathematical techniques to investigate observed phenomena. Statistical analysis can provide reassurance as to whether differences between study cohorts are real or occur by chance and determine the size of an intervention effect. There are some notable studies which have derived quantitative instruments to examine the effect of treatments in terms of patient-centred outcomes where the quantitative instrument has been built using qualitative methodologies. Patient satisfaction indices for mandibular implant overdentures are a notable example.

Specifically designed for edentulous individuals, the 'patient satisfaction' index developed by researchers at McGill University uses visual analogue scales anchored at either end by extremes of response to quantify patients' satisfaction with various aspects of their mandibular prostheses. Previous qualitative work identified a number of themes that were important to patients in terms of their satisfaction with their dental rehabilitation. This tool has since been used in many studies that compare pre- and post-rehabilitation with either conventional dentures or implant-assisted mandibular overdentures. In turn this allows meaningful comparison between studies.

Other quantitative instruments have been designed on the basis of a theoretical model. Perhaps the best known and most widely used in this field is the Oral Health Impact Profile-49 (OHIP-49) which assesses seven conceptual dimensions of 'oral health'. The 49 questions again incorporate the use of a Likert scale to record the impact of a patient's oral health on their quality of life (Oral Health Impact); the lower the score, the less the impact and the better the patient's quality of life. Since its inception variations of the OHIP-49 have been developed to allow a more focussed or specific assessment of particular dimensions of oral health. Of relevance to our discussion are the OHIP-20, OHIP-14 and OHIP-EDENT which are all relevant to the edentulous condition and its subsequent management with dentures.

There is a longer history of studies that have used such quantitative patient-oriented outcomes compared with those using qualitative outcomes, and whilst the numbers remain relatively small, this is now sufficient to begin to take strong messages from their outcomes. The first systematic review undertaken identified seven randomised controlled trials published between 1996 and 2006 comparing wearers of implant-supported mandibular overdentures and complete maxillary denture with conventional complete mandibular and maxillary denture wearers. These studies were reported in 18 papers [11]. A series of different instruments were used to assess the outcomes in terms of both satisfaction and the impact on quality of life. Their commonality was that these instruments recorded the patient's assessment of their position before treatment and after treatment allowing an assessment of the effect of treatment on aspects of their satisfaction with the prosthesis or the impact of the prosthesis on their quality of life. The conclusion of the systematic review was that patients are more satisfied with implant-assisted mandibular overdentures than conventional dentures and that patients' oral health-related quality of life can be significantly improved using implant-supported mandibular overdentures.

One major advantage of studies developing quantitative data such as this is the opportunity to collate studies of similar design to provide increased power, by bringing various results together in the form of a meta-analysis. Emami and colleagues compared all randomised controlled trials published in English or French up until April 2007 [12]. The outcomes they considered were both patient satisfaction and oral and general health-related quality of life. They identified seven RCTs discussed in ten publications and were able to use eight of these in their meta-analysis. Patients' general satisfaction was measured using either a 100 mm visual analogue or a Likert-type response scale. Of the six studies they were able to combine for this, the pool effect size was 0.80 and significantly ($p = 0.0004$) favoured the implant group.

To look at the effect of the mandibular prostheses on oral health-related quality of life, only the three studies using OHIP as the outcome were included. The pooled effect size was -0.41 and so was again consistent with a positive effect produced by the implant-supported overdenture (with OHIP a larger positive number on the scoring scale indicates a greater negative impact). Interestingly within the meta-analysis paper, the authors commented on the one study identified that used a measure to identify the impact of treatment on perceived general health QoL. This study used the SF-36 questionnaire but no difference was shown between groups for any of the subscales [12]. The SF-36 is a general health questionnaire, and it is unclear if there was really no impact or if this impact could not be measured for the reasons described previously whereby changes may be masked by the other conditions that the patient may have and their impact on the patient's general quality of life.

An updated meta-analysis undertaken by Kodama et al. [13] was able to include 11 RCTs which assessed the efficacy of implant-supported mandibular overdentures. The analysis was limited to RCTs involving patients over the age of 18 years, wearing maxillary conventional dentures and either mandibular two implant-supported overdentures or conventional dentures, and included general satisfaction and general health and/or oral health-related quality of life as the primary outcome measures. Studies had to include a follow-up period of at least 2 months.

Fifteen papers published since 1995 were identified that met the inclusion criteria (of which seven undertaken in Canada, three in the Netherlands, two in the UK (and Republic of Ireland), two in South America and one in North America). Whilst not strictly, limited to geriatric populations all studies contained individuals ≥65. Recruitment of patients varied, but largely fell into two different approaches: studies which recruited patients referred to implant services because of problems with conventional dentures and those where patients were actively recruited from the general population.

Nine studies considered patient satisfaction and analysis demonstrated a pooled ES 0.87 in favour of IOD. If the results are considered with respect to the method of recruitment, the ES was much greater in favour of IOD for those patients referred with initial problems (ES 1.09) compared to those studies who recruited from general population (ES = 0.76). With respect to oral health-related quality of life, 15 studies used either OHIP-49 or 1 of its derivatives. The 15 studies included for analysis demonstrated a combined ES of −0.66 (in favour of IODs).

When the analysis was restricted to studies with participants recruited from the general population, the ES was 0.71, compared to an ES of 0.72 seen in studies where patients were referred due to previous problems with conventional dentures. At this point it is important to reflect that these studies have been based on populations with age ranges that cover not just the geriatric population but much younger patients too.

There are very few studies which have targeted the over 65-year-old patient; however, an example would be the study by Awad and colleagues [14] and further reported by Heydecke and colleagues in 2003 [15]. This study suggests that the geriatric population enjoys similar positive outcomes in favour of implant-supported prostheses as the younger cohort (35–65) reported by the same group [14, 16].

17.1.5 Patients' Expectations

The general population's recognition of dental implants, as a type of tooth replacement, is growing. For instance, in 2013, the percentage of patients who were aware of dental implants was 77% in the USA, 72% in Austria and 96% in Jordan [17]. Whilst multiple sources of information may contribute to patients' knowledge and understanding of dental implants, previous studies indicate that the main sources of patient information regarding dental implants in the UK, Austria and Jordan are family and friends, with reference to dentists only made when extra information is needed [18].

Patients' expectations of health care are an important aspect of the human experience of any treatment and as such can be crucial and decisive in subsequently evaluating care provision. Thus when attempting to model patient satisfaction, their expectations are defined as one of the determinants [19].

In the UK, patients' expectations of implant-retained prostheses have been reported as being 'high' [20], and patients' belief in dental implants seems to be undiminished with passing time and potentially greater exposure [21]. Patients' anticipation of treatment outcomes has been considered unrealistic in some studies, with some in particular identifying that patients perceive implants as a panacea for all [22, 23]. Crucially negative patient-based outcomes have been observed when initial expectations are high, particularly in relation to the function and comfort of overdentures with an adverse relation that was between age and expectation of outcomes [24].

In light of these findings, it is clear that having an understanding of all aspects of the patients' lived experience of implant-assisted overdentures is becoming more important. From a medicolegal perspective, it is essential to provide prospective patients with accurate information thus enabling them to give truly informed consent, particularly as we see increasingly high success rates reported using clinician- or technique-centred outcomes.

For whilst it is important for patients to know that their implant has a 98% chance of surviving for 5 years after placement, it is possibly even more important for patients to understand the likely effects of implant-assisted overdentures on their quality of life and in particular the limitations of the final rehabilitation and the long-term maintenance and replacement implications *as reported by patients*.

Moreover, in terms of improving the patient experience and subsequently their satisfaction with the outcome, studies reporting patient-centred outcomes are best placed to counter unrealistic patient expectations.

References

1. Hadi M, Locock L, Fitzpatrick R. Understanding health care needs of people with chronic conditions: patient experiences, outcomes and quality of life. Qual Life Res. 2013;22(Supp 1):57.
2. Ziebland S, Coulter A, Calabrese JD, Locock L. Understanding and using health experiences. Oxford: Oxford University Press; 2013.
3. Maslow AH. A theory of human motivation. Psychol Rev. 1943;50(4):370–96.
4. Schipper H, Clinch JJ, Olweny CLM. Quality of life studies: definitions and conceptual issues. In: Spilker B, editor. Quality of life and pharmacoeconomics in clinical trials. Philadelphia: Lippincott-Raven Publishers; 1996. p. 11–23.
5. Bennadi D, Reddy CVK. Oral health related quality of life. J Int Soc Prev Community Dent. 2013;3(1):1.
6. Bourgeault I, Dingwall R, Vries R. The SAGE handbook of qualitative methods in health research. London: Sage Publishing Ltd.;2010. Section b, p. 125–56, 174–93.
7. Ellis JS, Levine A, Bedos C, Mojon P, Rosberger Z, Feine J, Thomason JM. Refusal of implant supported mandibular overdentures by elderly patients. Gerodontology. 2011;28(1):62–8.
8. Hyland R, Ellis J, Thomason M, El-Feky A, Moynihan P. A qualitative study on patient perspectives of how conventional and implant-supported dentures affect eating. J Dent. 2009;37(9):718–23.
9. Osman RB, Morgaine KC, Duncan W, Swain MV, Ma S. Patients' perspectives on zirconia and titanium implants with a novel distribution supporting maxillary and mandibular overdentures: a qualitative study. Clin Oral Implants Res. 2012;25:587–97.
10. Kashbour WA. Patients' experiences and clinicians' views of dental implant treatment; a qualitative study, PhD Thesis, Newcastle University; 2016.
11. Thomason JM, Heydecke G, Feine JS, Ellis JS. How do patients perceive the benefit of reconstructive dentistry with regard to oral health-related quality of life and patient satisfaction? A systematic review. Clin Oral Implants Res. 2007;18(Suppl 3):168–88.
12. Emami E, Heydecke G, Rompre PH, de Grandmont P, Feine JS. Impact of implant support for mandibular denture on satisfaction, oral and general health-related quality of life: a meta-analysis of randomized–controlled trials. Clin Oral Implants Res. 2009;20(6):533–44.
13. Kodama N, Singh BP, Cerutti-Kopplin D, Feine J, Emami E. Efficacy of mandibular 2-implant overdenture. An updated meta-analysis on patient-based outcomes. J Dent Res Clin Trans Res. 2016;1(1):20–30.
14. Awad MA, Manal A, Lund JP, Dufresne E, Feine JS. Comparing the efficacy of mandibular implant-retained overdentures and conventional dentures among middle-aged edentulous patients: satisfaction and functional assessment. International. J Prosthodont. 2003;16(2):117–22.
15. Heydecke G, Locker D, Awad MA, Lund JP, Feine JS. Oral and general health-related quality of life with conventional and implant dentures. Community Dent Oral Epidemiol. 2003;31(3):161–8.
16. Awad MA, Locker D, Korner-Bitensky N, Feine JS. Measuring the effect of intra-oral implant rehabilitation on health-related quality of life in a randomized controlled clinical trial. J Dent Res. 2000;79(9):1659–63.
17. Al-Dwairi ZN, El Masoud BM, Al-Afifi SA, Borzabadi-Farahani A, Lynch E. Awareness, attitude, and expectations toward dental implants among removable prostheses wearers. J Prosthodont. 2014;23(3):192–7.

18. Pommer B, Zechner W, Watzak G, Ulm C, Watzek G, Tepper G. Progress and trends in patients' mindset on dental implants. I: level of information, sources of information and need for patient information. Clin Oral Implants Res. 2011;22(2):223–9.
19. Thompson AGH, Sunol R. Expectations as determinants of patient satisfaction: concepts, theory and evidence. Int J Qual Health Care. 1995;7(2):127–41.
20. Allen PF, McMillan AS, Walshaw D. Patient expectations of oral implant-retained prostheses in a UK dental hospital. Br Dent J. 1999;186(2):80–4.
21. Grey EB, Harcourt D, O'Sullivan D, Buchanan H, Kilpatrick NM. A qualitative study of patients' motivations and expectations for dental implants. Br Dent J. 2013;214(1):E1.
22. Yao J, Tang H, Gao XL, McGrath C, Mattheos N. Patients' expectations to dental implant: a systematic review of the literature. Health Qual Life Outcomes. 2014;12(1):153.
23. Wang G, Gao X, Lo ECM. Public perceptions of dental implants: a qualitative study. J Dent. 2015;43(7):798–805.
24. Baracat LF, Teixeira AM, dos Santos MB, da Cunha Vde P, Marchini L. Patients' expectations before and evaluation after dental implant therapy. Clin Implant Dent Rel Res. 2011;13(2):141–5.